COGNITIVE
THERAPY
OF
DEPRESSION

The Guilford Clinical Psychology and Psychotherapy Series
Editor: Michael J. Mahoney, The Pennsylvania State University

COGNITIVE THERAPY OF DEPRESSION

AARON T. BECK
University of Pennsylvania

A. JOHN RUSH
Southwestern Medical School

BRIAN F. SHAW
University of Western Ontario

GARY EMERY
University of Southern California

THE GUILFORD PRESS   NEW YORK

© 1979 Aaron T. Beck, A. John Rush, Brian F. Shaw, and Gary Emery
Published by The Guilford Press, 72 Spring Street,
New York, N.Y. 10012
All rights reserved

Manufactured in the United States of America

Last digit is print number: 30 29 28 27 26 25 24 23 22

Library of Congress Cataloging in Publication Data

Main entry under title:

Cognitive therapy of depression.

(The Guilford clinical psychology and psycho-
therapy series)
    Bibliography:
    Includes index.
    1. Depression, Mental.   2. Cognitive
therapy.   I. Beck, Aaron T.   II. Series:
Guilford clinical psychology and psychotherapy
series.
RC537.C63   616.8'52   79-19967
ISBN 0-89862-000-7 (cloth)
ISBN 0-89862-919-5 (paperback)

This book is dedicated to our children, and children to be; Roy, Judith, Daniel, and Alice Beck; Matthew Rush; and Stephen Shaw.

PREFACE

A monograph that introduces a new approach to the understanding and psychological therapy of depression warrants some account of its historical development.

This work represents a combination of many years of research and clinical practice. In many ways, it is the end product of the direct contributions of numerous individuals: clinicians, researchers, and patients. In addition to these specific contributions, cognitive therapy probably reflects gradual changes that have been occurring in the behavioral sciences for many years but have only recently emerged as a major trend. It is not possible to assay at this time how much impact the so-called "cognitive revolution in psychology" has had on the development of cognitive therapy.

In order to place this volume in its personal perspective, I would refer the reader to the early evolution of the cognitive model and cognitive therapy of depression and other neuroses summarized in my previous volume, *Depression*, published in 1967. My next work, *Cognitive Therapy and the Emotional Disorders*, published in 1976, presented a broad extension of the specific cognitive aberrations in each of the neuroses, a detailed description of the general principles of cognitive therapy, and a more comprehensive outline of the cognitive therapy of depression.

The early origins of my formulations regarding cognitive therapy of depression are not completely clear to me at present. As far as I can recall, the first stirrings became manifest in my venture beginning in 1956 to validate certain psychoanalytic concepts of depression. I believed that these psychoanalytic formulations were correct but had failed to gain wider acceptance because of certain natural "resistances" of the academic psychologists and psychiatrists, attributable, in part, to the lack of supporting empirical data. Believing that the techniques could be developed to carry out the necessary controlled studies, I embarked on a series of investigations designed to provide convincing data. A second and perhaps stronger motive was my desire to pinpoint the precise psychological configuration characteristic of depression in order to develop a brief form of psychotherapy specifically directed toward alleviating this focal psychopathology.

Although the initial findings of my empirical studies seemed to support my belief in the specific psychodynamic factors in depression, namely, retroflected hostility, expessed as "a need to suffer," later experiments presented a number of unexpected findings that appeared to contradict this hypothesis. These anomalies led me to a critical evaluation of the psychoanalytic theory of depression and ultimately of the entire structure of psychoanalysis. The anomalous research findings led ultimately to the conclusion that depressed patients do *not* have a need to suffer. In fact, the experimental manipulations indicated that the depressed patient was more likely than the nondepressed to avoid behaviors evoking rejection or disapproval in favor of responses eliciting acceptance and approval by others. This marked discrepancy between laboratory findings and clinical theory led to an "agonizing reappraisal" of my own belief system.

Concurrently, I became somewhat painfully aware that the early promise of psychoanalysis that I had observed in the early 1950's was not borne out by the middle and late fifties—as my fellow psychoanalytic students and other colleagues entered their sixth and seventh years of psychoanalysis with no striking improvement in their behavior or feelings! Furthermore, I noted that many of my depressed patients reacted adversely to therapeutic interventions based on the "retroflected hostility" or "need to suffer" hypotheses.

My total reformulation of the psychopathology of depression as well as the other neurotic disorders derived from fresh clinical observations and experimental and correlational studies and repeated attempts on my part to try to make sense out of the evidence that appeared to contradict psychoanalytic theory. The research finding that depressed patients did not have a need to suffer prompted me to look for other explanations for their behavior, which at least on the surface *appeared* to reflect the need to suffer. How else could one explain their harsh self-criticisms, their misreading of positive experience in a negative way, and what appeared to be the ultimate of expression of self-directed hostility, namely, suicidal wishes?

Returning to my observations of the "masochistic" dreams that formed the basis for my original study, I searched for a variety of alternative explanations for the persistent or frequent themes in which the depressed dreamer appeared as a loser: thwarted in an attempt to achieve some important goal, losing something of value, or appearing diseased, defective, or ugly. Indeed, as I focused more on the patient's descriptions of himself and his experiences, I noted that he consistently embraced a negative construction of himself and his life experiences. These constructions—similar to the imagery in his dreams—seemed to be distortions of reality.

Further systematic research involving the development and testing of new instruments validated the notion that the depressed patient systematically distorted his experiences in a negative way. We found that the depressed patient had a global negative view of himself, the outside world, and the future which apparently was expressed in the wide range of negative cognitive distortions. As the evidence accumulated to support the prominent role of negative cognitive distortions, I concomitantly attempted to alleviate the individual's depressive symptomatology by developing techniques to correct his distortions through the application of logic and rules of evidence and to adjust his information-processing to reality.

Several additional studies expanded our knowledge of how a depressed patient evaluates his performance and makes predictions about future performance. These experiments showed that under specific conditions a graded series of successes in attaining a tangible goal could have a powerful effect in reversing the negative self-concept and expectations and thus directly ameliorate his depressive symptomatology.

This study thus added a powerful new approach to the techniques I had previously described for correcting cognitive distortions; namely, the use of actual experiments to test the patient's erroneous or exaggeratedly negative beliefs. This notion of testing hypotheses in a real life situation crystallized into the general concept of "collaborative empiricism."

By treating the patient's everyday experiences as a testing ground for checking his various beliefs about himself, we were able to extend enormously the therapeutic process: Almost every experience or interaction presented a potential opportunity for the patient to test his negative predictions and interpretations. Thus, the concept of homework or, as we later called it, "extended self-therapy" greatly expanded the impact of the therapy sessions.

The behavior therapy movement contributed substantially to the development of cognitive therapy. Methodological behaviorism, with its emphasis on specifying discrete goals, delineating the concrete procedures instrumental for achieving these goals and providing prompt tangible feedback, added new dimensions to cognitive therapy (and, in fact, led some writers to relabel our approach as "cognitive behavior therapy").

The writing of this monograph is largely the outgrowth of weekly conferences held for many years at the Department of Psychiatry of the University of Pennsylvania. The conferences consisted of presentations of specific problems with the patients; the participants drew freely on their own experience and collaborated in offering suggestions. These suggestions were formalized in a sequence of treatment manuals which culminated in the present volume. So many participants in these conferences made valuable contributions to our gradually accumulating body of knowledge that it would be impossible to acknowledge even the major contributors. We are grateful to the participants, who I am sure are well aware of their invaluable help.

We want especially to thank our colleagues who provided material, suggestions, and comments relevant to the various treatment manuals preceding this monograph. Among the most active were Marika Kovacs, David Burns, Ira Herman, and Steven Hollon. We are also most appreciative to Michael Mahoney who read the entire mauscript and made numerous editorial suggestions. We would also like to thank Stirling Moorey for his diligent assistance in the final stages of preparation of this book.

The contribution of Ruth L. Greenberg from the inception to the completion of this endeavor has been so vast that we cannot find adequate words to express our appreciation.

Finally the authors offer their sincere thanks to the typists, Lee Fleming, Marilyn Starr, and Barbara Marinelli.

A note about "sexist" language: When speaking in general terms about "the therapist" or "the patient," we have used masculine pronouns ("he," "his"). This usage by no means implies that we refer only to therapists and patients of the masculine sex. We have retained the traditional usage because of the simplicity and flexibility it affords.

Aaron T. Beck, M.D.
May, 1979

CONTENTS

Appendix: Materials

Chapter 1

AN OVERVIEW

THE PROBLEM OF DEPRESSION

Some authorities have estimated that at least 12% of the adult population have had or will have an episode of depression of sufficient clinical severity to warrant treatment (Schuyler and Katz, 1973). In the past 15 years, hundreds of systematic studies relevant to the biological substrate of depression and to the chemotherapy of depression have been published. Various publications from governmental agencies, as well as from the private sector, have suggested that definite breakthroughs have occurred in the understanding of the psychobiology of depression and in the treatment of this disorder through chemotherapy.

Despite this somewhat rosy picture, the clinician is confronted with a puzzling situation. Although there have been advances in the chemotherapy of depression, there is no evidence that the prevalence of depression has diminished. Moreover, the suicide rate, which has generally been regarded as an index of the prevalence of depression, has not decreased and in fact has shown an increase over the past years. Moreover, the lack of response of the suicide rate is all the more significant when one considers the enormous output of effort devoted to the setting up and maintenance of suicide prevention centers throughout the country.

A special National Institute of Mental Health report on *The Depressive Disorders* in 1973 by Secunda, Katz, Friedman, and Schuyler stated that depression accounts for 75% of all psychiatric hospitalizations and that during any given year 15% of all adults between 18 and 74 may suffer significant depressive symptoms. In terms of dollar costs, the authors suggested a range between 0.3 billion and 0.9 billion dollars. These authors also reiterated that "the burden for therapy for the large proportion of the depressive illnesses (75% of all psychiatric hospitalizations) falls squarely upon psychosocial therapeutic modalities."

VALUE OF PSYCHOTHERAPY IN DEPRESSION

The value of developing an effective psychotherapy for depression, determining its indications and contraindications, and establishing its role in the overall management of the depressed patient would seem to be self-evident. Since it appears that psychotherapy is practiced to varying degrees and in various forms in the treatment of almost all depressed patients, it is crucial to define specific forms of psychotherapy and to determine their effectiveness—so that the consumer can know whether this expensive service is achieving any beneficial results. There are, in addition, other reasons for defining and testing specific psychotherapeutic modalities.

1. Although antidepressant drugs are obviously less expensive than psychotherapy, not all depressed patients respond to this medication. The best estimates, based on a review of numerous controlled studies of the chemotherapy of depression, indicate that only about 60 to 65% show a definite improvement as a result of treatment with a common tricyclic drug (see Beck, 1973, p. 86). Hence, methods must be developed to help the 35 to 40% of the depressed people who are not helped with their first trial with an antidepressant drug.

2. Many patients who might be drug responsive either refuse to take the medication because of personal objections or develop side effects which cause them to terminate taking the drug.

3. It is possible that in the long run the reliance on chemotherapy might indirectly undermine the patient's utilization of his own psychological methods of coping with depression. The large literature on "attribution" suggests the possibility that patients treated with drugs will attribute their problem to a chemical imbalance and will attribute their improvement to the drug effects (Shapiro and Morris, 1978). Consequently, as social-psychological research indicates, the patients may be less likely to draw on or develop their own coping mechanisms to deal with the depression. The relatively high relapse

rate of patients previously treated with drugs (as high as 50% in the year following termination of drug treatment) suggests that this contention may be valid.

Conventional wisdom suggests that an effective course of psychotherapy might be more beneficial than chemotherapy in the long run because the patient can *learn from his or her psychotherapeutic experience.* Thus, such patients might be expected to cope with subsequent depressions more effectively, to abort incipient depressions, and conceivably might even be able to prevent subsequent depressions.

The fact that the suicide rate has not declined despite the very widespread use of antidepressant drugs suggests that even though chemotherapy may temporarily resolve suicidal crises, it has no sustaining effect that will inoculate the patient against making a suicidal attempt at some future time. Research indicates that there is a central psychological core in the suicidal patient—namely, hopelessness (or "generalized negative expectancies"). Positive results from using a direct approach to the hopelessness in depressed patients suggests that cognitive therapy might have longer range "antisuicidal effects" than the use of chemotherapy (see Chapter 10).

DEFINITION OF COGNITIVE THERAPY

Cognitive therapy is an active, directive, time-limited, structured approach used to treat a variety of psychiatric disorders (for example, depression, anxiety, phobias, pain problems, etc.). It is based on an underlying theoretical rationale that an individual's affect and behavior are largely determined by the way in which he structures the world (Beck, 1967, 1976). His cognitions (verbal or pictorial "events" in his stream of consciousness) are based on attitudes or assumptions (schemas), developed from previous experiences. For example, if a person interprets all his experiences in terms of whether he is competent and adequate, his thinking may be dominated by the schema, "Unless I do everything perfectly, I'm a failure." Consequently, he reacts to situations in terms of adequacy even when they are unrelated to whether or not he is personally competent.

3

The specific therapeutic techniques employed are utilized within the framework of the cognitive model of psychopathology, and we do not believe that the therapy can be applied effectively without knowledge of the theory. The therapeutic techniques are designed to identify, reality-test, and correct distorted conceptualizations and the dysfunctional beliefs (schemas) underlying these cognitions. The patient learns to master problems and situations which he previously considered insuperable by reevaluating and correcting his thinking. The cognitive therapist helps the patient to think and act more realistically and adaptively about his psychological problems and thus reduces symptoms.

A variety of cognitive and behavioral strategies are utilized in cognitive therapy. Cognitive techniques are aimed at delineating and testing the patient's specific misconceptions and maladaptive assumptions. This approach consists of highly specific learning experiences designed to teach the patient the following operations: (1) to monitor his negative, automatic thoughts (cognitions); (2) to recognize the connections between cognition, affect, and behavior; (3) to examine the evidence for and against his distorted automatic thought; (4) to substitute more reality-oriented interpretations for these biased cognitions; and (5) to learn to identify and alter the dysfunctional beliefs which predispose him to distort his experiences.

Various verbal techniques are used to explore the logic behind and basis for specific cognitions and assumptions. The patient is initially given an explanation of the rationale for cognitive therapy. Next, he learns to recognize, monitor, and record his negative thoughts on the Daily Record of Dysfunctional Thoughts (see Appendix). The cognitions and underlying assumptions are discussed and examined for logic, validity, adaptiveness, and enhancement of positive behavior versus maintenance of pathology. For example, the depressed person's tendency to feel responsible for negative outcomes while consistently failing to take credit for his own success is identified and discussed. The therapy focuses on specific "target symptoms" (for example, suicidal impulses). The cognitions supporting these symptoms are identified (for example, "My life is worthless and I can't change it.") and then subjected to logical and empirical investigation.

One of the powerful components of the learning model of psychotherapy is that the patient begins to incorporate many of the therapeutic techniques of the therapist. For example, patients frequently find themselves spontaneously assuming the role of the therapist in questioning some of their conclusions or predictions. Some examples of self-questioning that we have observed are: What is the evidence for my conclusion? Are there other explanations? How serious is the loss? How much does it actually subtract from my life? What is the degree of harm to me if a stranger thinks badly of me? What will I lose if I try to be more assertive?

Such self-questioning plays a major role in the generalization of cognitive techniques from the interview to external situations. Without such questioning, the depressed individual is pretty much bound by stereotyped automatic patterns, a phenomenon we might label "thoughtless thinking."

Behavioral techniques are used with more severely depressed patients not only to change behavior, but also to elicit cognitions associated with specific behaviors. Since the patient generally requires these more active techniques at the beginning of treatment, we will present the material on behavioral strategies (Chapter 7) prior to the exposition of cognitive techniques (Chapter 8). A sampling of these behavioral strategies include a Weekly Activity Schedule in which the patient logs his hourly activities; a Mastery and Pleasure Schedule, in which the patient rates the activities listed in his log; and Graded Task Assignments in which the patient undertakes a sequence of tasks to reach a goal which he considers difficult or impossible. Furthermore, behavioral assignments are designed to help the patient test certain maladaptive cognitions and assumptions.

An important problem confronting the therapist is making decisions regarding the choice and timing of particular types of interventions. As will be noted in Chapters 7 and 8, both behavioral and cognitive techniques have their own particular sets of advantages and applications in cognitive therapy. The retarded, preoccupied patient with a short attention span finds it very difficult to engage in introspection. In fact his preoccupations and perseverating ideation may become aggravated by such a procedure. Furthermore, behavioral methods are relatively powerful in counteracting his inertia and mobilizing him into constructive activity. Further, a successful experience in achieving a behavioral goal is likely to be more powerful than cognitive methods in contradicting erroneous beliefs such as "I am incapable of doing anything."

Although behavioral assignments may be more dramatic in disconfirming faulty *beliefs*, cognitive techniques may be the optimal kind of intervention to correct the patient's tendency to make incorrect inferences regarding the specific events. Consider a patient who has concluded that her friends dislike her because they did not call her for the past few days. This patient would be urged to practice cognitive skills such as identifying the "logical" processes that led to this conclusion, examining all the evidence, and considering alternative explanations. A behavioral task would be irrelevant for dealing with this type of cognitive problem.

These principles will be of utmost importance in the implementation of a coherent therapy. As the therapist gains experience, he is able to utilize a "decision tree" in conducting the interviews. Rather than selecting strategies in a hit-or-miss fashion, he will choose that technique most applicable to the particular symptom or problem.

Therapy generally consists of 15–25 sessions at weekly intervals. The moderately to severely depressed patients usually require interviews on a twice-weekly basis for at least 4 to 5 weeks and then weekly for 10–15 weeks. We generally taper the frequency to once every 2 weeks for the last few visits and recommend "booster therapy" after the completion of the regular course of treatment. These follow-up visits may be scheduled on a regular basis or may be left to the discretion of the patient. We have found that the average patient returns for three or four "booster" visits during the year following termination of formal therapy.

NEW FEATURES OF COGNITIVE THERAPY

What is new about this type of psychotherapy? Cognitive therapy differs from conventional psychotherapy in two important respects: in the formal structure of the interviews and in the kinds of problems that are focused upon.

"Collaborative Empiricism": In contrast to the more traditional psychotherapies such as psychoanalytic therapy or client-centered therapy, the therapist applying cognitive therapy is continuously active and deliberately interacting with the patient. The therapist structures the therapy according to a particular design which engages the patient's participation and collaboration. Since the depressed

patient is initially confused, preoccupied, or distracted, the therapist helps him to organize his thinking and his behavior—in order to help him to cope with the requirements of everyday living. Although the patient's collaboration in formulating the treatment plan may be seriously impeded by his symptoms at this stage, the therapist needs to use his ingenuity and resourcefulness to stimulate the patient to become *actively engaged* in the various therapeutic operations. We have found that classical psychoanalytic techniques such as free association and minimal activity by the therapist adversely affect the depressed patient because they allow him to sink further into the morass of his negative preoccupations.

In contrast to psychoanalytic therapy, the content of cognitive therapy is focused on "here-and-now" problems. Little attention is paid to childhood recollections except to clarify present observations. The major thrust is toward investigating the patient's thinking and feeling during the therapy session and between therapy sessions. We do not make interpretations of unconscious factors. The cognitive therapist actively collaborates with the patient in exploring his psychological experiences, setting up schedules of activities, and making homework assignments.

Cognitive therapy contrasts with behavior therapy in its greater emphasis on the patient's internal (mental) experiences, such as thoughts, feelings, wishes, daydreams, and attitudes. The overall strategy of cognitive therapy may be differentiated from the other schools of therapy by its emphasis on the *empirical investigation* of the patient's automatic thoughts, inferences, conclusions, and assumptions. We formulate the patient's dysfunctional idea and beliefs about himself, his experiences, and his future into hypotheses and then attempt to test the validity of these hypotheses in a systematic way. Almost every experience, thus, may provide the opportunity for an experiment relevant to the patient's negative views or beliefs. If the patient believes, for example, that everybody he meets turns away from him in disgust, we might help him to set up a system for judging other people's reactions and then motivate him to make objective assessments of the facial expressions and bodily movements of other people. If the patient believes he is incapable of carrying out simple hygienic procedures, we might jointly devise a checklist or graph which he can use to record the degree of success in carrying out these activities.

Cognitive Models: Historical Perspective

The general assumptions on which cognitive therapy is based include the following:

1. Perception and experiencing in general are *active* processes which involve both inspective and introspective data.
2. The patient's cognitions represent a synthesis of internal and external stimuli.
3. How a person appraises a situation is generally evident in his cognitions (thoughts and visual images).
4. These cognitions constitute the person's "stream of consciousness" or phenomenal field, which reflects the person's configuration of himself, his world, his past and future.
5. Alterations in the content of the person's underlying cognitive structures affect his or her affective state and behavioral pattern.
6. Through psychological therapy a patient can become aware of his cognitive distortions.
7. Correction of these faulty dysfunctional constructs can lead to clinical improvement.

The philosophical origins of cognitive therapy can be traced back to Stoic philosophers, particularly Zeno of Citium (fourth century B.C.), Chrysippus, Cicero, Seneca, Epictetus, and Marcus Aurelius. Epictetus wrote in *The Enchiridion:* "Men are disturbed not by things but by the views which they take of them." Like Stoicism, Eastern philosophies such as Taoism and Buddhism have emphasized that human emotions are based on ideas. Control of most intense feelings may be achieved by changing one's ideas.

Freud (1900/1953) initially presented the concept that symptoms and affect are based on unconscious ideas. Alfred Adler's Individual Psychology emphasized the importance of understanding the patient within the framework of his own conscious experiences. For Adler, therapy consisted of attempting to unravel how the person perceived and experienced the world. Adler (1931/1958) stated,

> We do not suffer from the shock of our experiences—the so-called *trauma*—but we make out of them just what suits our purposes. We

are *self-determined* by the meaning we give to our experiences; and there is probably something of a mistake always involved when we take particular experiences as the basis for our future life. Meanings are not determined by situations, but we determine ourselves by the meanings we give to situations. (p. 14)

A number of other writers whose work emerged from or was influenced by the psychoanalytic tradition have contributed important concepts to the development of cognitive psychotherapy. (For a comprehensive review, see Raimy, 1975.) Some of the new influential writers in this group are Alexander (1950), Horney (1950), Saul (1947), and Sullivan (1953).

Philosophical emphasis on conscious subjective experience stems from the works of Kant, Heidegger, and Husserl. This "phenomenological movement" has substantially influenced the development of modern psychology in this group of psychotherapies. The application of the phenomenological approach to specific pathological states is exemplified by the works of Jaspers (1913/1968), Binswanger (1944–45/1958), and Straus (1966). The influence of developmental psychologists such as Piaget (1947/1950, 1932/1960) is also apparent in the formulation of cognitive psychotherapy.

Recent developments in behavioral psychology have also emphasized the importance of the patient's cognitions. Bowers (1973) has argued for an interactional model of subject and environment events and against the "situationism" of classical behavioral approaches. Increasing emphasis on cognitive restructuring or modifying cognitions is reflected in the work of Arnold Lazarus (1972) who states "the bulk of psychotherapeutic endeavors may be said to center around the correction of misconceptions" (p. 165). This correction of misconceptions, Lazarus argues, may precede or follow behavioral change.

A growing number of American psychotherapists have outlined more specifically how the therapist might modify cognitions in a systemic manner during psychotherapy. Kelly (1955) developed personal construct therapy to alter the patient's ongoing conscious daily experience. In "fixed role" therapy, the patient assumes a role based on assumptions about the world or himself which are not congruent with his usual beliefs. In this new role the patient is brought face to face with assumptions he had been making about himself and his interaction with others. Kelly referred to these underlying assumptions or beliefs as "personal constructs."

9

More recently, Berne (1961, 1964) and Frank (1961) added different methods and conceptualizations to therapies designed to alter the ongoing conscious experience or cognitions of the patient.

The work of Ellis (1957, 1962, 1971, 1973) provided a major impetus in the historical development of cognitive–behavioral therapies. Ellis links the environmental or Activating event (A) to the emotional Consequences (C) by the intervening Belief (B). Thus, his Rational–Emotive Psychotherapy aims at making the patient aware of his irrational beliefs and the inappropriate emotional consequences of these beliefs. Rational–Emotive Psychotherapy is designed to modify these underlying irrational beliefs. The use of other techniques to raise these beliefs into awareness and modify them have been emphasized by Maultsby (1975).

Recent contributions to the development of cognitive therapy by behaviorally oriented writers (Mahoney, 1974; Meichenbaum, 1977; Goldfried and Davison, 1976; and Kazdin and Wilson, 1978) have provided a firmer empirical and theoretical basis for further growth in this area.

Cognitive therapy of depression includes a group of interrelated techniques which have been distilled in the crucible of clinical experience with depressed patients. The specific techniques are applied within the framework of a theory about psychological structuring of depression (Beck, 1976). As indicated previously, it is necessary to understand the cognitive model theory of depression in order to apply the specific techniques of cognitive therapy.

The Cognitive Model of Depression

The cognitive model of depression evolved from systematic clinical observations and experimental testing (Beck, 1963, 1964, 1967). This interplay of a clinical and experimental approach has allowed for a progressive development of the model and of the psychotherapy derived from it (see Beck, 1976).

The cognitive model postulates three specific concepts to explain the psychological substrate of depression: (1) the cognitive triad, (2) schemas, and (3) cognitive errors (faulty information processing).

Concept of Cognitive Triad

The cognitive triad consists of three major cognitive patterns that induce the patient to regard himself, his future, and his experiences in an idiosyncratic manner. The first component of the triad revolves around the patient's negative view of himself. He sees himself as defective, inadequate, diseased, or deprived. He tends to attribute his unpleasant experiences to a psychological, moral, or physical defect in himself. In his view, the patient believes that *because* of his presumed defects he is undesirable and worthless. He tends to underestimate or criticize himself because of them. Finally, he believes he lacks the attributes he considers essential to attain happiness and contentment.

The second component of the cognitive triad consists of the depressed person's tendency to interpret his ongoing experiences in a negative way. He sees the world as making exorbitant demands on him and/or presenting insuperable obstacles to reaching his life goals. He misinterprets his interactions with his animate or inanimate environment as representing defeat or deprivation. These negative misinterpretations are evident when one observes how the patient negatively construes situations when more plausible, alternative interpretations are available. The depressed person may realize that his initial negative interpretations are biased if he is persuaded to reflect on these less negative alternative explanations. In this way, he can come to realize that he has tailored the facts to fit his preformed negative conclusions.

The third component of the cognitive triad consists of a negative view of the future. As the depressed person makes long-range projections, he anticipates that his current difficulties or suffering will continue indefinitely. He expects unremitting hardship, frustration, and deprivation. When he considers undertaking a specific task in the immediate future, he expects to fail.

The cognitive model views the other signs and symptoms of the depressive syndrome as consequences of the activation of the negative cognitive patterns. For example, if the patient incorrectly *thinks* he is being rejected, he will react with the same negative affect (for example, sadness, anger) that occurs with *actual* rejection. If he erroneously believes he is a social outcast, he will feel lonely.

The motivational symptoms (for example, paralysis of the will, escape and avoidance wishes, etc.) can be explained as consequences of negative cognitions. Paralysis of the will results from the patient's pessimism and hopelessness. If he expects a negative outcome, he will not commit himself to a goal or undertaking. Suicidal wishes can be understood as an extreme expression of the desire to escape from what *appears* to be insoluble problems or an unbearable situation. The depressed person may see himself as a worthless burden and consequently believe that everyone, himself included, will be better off when he is dead.

Increased dependency is also understandable in cognitive terms. Because he sees himself as inept and helpless and unrealistically overestimates the difficulty of normal tasks, he expects his undertakings to turn out badly. Thus, the patient tends to seek help and reassurance from others, whom he considers more competent and capable.

Finally, the cognitive model may also explain the physical symptoms of depression. Apathy and low energy may result from the patient's belief that he is doomed to failure in all efforts. A negative view of the future (a sense of futility) may lead to "psychomotor inhibition."

Structural Organization of Depressive Thinking

A second major ingredient in the cognitive model consists of the concept of schemas. This concept is used to explain why a depressed patient maintains his pain-inducing and self-defeating attitudes despite objective evidence of positive factors in his life.

Any situation is composed of a plethora of stimuli. An individual selectively attends to specific stimuli, combines them in a pattern, and conceptualizes the situation. Although different persons may conceptualize the same situation in different ways, a particular person tends to be consistent in his responses to similar types of events. Relatively stable cognitive patterns form the basis for the regularity of interpretations of a particular set of situations. The term "schema" designates these stable cognitive patterns.

When a person faces a particular circumstance, a schema related to the circumstance is activated. The schema is the basis for molding data into cognitions (defined as any ideation with verbal or pictorial content). Thus, a schema constitutes the basis for screening out, differentiating, and coding the stimuli that confront the individual. He categorizes and evaluates his experiences through a matrix of schemas.

The kinds of schemas employed determine how an individual will structure different experiences. A schema may be inactive for long periods of time but can be energized by specific environmental inputs (for example, stressful situations). The schemas activated in a specific situation directly determine how the person responds. In psychopathological states such as depression, patients' conceptualizations of specific situations are distorted to fit the prepotent dysfunctional schemas. The orderly matching of an appropriate schema to a particular stimulus is upset by the intrusion of these overly active idiosyncratic schemas. As these idiosyncratic schemas become more active, they are evoked by a wider range of stimuli which are less logically related to them. The patient loses much of his voluntary control over his thinking processes and is unable to invoke other more appropriate schemas.

In milder depressions the patient is generally able to view his negative thoughts with some objectivity. As the depression worsens, his thinking becomes increasingly dominated by negative ideas, although there may be no logical connection between actual situations and his negative interpretations. As the prepotent idiosyncratic schemas lead to distortions of reality and consequently to systematic errors in the depressed person's thinking, he is less able to entertain the notion that his negative interpretations are erroneous. In the more severe states of depression, the patient's thinking may become completely dominated by the idiosyncratic schema: he is completely preoccupied with perseverative, repetitive negative thoughts and may find it enormously difficult to concentrate on external stimuli (for example, reading or answering quesions) or engage in voluntary mental activities (computations, problem-solving, recall). In such instances we infer that the idiosyncratic cognitive organization has become autonomous. The depressive cognitive organization may become so independent of external stimulation that the individual is unresponsive to changes in his immediate environment.

Faulty Information Processing

These systematic errors in the thinking of the depressed person maintain the patient's belief in the validity of his negative concepts despite the presence of contradictory evidence (see Beck, 1967).

1. *Arbitrary inference* (a response set) refers to the process of drawing a specific conclusion in the absence of evidence to support the conclusion or when the evidence is contrary to the conclusion.
2. *Selective abstraction* (a stimulus set) consists of focusing on a detail taken out of context, ignoring other more salient features of the situation and conceptualizing the whole experience on the basis of this fragment.
3. *Overgeneralization* (a response set) refers to the pattern of drawing a general rule or conclusion on the basis of one or more isolated incidents and applying the concept across the board to related and unrelated situations.
4. *Magnification and minimization* (a response set) are reflected in errors in evaluating the significance or magnitude of an event that are so gross as to constitute a distortion.
5. *Personalization* (a response set) refers to the patient's proclivity to relate external events to himself when there is no basis for making such a connection.
6. *Absolutistic, dichotomous thinking* (a response set) is manifested in the tendency to place all experiences in one of two opposite categories; for example, flawless or defective, immaculate or filthy, saint or sinner. In describing himself, the patient selects the extreme negative categorization.

A way of understanding the thinking disorder in depression is to conceptualize it in terms of "primitive" vs. "mature" modes of organizing reality. As is apparent, depressed persons are prone to structure their experiences in relatively primitive ways. They tend to make broad global judgments regarding events that impinge on their lives. The meanings that flood their consciousness are likely to be extreme, negative, categorical, absolute, and judgmental. The emotional response, thus, tends to be negative and extreme. In contrast to this primitive type of thinking, more mature thinking automatically integrates life situations into many dimensions or qualities (instead of a single category), in quantitative rather than qualitative terms, and according to relative rather than absolutistic standards. In primitive thinking, the complexity, variability, and diversity of human experiences and behavior are reduced into a few crude categories.

The characteristics of the typical depressive thinking appear to be analogous to those described by Piaget (1932/1960) in his descriptions of the thinking of children. We have applied the label "primitive" to this kind of thinking to distinguish it from the more adaptive thinking observed in later stages of development. The differentiating characteristics of these forms of thinking are schematized below.

"PRIMITIVE" THINKING	"MATURE" THINKING
1. *Nondimensional and global:* I am fearful.	*Multidimensional:* I am moderately fearful, quite generous, and fairly intelligent.
2. *Absolutistic and moralistic:* I am a despicable coward.	*Relativistic and nonjudgmental:* I am more fearful than most people I know.
3. *Invariant:* I always have been and always will be a coward.	*Variable:* My fears vary from time to time and from situation to situation.
4. *"Character diagnosis":* I have a defect in my character.	*"Behavioral diagnosis":* I avoid situations too much and I have many fears.
5. *Irreversibility:* Since I am basically weak, there's nothing that can be done about it.	*Reversibility:* I can learn ways of facing situations and fighting my fears.

According to this schematic representation, we observe that the depressed patient tends to view his experienes as total deprivations or defeats (nondimensional) and as irreversible (fixed). Concomitantly, he categorizes himself as a "loser" (categorical, judgmental) and doomed (irreversible character deficits).

The bulk of this monograph is devoted to a description of ways in which to identify such idiosyncratic thinking patterns and strategies to counteract them. Specific suggestions for dealing with the absolutistic, dichotomous thinking may be found in the section on Cognitive Symptoms in Chapter 9.

Predisposition to and Precipitation of Depression

The cognitive model offers a hypothesis about predisposition to depression. Briefly, the theory proposes that early experiences provide the basis for forming negative concepts about one's self, the future, and the external world. These negative concepts (schemas) may be latent but can be activated by specific circumstances which are analogous to experiences initially responsible for embedding the negative attitude.

For example, disruption of a marital situation may activate the concept of irreversible loss associated with death of a parent in childhood. Alternatively, depression may be triggered by a physical abnormality or disease that activates a person's latent belief that he is destined for a life of suffering. Unpleasant—even extremely adverse—life situations do not necessarily produce a depression unless the person is particularly sensitive to the specific type of situation because of the nature of his cognitive organization.

In response to traumatic situations the average person will still maintain interest in and realistically appraise other nontraumatic aspects of his life. On the other hand, the thinking of the depression-prone person becomes markedly constricted and negative ideas develop about every aspect of his life.

There is substantial empirical support for the cognitive model of depression. Naturalistic studies, clinical observations and experimental studies have recently been reviewed (Beck and Rush, 1978). Studies have documented the presence and intercorrelation of the constituents of the "cognitive triad" in association with depression. Several studies support the presence of specific cognitive deficits (for example, impaired abstract reasoning and selective attention) in depressed or suicidal persons.

A Reciprocal Interaction Model

Our discussion of the cognitive theory of depression may appear one-sided up to this point; it may appear that the patient may develop depression independently of his interpersonal experiences. Part of this apparent overemphasis on the "intrapsychic" aspects of depression is the result of the deliberate focus on the individual and his construction of reality. Expanding the unit of observation to the important aspects of his environment (for example, family, friends, peers, employer, etc.).

As pointed out by Bandura (1977), a person's behavior influences other people whose actions in turn influence the individual. A person slipping into depression may withdraw from significant other people. Thus alienated, the "significant others" may respond with rejections or criticisms, which in turn, activate or aggravate the person's own self-rejection and self-criticism. (Alternatively, rejection from others may be the first link in the chain leading to clinical depression.) The resulting negative conceptualizations lead the patient (who may by now be clinically depressed) to further isolation. Thus the vicious cycle can continue until the patient is so depressed that he may be impervious to attempts by others to help him and show him love and affection.

A harmonious interpersonal relationship, on the other hand, may provide buffers against the development of a full-blown depression. Thus a strong social support system may provide such powerful evidence of acceptance, respect, and affection that it neutralizes the patient's tendency to downgrade himself. Further, the treatment of the depressed patient is often greatly facilitated by utilizing a family member or close friend to serve as a representative of social reality, to help the patient to test the validity of his negative thinking. When counterproductive interactions with significant other persons contribute to the maintenance of the depression, then a form of "couples therapy," marriage counseling, or family therapy may be indicated.

It should be emphasized that depressed patients may vary considerably in the extent to which their depressions are aggravated or alleviated by other persons. Some depressions are relatively nonreactive and proceed along an inexorable path despite favorable environmental influences.

Primacy of Cognitive Factors in Depression

Important questions have been raised regarding the *primacy* of cognitive factors in the syndrome of depression. As Schreiber (1978) points out, negative distortions could be regarded on a par with affective, motivational, behavioral, and vegetative symptoms simply as a manifestation or symptom of depression. In fact, many contemporary descriptions regard depression as an affective disorder, pure and simple, and ignore the cognitive aspects completely.

In our conceptualization of depression, we have attempted to make some sense out of the highly diverse phenomena of depression by arranging them in a coherent logical sequence. The way the signs and symptoms of a disorder may be fitted together in order to construct meaningful (although hypothetical) relationships may be illustrated by an analogy.

Let us consider a patient who presents himself to his physician with generalized weakness, chest pain, labored and noisy breathing, chronic cough, and bloody sputum. In order to place these phenomena in a comprehensible sequence, we would be bound to focus our attention on his chest pain as the first link in the chain reaction. We could then chart the following sequence: chest pain $\longrightarrow$ breathing difficulty + cough $\longrightarrow$ bloody sputum and generalized weaknesses. The working hypothesis would be that he has a lesion in his lungs that would account for the respiratory symptoms and chest pain. Assume the physician has to rely completely on the patient's reports and his own physical examination. If he were then able to demonstrate (after percussion and auscultation of the chest) some abnormality in the relevant portion of the lung, for example, an area of increased density, we would have some supporting evidence for the preliminary formulation. Further, if the physician could reverse the illness by reducing or eliminating the increased density in the lung (for example, through breathing exercises, bed rest, or artificially collapsing the lung) we would obtain further support for the notion of the pathogenesis of the illness.

At this point, however, one could not make any definite statement regarding the immediate cause of the illness (possibly a lung infection or a tumor) nor the ultimate cause (possibly a bacterium, a toxin, or a carcinogenic agent). We could only state

18

that within the constraints of the available data provided by the patient and the limited data elicited by direct examination, we could reasonably ascribe *primacy* in the sequence of symptoms to pathology in the lung. We would have to be content with the evidence that the lesion in the lung is a contributing factor to or a mechanism for maintaining the illness. In many ways, our formulation regarding depression is analogous to this hypothetical sign-and-symptom configuration.

Thus, in taking a "cross section" of the symptomatology of depression, we have arrived at the position that we should look for the primary psychopathology in the peculiar way the individual views himself, his experiences, and his future (the "cognitive triad") and his idiosyncratic way of processing information (arbitrary inference, selective recall, overgeneralization, etc.). Our clinical experience and experimental work suggests that the parallel to a lung lesion may be useful. The most florid manifestations of depression may distract the clinician (as well as the patient) from even noting the locus of significant pathology. Just as in the case of a "silent tumor" of the lung, the most dramatic symptoms may be physical pain, cough, and weakness, so in depression the overriding symptoms may be psychic pain, agitation, and loss of energy. If the diagnostician does not search for other pathology, he may miss the primary phenomenon in the chain of events, namely the thinking disorder.

It should be emphasized that our explanation up to this point is based on the analysis of the *phenomena* of depression. Our observational tools at this level of analysis do not provide data regarding the ultimate "cause." The patient's negative constructions of reality can be postulated to be the first link in the chain of symptoms (or "phenomena"). Such a formulation provides a whole range of testable hypotheses. Recent reviews of the literature have cited over 35 correctional and experimental studies that support these hypotheses (Beck and Rush, 1978; Hollon and Beck, in press).

As mentioned previously, the cognitive model, however, does not address itself to the question of the possible *ultimate etiology* or cause of unipolar depression: for example, hereditary predisposition, faulty learning, brain damage, biochemical abnormalities, etc., or any combination of these.

Another challenge to the cognitive model is related to the question of predisposition to depression. This issue regarding the cognitive model focuses on how peculiarities in the cognitive organization contribute to the susceptibility to and the precipitation of the disorder. Our formulation of the role of predisposing maladaptive cognitive structures is based partly on long-term clinical observation as well as logical speculation. It does not seem plausible to us that the aberrant cognitive mechanisms are created *de novo* every time an individual experiences a depression. It appears more credible that he has some relatively enduring anomaly in his psychological system. Thus, we need to make our longitudinal analysis in structural terms. A set of dysfunctional "cognitive structures" (schemas) formed at an earlier time becomes activated when the depression is precipitated (whether by psychological stress, biochemical imbalance, hypothalamic stimulation, or some other agent). The formation and manner of activation of the depressogenic schemas has been formulated previously (Beck, 1967).

COGNITIVE REVOLUTIONS: SCIENTIFIC AND DEPRESSIVE PARADIGMS

In a sense, the cognitive therapy of depression presents an attempted solution to the "paradoxes of depression" (Beck, 1976, pp. 102–05). The phenomena of depression are characterized by a reversal or distortion of many of the generally accepted principles of human nature: the "survival instinct," sexual drives, need to sleep and eat, the "pleasure principle," and even the "maternal instinct." These paradoxes may become comprehensible within the framework of what contemporary writers in psychology have referred to as "the cognitive revolution in psychology" (Dember, 1974; Mahoney, 1977; Weimer and Palermo, 1974). Although the shift toward the study of cognitive processes may be regarded as a continuation of the long dialectic between intrapsychic psychology and situationism or the broader philosophical conflicts between mentalism and physicalism, there is evidence that a new scientific paradigm may be emerging.

The scientific paradigm—(in the sense used by Kuhn, 1962)—that encompasses the Cognitive Model of Depression includes much more than a theory and a therapy. It also includes a previously neglected domain (the cognitive organization), a technology and conceptual tools used for obtaining data in this domain, a set of

20

generally acceptable principles for constructing the theory, and, finally, a specialized technology to collect and evaluate evidence to support the theory. As with other paradigms, "rules of evidence" have been established to determine what data are admissible and how these may be credibly interpreted. In addition, since we are dealing with the practical application of the theory, the paradigm also extends to a system of psychotherapy with its particular set of rules for obtaining and interpreting data and a well developed research design for evaluating improvement attributable to the therapeutic procedures.

What is revolutionary about the new scientific paradigm of depression? First, it focuses on the personal paradigm of the patient (see Chapter 4, p. 61). Secondly, it conceptualizes this depressive paradigm in terms of a "cognitive revolution." Specifically, the cognitive organization of the depressed person has undergone a revolution (or perhaps "convolution") which produces a marked *reversal* in the way the patient construes reality. In contrast to the usual notion of a scientific revolution, which is generally regarded as representing progress, the "depressive revolution" constitutes a regression.

Our new *scientific* paradigm of depression states: The *personal* paradigm of the patient when he is in a depressed state produces a distorted view of himself and his world. His negative ideas and beliefs appear to be a veridical representation of reality to him even though they appear farfetched to other people and also to himself when he is not depressed. His observations and interpretations of events are molded by his conceptual framework—equivalent to Kuhn's description of a scientific paradigm. The gross changes in his cognitive organization lead to incorrect information processing, as a result of which he suffers a wide variety of painful symptoms. We utilize our scientific paradigm first to understand and secondly to modify the incorrect personal paradigm so it no longer provides spurious observations and interpretations. We propose, furthermore, that when the patient's personal paradigm is reversed and realigned with reality (a kind of "counter-revolution") his depression starts to disappear.

The concept of a cognitive revolution in depression has implications for research in the psychopathology (as well as the psychotherapy) of this condition. Much of the analogue research and studies of "subclinical" depression have assumed a *continuity* from normal to pathological states. If the clinical state of depression is qualitatively different from the nondepressed state, researchers may need to set aside their working principles (e.g., conditioning theory, information processing) that are applicable to the study of normals and adopt a different paradigm for studying depression. This shift in the kind of theory applicable to the normal vs. the abnormal personality may be illustrated in the following example.

One of the primary characteristics of the severely depressed patient is his relative obliviousness to environmental inputs. Irrespective of what is transpiring around him, he tends to perseverate about themes of deprivation, defectiveness, or disease. In metaphorical terms, the cognitive organization has become relatively autonomous and grinds out a continuous stream of repetitive, negative ideas. These cognitions consist to some extent of stereotyped negative constructions of immediate external events, but for the most part represent reverberations of the repetitive negative ideation that is divorced from the current environmental situation. Hence formulations such as Bandura's reciprocal-interaction model would not be applicable to such psychopathological state. The "autonomous cognitive model" might be more suitable for developing hypotheses and devising relevant experiments for studying the psychologically disturbed person.

Prerequisites for Conducting Cognitive Therapy of Depression

1. The psychotherapist treating depressed patients must have a solid understanding of the clinical syndrome of depression. On the basis of his formal education and training, he needs grounding in the interviewing skills necessary to define the patient's "mental status" and to obtain an adequate history. He should be thoroughly familiar with the myriad clinical manifestations of the syndrome and the vicissitudes of the clinical course and outcome. These clinical features include a knowledge of spontaneous remissions, relapse rate, and suicidal risk.

The therapists should not be bound by some idiosyncratic definition of depression dictated by a particular "school" of psychiatry or psychology but should adhere to the widely accepted descriptions of the syndromes. For example, the description of the symptomatology, clinical course, and nosology of depression described in *Depression, Causes and Treatment* (Beck, 1967) has been generally accepted as definitive by researchers and clinicians, irrespective of their own theories regarding the nature and etiology of depression. Hence, this text (or an equivalent text) should be used by the investigator or therapist as a framework in dealing with this condition.

We believe that the tendency of many psychotherapists to ignore the traditional nosological categories and to concentrate simply on the patient's problems is restrictive and may lead to unfortunate consequences. Although we are sympathetic to the philosophy of "treating the patient rather than the disease," there are substantial reasons for separating psychological disturbances into classes and consequently for applying sensitive techniques for arriving at the correct diagnosis.

Depression, for example, has a number of highly differentiating characteristics. First, it has a particular set of discriminable symptoms and behaviors which set it apart from other neuroses. Secondly, it tends to run a particular course. A typical depression usually starts off mild, reaches a peak of severity, and then generally declines in intensity until its time-limited characteristic and "spontaneous remissions" have been observed repeatedly by clinicians. Depression tends to be episodic with periods of symptom-free intervals. The time-limited nature of depression distinguishes this syndrome from others such as phobias and obsessive compulsive neuroses and even chronic anxiety which may continue for a lifetime without any substantial change. Third, because of the lethal complication that is almost specific for this syndrome, namely, suicide, the diagnosis of depression is particularly important. Fourth, specific somatic treatments have been successfully applied to depression. The tricyclic drugs, for instance, have a highly selective application to this syndrome. Electroconvulsive treatment often produces highly dramatic results in selected cases of depression although it tends to make other conditions, such as anxiety neurosis, worse. Fifth, an accumulating body of evidence indicates that there is a particular type of biological derangement in depression, possibly related to a depletion of neurotransmitters. Sixth, there is some evidence that certain types of depressive illness (e.g., bipolar depressions) have a strong hereditary determinant. Seventh, we have found in our research studies that the specific content of the cognitive distortions and the underlying assumptions are different from those found in other disorders. Finally, the types of precipitating factors (when they are present) may differ in the various neurotic disorders. The precipitants of depression revolve around a perceived or actual loss; in other syndromes, such as anxiety, the specific precipitating factors are more related to threat or danger.

A concise summary of the symptomatology and differential diagnosis of depressive disorders may be found in Chapter 17 (Cognitive Therapy and Antidepressant Medications) in this monograph. Before making a decision regarding the choice of treatment for a depressed patient, the clinician should master the material in that chapter. Otherwise, he may discover to his consternation that he has been treating a continuously cycling manic depressive with an exclusively psychological approach when the patient should be receiving lithium. Similarly, the clinician must be sensitive to the presence of major affective disorders and psychotic depression lest he unwittingly withhold effective antidepressant medication. Furthermore, he needs to know how and when to combine antidepressant medication with cognitive therapy.

There is danger that an inexperienced clinician may fix attention on one facet of depression and ignore the numerous affective, motivational, cognitive, behavioral, and physiological components. We know of several instances in which a therapist, blinded by theory, proudly reported change in one area, for example, improved interpersonal relations, increased activity level, or an apparent reduction of sadness. Within a few days, the patient committed suicide!

2. Since suicide is *the* lethal complication of depression, the clinician requires specialized skills in recognizing the suicidal patient and determining suicidal risk. Even a mildly depressed patient may commit suicide; moreover, suicide attempts during psychotherapy are not uncommon. The clinician needs to be alert to indicators of increased suicidal risk during treatment to be prepared to make crucial decisions regarding such matters as notifying the patient's family of the suicidal risk, recommending hospitalization, prescribing special precautions within the hospital, etc.

Guidelines for assessing suicidal risk may be found in the monograph, *The Prediction of Suicide* (Beck, Resnik, and Lettieri,

24

1974) and also in the article describing the Scale for Suicidal Ideation (Beck, Kovacs, and Weissman, in press). Prompt psychological intervention, especially when the therapist is able to isolate and reverse the underlying hopelessness, is discussed in detail in Chapter 10.

3. The aspiring *cognitive therapist* must be, first, a good *psychotherapist*. He must possess necessary characteristics such as the capacity to respond to the patient in the atmosphere of a human relationship—with concern, acceptance, and sympathy. No matter how proficient he is in the technical application of cognitive strategies, he will be severely hampered if he is not adequately endowed with these essential interpersonal characteristics.

We have found that therapists with diverse backgrounds and experience can conduct cognitive therapy successfully. Therapists who have practiced psychodynamic therapy frequently are empathetic and sensitive to and skillful in dealing with transference reactions. Behavior therapists, on the other hand, are generally well qualified to apply the specific therapeutic techniques.

4. The knowledgeable, warm, empathetic, accepting therapist cannot expect to achieve good results in the cognitive therapy of depression simply on the basis of studying this monograph. He will need, in addition, to satisfy the following prerequisites:

a. A clear understanding of the cognitive model of depression as described in *Depression: Causes and Treatment* (Chapters 15, 17, 18) and in Chapter 5 of *Cognitive Therapy and the Emotional Disorders* (Beck, 1976).

b. A grasp of the conceptual framework of cognitive therapy as outlined in the latter volume (Chapters 2, 3, 4, 9, 10, and 12) as well as its special application to the treatment of depression (Chapter 11).

c. Formal training at a center for cognitive therapy. This should include supervision in the therapy of depressed patients. The importance of intensive training, including an extended period of supervision, is borne out by a recent study at the Center for Cognitive Therapy. We found that following a three-month crash course including supervision of the treatment of two or three depressed patients, fewer than 25% of the trainees (consisting of psychiatrists and psychologists) met even minimal criteria for competency in cognitive therapy. The 25% continued with weekly supervision of their cases and by the end of a year most were considered to have achieved a reasonable level of competency (see Competency Checklist for Cognitive Therapists in the Appendix). Our experience in general indicates a range of six months to two years in order to reach criteria for competency.

d. Training at workshops, group preceptoring, and institutes, and the utilization of videotapes and annotated transcripts. Such training also requires continual supervision by a qualified instructor on a weekly basis until the competency criteria are met.

Limitations of Cognitive Therapy

A number of systematic studies of cognitive therapy in the treatment of depression (see Chapter 18) indicate the promise of this approach. However, considerable additional research is necessary in order to corroborate the findings of the initial studies and to define the limits of applicability of the method in terms of the specific kinds of depression (for example, presence of "borderline" characteristics) and other patient characteristics (educational level, attitudes toward psychotherapy vs. chemotherapy, psychological-mindedness, "ego strength," and various demographic factors).

In view of the fact that a large body of information is necessary before the role of cognitive therapy in the treatment of depression is defined, we hope that this monograph will be used by investigators seeking to address the serious questions revolving around the applicability and utility of cognitive therapy.

The following *caveats* should be observed by professionals applying the strategies outlined in this manual.

1. Except for research purposes, the therapy should be confined to the kinds of patients who have been shown by research studies to be responsive to this approach. (The readers should review the original reports of the controlled studies summarized in Chapter 18.) These studies have shown the efficacy of cognitive therapy in the

treatment of depressed college students referred to a mental hygiene clinic, a community mental health clinic, or a university psychiatric outpatient department.

2. The effectiveness of this therapy has been demonstrated only with unipolar, nonpsychotic, depressed outpatients. Hence, standard treatment procedures should be used with severe or bipolar depressives, highly regressed or highly suicidal patients (for example, hospitalization and "somatic" therapies). The combination of cognitive therapy and antidepressant drugs is discussed in Chapter 17.

3. Antidepressant medication has established its efficacy in a large number of studies. Hence, cognitive therapy should be reserved for those cases of unipolar depressed patients for whom the clinician believes this approach is preferable to antidepressant medication: (a) The patient refuses drug medication, (b) prefers a psychological approach in the hope that the learning experience will reduce his proneness to depression, (c) has unacceptable side effects to antidepressant medication or has a medical condition that contraindicates the use of antidepressant drugs, (d) has proven to be refractory to adequate trials of antidepressant drugs.

COMMON PITFALLS IN LEARNING COGNITIVE THERAPY

In teaching cognitive therapy, we have observed certain common defects and errors in the therapeutic approach of the trainees.

1. *Slighting the Therapeutic Relationship.* The novice therapist often becomes so enamored of the techniques that he forgets the importance of establishing a sound therapeutic relationship with the patient. Interpersonal problems with the patient present one of the most common problems of therapists when they first begin to learn cognitive therapy. The therapist must never lose sight of the fact that he is engaged with another human being in a very complicated task. The therapist should be particularly sensitive to the following:

   a. The importance of discussion and expression of the patient's emotional reactions (Chapter 2).
   b. The patient's own habitual style of communicating. The therapist must adapt his own personal style so that it meshes with that of the patient. Fortunately, since cognitive therapy

is active, the therapist has the opportunity to develop a broad repertoire of styles. At times, for example, he may have to be very active and at other times, relatively restrained; some patients require considerable coaching, others require encouragement to take the initiative.

c. The disruption in the patient's adaptive interpersonal operations as a result of the depression. The therapist needs to recognize the enormous obstacles to communication posed by depression: difficulties in concentration, communicating and formulating the problems orally, forming an affective relationship. Some depressed patients are practically mute and the therapist needs to take the lead in guessing at what is troubling the patient and obtaining appropriate feedback from the patient in changing or sharpening his guesses. Other patients may feel such a pressure to be certain that they are understood that the therapist must remain relatively passive.

d. The patient's hypersensitivity to any action or statement that might be construed as rejection, indifference, or discouragement. The patient's exaggerated responses or misinterpretations may provide valuable insights but the therapist must be alert to their occurrence and prepare the framework for utilizing these distorted reactions constructively.

2. *Being Stylized, Capricious, or Overly Cautious.* Novice therapists are prone to slide into one of two opposing therapeutic stances. They are so eager to master the technical aspects that they parrot their role models ("The Masters") instead of integrating the therapeutic approach into their own natural style. They thus appear like robots, busily engaged in uttering clichés or employing "gimmicks" that the patients may readily identify from their own reading of material on cognitive therapy. At the other extreme, the therapist may stretch the elasticity of the cognitive model to "try out" whatever particular techniques appeal to him without regard to their appropriateness for this particular patient at this particular time. Such therapists also tend to jump from one technique to another without testing the effectiveness or limitations of any of the techniques.

On the other hand, the neophyte may be overly cautious lest he "do the wrong thing" and upset the patient. As a result, he may retreat into silence or mechanically follow the standard treatment protocol. Fortunately, the overall strategy of cognitive therapy provides a number of safeguards, such as obtaining feedback from the patient regarding his understandings of the therapist's communications and any counterproductive reactions he may have to the therapist's manner, techniques, or suggestions (Chapters 3 and 4).

3. *Being Overly Reductionistic and Simplistic.* Many trainees believe cognitive therapy involves *only* getting people to recognize and correct their negative thinking. Often the therapist is not well grounded in the cognitive model of emotional disorders. It is difficult, if not impossible, to do successful cognitive *therapy* without fully understanding the related *theory.*

Although it is true that the cognitive model attempts to reduce a highly complex disorder into a finite number of concepts, each patient presents a specific idiosyncratic pattern of psychopathology. Furthermore, there is no standard format that can be applied systematically to all patients to obtain the crucial data and change the idiosyncratic patterns.

Since the approach in this treatment monograph consists of operationalizing the techniques as well as the principles of cognitive therapy, the inexperienced therapist may attempt to conduct therapy "from a cookbook." The therapist needs to tread the line between being overly concrete and overly abstract; atomistic vs. global. Cognitive therapy is a holistic approach but it is applied in a sequence of discrete, readily understandable steps.

4. *Being Overly Didactic or Excessively Interpretive.* The use of questions is an important part of cognitive therapy. It may be easy for the therapist to point out that the patient has distorted his experiences, that there is an intervening thought between an event and an emotional experience. But very little progress may occur. It is important that the therapist ask questions that open up the patient's closed logic by using an inductive approach.

A further benefit of this inductive procedure is that the patient can practice this self-questioning behavior later when he is without a therapist. That is, he "hears" the therapist's voice asking questions such as "What is the evidence?" "What is the most adaptive thing for me to do right now?" Further, by learning to recognize and test his hypotheses, the patient develops a healthy empiricism that serves as a safeguard against forming unrealistic conclusions.

A paradoxical drawback of the therapist's preaching his own theories and telling the patient what he thinks the patient is thinking is that such an approach often produces positive results. Because of the demand characteristics of such an approach, the patient "produces" data that support the therapist's beliefs and this often leads to a spurious improvement. In the long run, however, the gains are generally lost and the patient is likely to relapse.

It is essential at times for the therapist to assume an educative role with the patient and explain some of the characteristics of depression and cognitive therapy. The therapist should be vigilant, however, that his explanation should not be accepted uncritically and should insure that they be tested by the patient at a later date.

5. *Being Too "Superficial."* It is crucial that the neophyte recognize the importance of fully ascertaining meanings. Although correcting unrealistic automatic thoughts is an important element in treating a patient, the *totality* of the meaning of the patient's experience is crucial. At times, the meanings people give to a situation may not be fully formulated but rather will have to be drawn out by the therapist.

For example: If a patient receives a rejection of a manuscript, his automatic thought may be "I've failed at this. It's been a waste. I'm never going to write anything again." However, if the therapist asks the patient "What does this mean to you in terms of your future, yourself, and your experiences?" he is likely to get even more salient material. The patient might say, "It means I am totally inadequate, I will never be able to do anything. I'll never advance in my career. . . . I will never be happy."

By relying exclusively on the immediate raw data of the automatic thoughts, the therapist misses the crucial—but unexpressed—meaning: namely, the patient's anticipated consequences in terms of the rest of his life. Furthermore, the therapist and patient must explore the assumptions underlying these meanings and anticipated consequences. In this case, for example, the patient operates on assumptions such as "A single failure predicts continued failure" and "I can never be happy unless I am a successful writer."

Along the same lines, the therapist should be on guard against accepting facile explanations and should check the reliability of the patient's reports of his introspections. The therapist can acquire confidence that he understands the totality of a particular experience by entering into the patient's "phenomenal world." He can then describe his vicarious experience to the patient and obtain feedback regarding the accuracy of his perceptions of the patient's experience. This participatory experience, a component of "empathy," is described more fully in Chapter 8.

6. *Reacting Negatively to Depressed Patients.* The therapist has to keep in mind that working with depressed patients is often hard, tedious work. He should guard against placing pejorative constructions on the depressed person's behavior (Chapter 4). He has to realize that the depressed person may truly believe that therapy has only a minimal chance of helping him, that his life really is difficult, and the future holds no hope. Often new therapists will

a. get caught up in the patient's belief that his life is hopeless and thus give up on the patient and believe he can't be helped;

b. label the patient as being resistant and make a motivational interpretation of the patient's behavior (instead of exploring the basis for the patient's "oppositionalism," nihilism, or skepticism, which are generally rooted in the patient's faulty assumptions). He may then react to the patient on the basis that he is being manipulated. On the other hand, the therapist could constructively view the patient's skepticism as a continuous stimulus to apply the inductive method to the patient's "personal paradigm" (Chapter 4).

One of the best antidotes to responding counterproductively to the patient's self-defeating reactions to therapy is the attempt to empathize with the patient, as described in the previous section. By entering into the patient's phenomenal world, the therapist can understand how the patient's "resistances" are inevitable consequences of the way he construes reality.

7. *Accepting "Intellectual Insight."* The therapist has to be on the guard that he is not misled by the patient's statements that he believes the therapist's formulations "intellectually" but not "emotionally." If the therapist's formulation is correct, the patient may gradually integrate the therapist's idea into his belief system. This is accomplished best through empirical demonstration.

When an individual holds an important belief, he usually has some subjective feeling about it. He has learned to "trust" this subjective feeling that the belief is right. (Of course, this feeling is often a misleading sign and thus leads to misinterpretations that produce serious difficulties.) Thus, when he says "I can believe what you are saying—intellectually," he is simply acknowledging the *possibility* that the therapist's statement is correct, but he has not attached much truth value to it. What is "real" to him is his own belief—not the therapist's declarations or pontifications.

Recommendations regarding the therapeutic approach to questions concerning "intellectual" vs. "emotional" insight will be found in the chapter on technical problems (Chapter 14).

MAXIMIZING THE IMPACT OF COGNITIVE THERAPY

The general principles and techniques of cognitive therapy will be explained in detail in the remaining chapters in this book. However, it is well to underscore at this point certain concepts relevant to enhancing the immediate and long-range effectiveness of this therapy.

1. *Importance of the Collaborative Enterprise with the Patient.* The more the therapist and patient work together, the greater the learning experience for both. The joint effort not only engenders a cooperative spirit but also a sense of exploration and discovery. These factors enhance motivation and help to overcome the many obstacles inherent in psychotherapy.

2. *Value of Capitalizing on the Variations and Fluctuations in the Patient's Depression.* When the patient shows an improvement, the therapist should encourage him to pinpoint what methods (if any) contributed to the improvement. Exacerbations of symptoms or relapses should be anticipated and "welcomed" as a valuable source of information for exploring the factors leading to intensification of depression *and* a valuable opportunity for the patient to practice his techniques for dealing with these problems. This approach is representative of the general philosophy of "turning every disadvantage into an advantage." The therapist should not become too enthusiastic by rapid improvements which are often the result of "nonspecific factors" such as the therapist–patient relationship and the patient's expectancies. The therapist should emphasize the

importance of the patient's *learning* methods to reverse the depression rather than passively getting better. Although appealing, the role of Dr. Sunshine is less effective than the model of serious, objective collaboration on problem solving.

3. *Continuing Emphasis on Self-Exploration.* The concentration on exploring the meaning of events throughout the course of therapy and, especially, after termination, should be encouraged. Even such events as the prospect of termination should be examined and the meanings teased out.

4. *"State-Dependent Learning" and the Collaboration of Significant Others.* We have found that patients learn best to analyze and deal with their difficulties when their problems are "hot." Thus, if they actually experience depressive feelings and the associated cognitions during a therapy session, they can be prepared to deal with the troublesome state when the therapist is not present. For this reason, it is sometimes advisable to attempt to "recreate" a quiescent situation during a therapy session. Moreover, appointments may be scheduled to fit into times when the problematic situation (for example, increased loneliness) is likely to occur, such as weekends or evenings. Sometimes, telephone interviews may be necessary in order to deal with the problem when it is activated. Rather than attempt to fit the patient's treatment into the "Procrustean Bed" of the arbitrarily scheduled treatment session, the therapist or a professional aide might make a home visit, in order to help the patient work out a problem (for example, handling housework or doing school homework) that is specifically related to a particular situation. We have found, for instance, that professional visits of this nature often achieve better results than office visits. Our findings, in this regard, appear to fit current concepts of "state-dependent learning": What a person learns in a particular state is more likely to generalize to that specific state than to other states. Thus, the best time for a patient to learn to deal effectively with suicidal impulses is when he is actively suicidal.

Since home visits are often inconvenient or impossible to schedule, the active collaboration of a family member or friend may be indicated. The "auxiliary therapist" can be trained to implement specific therapeutic strategies in the home situation.

Chapter 2

THE ROLE OF EMOTIONS IN COGNITIVE THERAPY

It is a truism that the richness of human experience is a blend of feelings and emotions. Most people will say that what seems most real or valid to them are their feelings or emotions. Without the free play of emotions, there would be no thrill of discovery, no entertainment over humorous situations, no excitement at seeing a beloved person. Human beings would operate purely at a "cerebral" level, devoid of the feeling tones that make their lives vibrant rather than mechanical.

In one respect the depressed person is like a purely "cerebral" being: He can see the point of a joke but is not amused. He describes the appealing features of his wife or child without a sense of satisfaction. He can recognize the appeal of a favorite food or musical piece—but without experiencing a sense of relish.

Paradoxically, although the depressed person's capacity to resonate with positive feelings is dulled, he experiences extreme vibrations of unpleasant emotions. It is as though his entire reservoir of feelings is channeled through the sluices of sadness, apathy, and unhappiness.

Thus, when we deal with the depressed patient, we must never lose sight of the gravity of his *loss*—the constriction of his capacity to feel pleasure, affection, gaiety, and amusement—and the intensity of his sadness. Not infrequently, depressed patients seek help primarily because they no longer feel love for members of their family or because they have lost their zest for life. On further exploration, of course, we find that the various other manifestations of depression are also present.

The use of terms such as Rational Therapy or Cognitive Therapy frequently convey the notion of an intellectualized set of rituals that ignore feelings and sensations and substitute a sterile dialectic for a human relationship. The rational—or cognitive—approach has been frequently confused with the philosophical school of rationalism and the movement of rationalism pioneered by Ayn Rand and Nathaniel Brandon. In fact, Albert Ellis changed the name of his approach from Rational Psychotherapy to Rational-Emotive Therapy in order to emphasize the importance of the emotions in the formulation of his theory and therapy.

The *goal* of cognitive therapy is to relieve emotional distress and the other symptoms of depression. The *means* is by focusing on the patient's misinterpretations, self-defeating behavior, and dysfunctional attitudes. However, the therapist must be sensitive to the patient's intensified unpleasant emotions. He needs to be able to empathize with the patient's painful emotional experiences as well as to be able to identify his faulty cognitions and the linkage between negative thoughts and negative feelings. Similarly, the therapist should continuously be alert to flickers of amusement and satisfaction in order to enhance these pleasant emotions. When possible, he should fan the embers of the patient's affection and gratification. People in our culture, not trained in the Stoic tradition, attach great meaning to their pleasant emotional experiences. The loss of these pleasant feelings conveys a sense of not being a "real person," of having one's existence dried up. From the standpoint of therapy, the patient's report and experience of these feelings provide a valuable indication of his progress and a guide to specific therapeutic strategies.

We should, however, note that cognitive therapy does not emphasize the *exclusive* value of the searching out and enhancement of emotional experience to the extent advocated by the experiential schools of psychotherapy (e.g., Primal Therapy, Janov, 1970). These "abreactive" therapies generally ignore the relevance of irrational or dysfunctional ideation to the production of excessive, inappropriate emotional reactions, and dismiss the value of the rational techniques in their alleviation.

From the standpoint of the theory of what gets people better, a number of writers have presented convincing arguments that therapeutic improvement produced by a number of diverse therapies can be attributed largely to cognitive modification. For example, clinical and empirical evidence has been adduced in support of the notion that improvement in the course of systematic desensitization is mediated by cognitive restructuring (for example, Breger and

McGaugh, 1965). Similarly, Ellis has indicated that the prime mover in the success of the "feeling" therapies, such as Gendlin's experiential therapy, is cognitive reorganization.

Specific types of "emotional problems" other than depression have been shown to consist of far more than evocation of pure emotion. Serious empirical work has demonstrated the crucial role of cognitive factors in the production and alleviation of anxiety (Lazarus, 1966; Meichenbaum, 1977) and of anger (Novaco, 1975). In fact, it would be less misleading if emotional disorders were relabeled "psychological disorders."

In addition to including a detailed formulation of the relationship of emotions to cognitive processes, cognitive therapy draws heavily on "emotional techniques" as part of the therapeutic repertoire. We have found that the spontaneous expression of emotions and intensification of emotions through techniques such as "sensory awareness" and "flooding" are important tools—as long as they are woven into the program of cognitive modification. In fact, since an essential part of the cognitive therapy of depression is to establish the connection between an unpleasant emotion and the antecedent cognitions or the prevailing attitude, it is obviously essential to focus on and discriminate the patient's emotional reactions.

IDENTIFICATION AND EXPRESSION OF EMOTIONS

We have already indicated the importance of assigning an appropriate role to the emotions in the cognitive model of personality and psychopathology (Chapter 1). We have previously emphasized the importance of designing the cognitive approach as a "humanistic" as opposed to a "mechanistic" therapy. It is, therefore, crucial that the inexperienced therapist have a continuing awareness and appreciation of vicissitudes of the patient's emotional reactions—and his own, as well. Moreover, the early identification of the patient's inappropriate or excessive emotional reactions is obviously crucial as a signal of a dysfunctional cognition.

Some patients (especially men) may initially reject the notion that they are feeling sad; however, they generally become aware of and acknowledge their feelings after clarification of other depressive symptoms. We have found, for instance, that some patients who endorse the statement "I am not sad or unhappy" in the first set of alternatives on the Beck Depression Inventory change their response to "I am very sad" after they have completed the rest of the questionnaire.

Occasionally a patient may present a variety of symptoms associated with depression (for example, loss of energy, sleep disturbance, loss of appetite, negative attitudes) but, instead of feelings of sadness, may complain of the loss of or diminution of positive feelings; for example, loss of affection for spouse, children, or friends; lack of zest for new activities; reduction of gratification from ordinarily satisfying activities. Such a patient may experience apathy but not be aware of sadness.

In ascertaining the patient's emotional reactions, the therapist should be careful not to fall into the semantic trap of accepting any phrase that follows the words "I feel" as an emotion. It is common for people to preface a wide assortment of opinions, beliefs, speculations, and other attributions with words such as "I feel." When a person makes statements such as "I feel I am worthless" or "I feel I have to be successful in order to be happy," he is verbalizing an *idea* that may be associated with a feeling. Or he may be expressing a concept tentatively—as though to say "I realize this may not be a defensible idea. So I will say 'I feel it' rather than 'I believe it.'"

A therapist of the experiential school may seize on the prefatory words ("I feel") and be misled into believing he will get closer to the patient's "true" feelings if he reflects back, "So you feel. . . . " It is desirable for the cognitive therapist to get an early start in making appropriate translations of "I feel . . ." into "You believe . . . ."

After reaching a consensus with the patient on the semantic distinction between *feelings* (sadness, joy, anger, anxiety) and *thoughts* or opinions, the therapist should attempt to assess the patient's capacity to recognize and label his feelings. In general, depressed patients do not have much difficulty in identifying their feelings and in linking the arousal or intensification of unpleasant feelings to specific situations. Occasionally, however, they seem to divorce their feelings from the rest of their behavior. One patient, for instance, would feel a lump in her throat after having a disappointing experience. She would then infer—and indeed experience—a feeling of sadness. Another patient would start to cry prior to recognizing any unpleasant feeling. She would state, "I am crying so I guess I feel sad." On further exploration, she discovered that she had experienced a twinge of sadness before she wanted to cry—which indicates that she was not simply inferring the presence of sadness from the fact that she was crying.

In the course of careful history taking, the patient may expand his or her sphere of awareness to encompass unpleasant feelings. A 35-year-old housewife, for example, complained of easy fatigability, lassitude, and general physical weakness of a year's duration but appeared cheerful and denied having had any feelings or sadness or unhappiness. She told the psychiatrist, "I just don't understand why I feel so tired all the time. I have a devoted husband and two nice kids. I don't have any problems in my marriage . . . actually, I have everything a person could want." The therapist then asked her to tell him more concretely about her relations with her husband. As she started to describe specific interactions with her husband, she began to sob—to her surprise and that of the therapist. She was at a loss to reconcile her feeling of sadness with her rosy view of her marriage.

As she described some of her husband's typical behavioral patterns, she started to cry uncontrollably. After she had regained her composure, she said, "You know . . . I think those things bother me more than I realized." She stated that *now* she was feeling very sad. As she began to grasp her problems with her husband, her sadness increased. From then on, her sadness provided an excellent barometer of the severity of her marital difficulties. Once she learned to focus on her feelings, she was able to tie her sad feelings to specific cognitions such as, "He is inconsiderate." "He always gets his own way." "He doesn't care about what I want." "He acts as though I'm an idiot child."

In the course of rapid counseling, she found that as she was able to modify the absolutistic quality of her evaluations of her husband, she experienced alleviation of sadness and other symptoms of depression. Prior to therapy, she had tended to label her husband as "all good" or "all bad" but would quickly dismiss (and forget) the "bad" labels. After implementing suggestions that she inform her husband more explicitly of her desires, she found he was surprisingly responsive. Almost simultaneously, she became as happy, energetic, and lively as she had been prior to the onset of her depression. Interestingly, in the 15 years since this consultation, she has been free of depressive symptoms.

This patient's central problems revolved around (a) her tendency to construe her experiences in extreme terms and (b) her rejection of any idea or feeling dissonant with her highly romanticized view of her world. Thus, before marriage, she had conceived of her husband as perfect and idealized their relationship. In actuality, although attractive and charming, her husband was egocentric and dominating. In order to preserve her dream of a harmonious relationship, she automatically subordinated her own wishes to his. Periodically, she would, however, have extremely negative thoughts about him, such as "He is cruel and unfeeling," and would feel sad and annoyed. Although she rapidly dismissed the thoughts, the unpleasant feelings persisted. She then struggled to suppress these dysphoric feelings since they were discordant with her view of herself as a happy-go-lucky person. Her loss of energy and fatigability in large part arose from her struggle to deny the existence of unpleasantness. Also, the wide discrepancy between her idealized expectancies and her actual satisfactions left her with a sense of chronic disappointment, which in turn, dampened her own feelings of vitality and curtailed her spontaneity.

After the patient was able to recognize and confront her sadness and irritations, she was then encouraged to see her husband more realistically—as neither the Knight in Shining Armor nor Simon Legree. The final step was restructuring her relationship with her husband. The therapist helped her to achieve this with varieties of assertive training, including role-playing (see Chapter 7).

This case illustrates the importance of skillful questioning in eliciting the patient's feelings prior to the exploration of dysfunctional thoughts and erroneous beliefs. It also underscores the necessity for ferreting out the specific details of a patient's current life situation and not accepting the patient's global statements—whether positive or negative—at face value. In contrast to this woman, however, most depressed patients are drawn to making only overblown *negative* generalizations, which usually collapse when the therapist explores the specific details.

As a final note in the context of the importance of encouraging a patient to express feelings, we have found on occasion that a patient is surprised to find that the therapist accepts and, indeed, empathizes with his feelings of sadness and unhappiness. A policeman, for instance, following a warm response to his expressions of despair, cried for about 5 minutes and then said, "This is the first time I have cried since I was a child." He felt immediate relief and began to emerge immediately from his long-standing depression.

ROLE OF EMOTIONS IN THE THERAPEUTIC RELATIONSHIP

Obviously, practically all components of the therapeutic relationship have emotional aspects. When the therapeutic relationship is going well, the patient generally experiences warm feelings toward the therapist, has optimism about being helped, is grateful to the therapist, has a comforting sense of security when he thinks of seeing the therapist, and looks forward to the therapeutic session. Similarly, the therapist may have a wide range of emotional reactions to the patient—he experiences empathy, concern, the desire to help, and satisfaction over being able to help the patient.

The efficacy of the therapeutic relationship is dependent to a large degree on the patient's capacity to experience and express his feelings during the therapy session. Depressed patients often describe a feeling of "not being genuine." They interpret as a sign of insincerity their difficulty in honestly telling other people how and what they feel and the fact that they maintain a social facade to conceal their loss of positive feelings. Hence, many depressed patients state that simply being able to behave emotionally—without restraint—helps to restore a sense of honesty and genuineness. The patient may say, for instance, "Even though I am probably weak for giving in to my feelings this way, at least I can be honest about it." Thus, the patient's liberty to "be himself" during the session relieves him of the burden of covering up his feelings and trying to put up a brave front.

The patient's shame about his feelings covers a wide range of emotionalized attitudes: his diminution of his ability to express love or even to experience it; his irritation, especially toward those who are important to him, and his ubiquitous anxiety. Above all, patients feel ashamed when their sadness seems to be excessive or inappropriate to their life situation. A patient will say, for instance, "I have everything that anybody could want and yet I am unhappy and displeased and dissatisfied with everything." Patients may be self-reproachful for their apparent lack of appreciation for their "blessings" and, indeed, may experience a good deal of guilt feelings because of this. Indeed, many state they feel guilty and unworthy "because people are so good to me." In fact, some depressives feel worse when friends and family show the patient special consideration or kindness.

Emotional reactions such as these and the not infrequent experience of diminution or loss of love or even irritation toward their circle of friends and relatives are topics that depressed patients practically never feel free to talk about except in the context of therapy. Even then, the patient is not likely to bring up these topics unless the therapist has established rapport with him and also is sensitive to his particular set of "shameful" reactions. "Opening up" relieves the patient of the strain of suppressing or concealing his feelings. The acceptance by the therapist of the patient's negative feelings and attitudes is likely to reduce guilty feelings and self-flagellation.

Many patients also seem to experience relief after being able to cry during the therapeutic session. Uninhibited crying seems to have some intrinsically therapeutic merit in many cases. The benefit is enhanced by the patient's sense of having a sanctuary for self-expression without being judged. However, some patients react badly if they cry during the session. Some patients (particularly men) may consider crying a sign of weakness. Other patients have problems in being able to control their crying and, indeed, would cry throughout the therapeutic session unless the therapist employed specific strategies (diversion or behavioral control) to deal with this problem. As will be discussed in the chapter on special problems, training the patient to control his crying may be a vital prerequisite to fostering constructive communication with him.

The therapist must always keep in mind that he is treating the patient and is not obtaining treatment for himself. In other words, it is particularly important that the therapist be careful not to use the therapy to solve his own problems. However, on occasion we have heard of therapists who were so empathetic with the patient that they started to cry along with the patient; this kind of interchange apparently had some therapeutic value in building a bridge with the patient. Nonetheless, this type of response occurred with highly experienced therapists who knew when to give vent to their own feelings.

EMOTIONAL RELEASE

When we talk about "the release of feelings," of course, we are using a metaphor. The metaphor is based on an image such as an inner well of emotion that is pressing to be released. In this imagery, the emotion flows out as water would from a reservoir. Many therapists, however, take the metaphor literally and induce the patient to express particular feelings that are not actually present. Some therapists of the "experiential school" proceed on the assumption that "the dammed-up feelings" are the source of all the problems and that the release of the feelings will magically get the patient better. While it is true that the patient may *feel* better after expressing his feelings, this experience may not in itself have any lasting effect on the therapy and in fact if it is the major or only component of the therapy, the patient may feel worse in the long run.

In contrast, some patients may regard the expression of feelings as shameful. Although they may be willing to give an intellectual description of their feelings, they may inhibit the overt expression of emotion (sobbing; loud, angry outbursts; tremulous verbalizations; clenching of fists). Hence, they do not gain the benefit of a true "catharsis." In such cases, it may be necessary to identify the patient's objections to expressing feelings before the patient can allow himself to express them.

The therapist should take the stance that any feelings the patient has may appropriately be discussed during the session. That is, all feelings are acceptable. However, it is important to structure the session in such a way that the entire time is not devoted to the patient's "emoting." Particularly when the patient's emotional reactions are excessive or based on irrational ideas, it is important to encourage the patient to explore the attitudes that seem to be generating the exaggerated feelings. Some therapists are particularly vulnerable to a patient's annoyance and criticisms of them. The therapist should remind himself that such negative expressions are part of the normal range of emotions and are generally accentuated in someone who has a psychological disorder, and thus should not be discouraged. Continuous haranguing by the patient, however, can be counterproductive. The therapeutic management of such a situation will be discussed in the chapter on special problems.

Similarly, while the experience of warm, grateful feelings toward the therapist often speeds the therapy, at times the patient may become so bogged down in his positive feelings toward the therapist that he does not move along in therapy. Furthermore, the patient may become involved in a very intense "transference" reaction to the therapist, which then poses a problem. Some patients may withdraw from therapy because of infatuation with the therapist and others may want to dominate the relationship with expressions of love; they may desire to fulfill their erotic desires toward the therapist, either inside or outside the therapy session. If the patient wishes to terminate treatment because of such reactions, then the therapist should encourage the patient to bring them out into the open so that they can be examined. In any event, a number of techniques are available for dealing with such reactions.

For example, when a female patient "falls in love" with a male therapist, it is useful to ask the patient to write out all the positive characteristics that she attributes to him. These reactions can then be examined against the evidence to support them. It usually becomes apparent that the patient's conception of the therapist embodies rather grandiose images of him and expectations of having some kind of idyllic life together outside of therapy.

Similarly, unremitting anger toward the therapist can be dealt with by having the patient list the various negative attributes assigned to the therapist and consequently examine the evidence for these. These particular techniques are part of the process of "reality-testing" that is intrinsic to cognitive therapy.

Timing just when to interrupt the patient's outbursts is essential so that the patient has an opportunity to express his negative feelings but does not reach the point that the anger "gets out of hand" and becomes self-perpetuating. After expressing anger toward the therapist or toward some other person, many patients can then sit back and evaluate their feelings; that is, they spontaneously begin to examine whether there is a valid basis for their reactions. Other patients require judicious monitoring in order to achieve a therapeutic balance between emotional expression and rational discussion. Some experimental work by Robert Green and Edward Murray (1975) suggests that rational restructuring is facilitated by emotional release.

If the patient begins to feel better after the expression of feeling, this may then set up a favorable cycle. Since the depressed patient may have lost hope that he would ever be able to feel better again, this positive experience helps to restore his morale and also his motivation to cooperate in the therapy. Any evidence of feeling better is likely to increase the patient's motivation for therapy and thus contribute to its efficacy.

Chapter 3

THE THERAPEUTIC RELATIONSHIP: APPLICATION TO COGNITIVE THERAPY

Cognitive psychotherapy consists of a number of specific treatment techniques, each of which is applied in a planned and logical fashion and tailored to the individual patient. As with other psychotherapies, the cognitive therapist applies the specific techniques in the context of a particular kind of interpersonal relationship. The way in which the therapist applies these techniques directly influences the nature of the therapist–patient relationship and vice versa.

This chapter describes the general nature of the therapeutic collaboration in cognitive therapy and characteristics of the therapist which we believe facilitate the application of specific techniques for cognitive therapy. These principles provide a standard against which the therapist might assess his own attitudes and techniques. Finally, the specific details of preparing the patient for treatment, formulating a treatment plan, and conducting goal-oriented treatment sessions are presented.

DESIRABLE CHARACTERISTICS OF THE THERAPIST

The general characteristics of the therapist which facilitate the application of cognitive therapy (as well as other kinds of psychotherapies), include warmth, accurate empathy, and genuineness. These characteristics affect the therapist's attitudes and behaviors during treatment. If these attributes are overemphasized or applied artlessly, they may become disruptive to the therapeutic collaboration. On the other hand, a therapist with these qualities who carefully utilizes them can substantially increase his effectiveness.

We believe that these characteristics in themselves are necessary but not sufficient to produce an optimum therapeutic effect.

However, to the degree that the therapist is able to demonstrate these qualities, he is helping to develop a milieu in which the specific cognitive change techniques can be applied most efficiently.

A word of caution is in order. Cognitive and behavioral techniques often *seem* deceptively simple. Consequently, the neophyte therapist may become "gimmick-oriented" to the point of ignoring the human aspects of the therapist–patient interaction. He may relate to the patient as one computer to another rather than as one person to another. Some of the younger therapists who are most skilled in applying the specific techniques have been perceived by their patients as mechanical, manipulative, and more interested in the techniques than in the patient. It is important to keep in mind that the techniques detailed in this book are intended to be applied in tactful, therapeutic, and human manner by a fallible person—the therapist.

Warmth

A warm attitude, a caring concern for and interest in the patient, can help to counteract the patient's predilection to perceive the therapist as indifferent or distant or to view himself as an unwelcome burden on the therapist. Thus, the therapist's warm attitude may help to correct specific negative cognitive distortions which the depressed person brings to the therapeutic relationship and to other relationships as well. It is crucial to bear in mind that the determinative factor in the patient's response is his *perception of warmth* rather than the actual degree of warmth expressed by the therapist.

On the other hand, the therapist is well-advised to exercise caution and vigilance in displaying this warm attitude. If the therapist is too active in demonstrating a warm, caring concern (or more importantly, if the patient thinks the warm attitude is too intense), the patient may react negatively. For example, the patient may think, "I am undeserving of such caring," or "I am deceiving the therapist because he appears to like me and I know I am worthless." Or the patient may misconstrue the therapist's motives: "He's insincere," or "How can he like a worthless person like me?" Occasionally, the patient may interpret expressions of warmth as signs of deep affection or love and may become infatuated with the therapist (see Chapter 2). Thus, the therapist is advised to display an open and caring attitude while avoiding being effusive or overly solicitous.

In essence, the therapist must strike an appropriate balance in displaying warmth. The patient may construe minimal warmth as rejection, while too hearty a display of caring may be misinterpreted in either a negative or overly positive way. Thus, the therapist must carefully attend to signs that suggest that his attitudes are counterproductive.

The safeguard consists of directly asking the patient how he perceives the therapist; for example, as distant, overbearing, or insincere; or as too emotionally involved with him. Often the patient's responses will offer useful guides as to the best way for the therapist to relate himself to the patient as well as provide concrete information regarding the patient's specific sensitivities and cognitive distortions.

The therapist generally conveys his acceptance and warmth in his manner, tone of voice, and way of phrasing his words. These styles are best learned by observing experienced clinicians. The experienced therapist will often vary the degree to which he demonstrates a warm, caring attitude depending on the phase of therapy. Early in treatment the patient may need more active expressions of warmth. Later in treatment, the patient may assume that the therapist is caring and require less overt demonstrations of warmth.

Accurate Empathy

Accurate empathy refers to how well the therapist can step into the patient's world and see and experience life the way the patient does. In fact, the therapist will, to some degree, experience the patient's feelings. To the extent that his empathy is reasonably accurate, the therapist will be able to understand how the patient structures and responds to certain events. Furthermore, the therapist can convey that he can share some of the patient's distress. This expression helps the patient regard the therapist as understanding and, thereby, facilitates further disclosure of feelings and cognitions. In this respect, accurate empathy facilitates therapeutic collaboration (see Rogers, 1951).

Other obvious benefits are derived from such empathy. If the therapist can accurately perceive and share the patient's expectancies, he is more likely to be able to make sense out of the patient's unproductive behaviors and to be less judgmental about them. For example, the therapist may realize that a "resisting" or "negativistic" patient is actually a person who regards himself as so incompetent and hopeless that he doesn't believe he can answer questions or follow out homework assignments well enough even to try. The empathic therapist may be able to understand that the "cynical patient" is a person who has felt "let down" so often in the past that he is wary and angry at the prospect of further frustration.

The irritation evoked in the therapist by the patient's cynicism or apparent negativism may be damped down by an empathic understanding of how this patient's negative expectations have made him mistrustful or nihilistic. By trying to project himself into the patient's microcosm, the therapist is less prone to react in an antitherapeutic way. Moreover, by "trying on" the patient's negative attitudes and cognitions the empathic therapist can then begin to develop antidotes or counterarguments to these negative ideas. As he begins to "enter" the patient's world, the therapist can check on how accurately he is approximating the patient's view by *testing whether his evoked feelings correspond with the patient's feelings.* (Therapists can improve their empathic responses through various training procedures such as "role-playing" the patient in a simulated interview.)

The therapist must be careful not to project his own attitudes or expectations onto the patient and thereby to distort the patient's report. For example, a depressed patient whose mother just died may not necessarily feel sad or upset. Some patients regard such a death in positive terms—as an escape from a harsh, cruel world. The therapist must carefully map out with each patient just how he reacts to such events.

On the other hand, an overreliance on empathy may mislead the therapist into accepting the veridicality of the patient's automatic negative representation of himself and the world. If the therapist does not seek other data not spontaneously reported by the patient, he may begin to believe that the patient's views are an accurate representation of his real life situation. Thus, he should balance his empathic understanding by objective checking of the patient's introspections against other sources of information and testing the logic involved in the patient's inferences and conclusions.

It is important to maintain the distinction between empathy and sympathy. Sympathy refers more to a feeling of compassion for and an active sharing of the patient's pain. An overly sympathetic response may vitiate the therapist's attempts to relieve the sources of the patient's distress. Empathy, on the other hand, includes an intellectual (as well as an emotional) component, namely, understanding the cognitive basis for the patient's feelings; it also implies the ability to detach oneself from the patient's feelings (which may include anger or anxiety as well as sadness) in order to maintain objectivity toward his problems. Although the empathic therapist may realize how the patient's thinking leads to a specific feeling, he need not concur in such thinking if it is erroneous or illogical or if it accentuates rather than resolves problems. We should emphasize, however, the value of the therapist's accepting that the patient's thinking, feelings, and wishes seem valid to the patient and he should not ignore them, dismiss them, or attempt to "talk the patient out of having them."

Genuineness

Genuineness is an important ingredient in all types of psychotherapy. A genuine therapist is honest with himself as well as with the patient. However, he need not be blunt or disruptive with his directness. In view of the depressed patient's tendency to attend selectively to the negative and to extract evidence of his own deficiencies, the therapist needs to mix diplomacy with honesty. The patient may misperceive directness as criticism, hostility, or rejection. Moreover, a strongly positive statement—even though genuine—may evoke antitherapeutic reactions.

It is not sufficient for the therapist to be genuine; he must have the *skill* to communicate this genuineness to the patient; he needs to penetrate or circumvent the patient's system of distortions in order to convey a realistic image of himself. An inexperienced therapist, for example, may extend himself to assure the patient that he will recover. Such a "promise" generally makes the hopeless patient regard the therapist as insincere, lacking in understanding, or foolish. (The more effective kind of reassurance comes from demonstrating to the patient that his painful symptoms may be reversed by correcting his unrealistic ideas and self-defeating behavior.) Stressing his dedication to the patient similarly may evoke suspicious or guilt-laden thoughts, such as "Why does he claim he cares so much for me?" or "I don't deserve so much attention."

THE THERAPEUTIC INTERACTION

Having considered the therapeutically valuable attributes of the therapist, let us focus on the development and maintenance of a therapeutic relationship. The relationship involves both the patient and the therapist and is based on trust, rapport, and collaboration. Cognitive and behavior therapies probably require the same subtle therapeutic atmosphere that has been described explicitly in the context of psychodynamic therapy.

Basic Trust

The importance of *basic trust* in the therapeutic relationship is nicely illustrated in the following description by Chassell (1977).

> An *obscuring factor* is introduced by the existence of basic trust, basic pseudo-trust, and basic distrust in patients. Patients with genuine basic trust tend to exhibit a workable positive transference favoring progress, because they want to have a good object to help them in their difficulties and will utilize the therapist with great tolerance, provided he does not too grossly contradict this image. Patients with pseudo-trust may exhibit many puzzling transference phenomena: emphasizing their dependency needs, testing the limits of the therapist's patience, raising him on a pedestal—and all the while nursing suspicion of his *good faith* [italics ours]. Patients with basic distrust may well make no genuine progress until this problem has been partly solved, and certainly will be most acutely aware of unconscious indications of discrepancies in the therapist's attitude, as well as attributing to him many attitudes which are not there. Very likely the hysterical characters belong to the pseudo-trust group; I am sure that the obsessionals do. (p. 11)

In attempting to develop or elicit trust in the relationship, the cognitive therapist carefully balances the importance of autonomy (letting the patient do the talking, planning, etc.) against the need for structure (the therapist's being directive, taking the initiative, etc.); dependability and responsiveness (being punctual, responding to phone calls, etc.) against the value of setting limits (deciding not to do for the patient what he can do for himself); and being a "real person" (that is, displaying friendly and human qualities) against being unobtrusive and objective. In general, in the initial parts of treatment, the therapist tends to provide more structure and to be more responsive and more "involved" in the patient's problems. In the latter half of treatment, the therapist spurs the patient to take the initiative (for example, to plan the agenda for the interview and homework assignments); he expects the patient to do more for himself and inserts less of himself into the therapy than in earlier phases.

Importance of Rapport

Although often of relatively minor importance in treating delimited disabilities such as specific phobias, rapport is a crucial ingredient in treating depressed patients. The term *rapport*, in general, refers to harmonious accord between people. In the therapeutic relationship, rapport consists of a combination of emotional and intellectual components. When this type of relationship is established, the patient perceives the therapist as someone (a) who is tuned in to his feelings and attitudes, (b) who is sympathetic, empathic, and understanding, (c) who is accepting of him with all his "faults," (d) with whom he can communicate without having to spell out his feelings and attitudes in detail or to qualify what he says. When rapport is optimal, the patient and therapist feel secure and reasonably comfortable with each other. Neither is defensive, overly cautious, tentative, or inhibited.

By "acceptance" we do not mean that the therapist approves of or agrees with everything the patient says, but rather that he is not judgmental. This enables the patient to drop his social mask and pretenses and provides a basis for a more genuine relationship with the therapist.

The therapist who experiences a sense of rapport feels concern for and cares about the patient. Like the patient, he feels a certain freedom in communication. He experiences empathy and senses that they are operating on the same wavelength and feels confident that he can speak spontaneously without being misunderstood.

The free expression of feelings by the patient, of course, facilitates the therapist's experiencing rapport as well as empathy. It is much easier to empathize when the patient is able to convey his feelings with clarity than when the therapist has to strain to ferret out the patient's feelings. In addition to having the sense of being accepted and understood, the patient experiences the therapist as somebody who wants to help him and is able to help him.

It is generally therapeutic for the therapist to express, *judiciously*, feelings such as concern, appreciation, warmth, and encouragement. Moreover, it is sometimes therapeutic if he acknowledges some of his own "negative" feelings, such as disappointments, frustrations, irritations. However, he must exercise caution in how much of his own feelings he expresses toward the depressed patient. He must realize that a genuine expression of feeling on his part may be misinterpreted by the patient. Because of their tendency to distort or magnify, depressed patients may interpret positive expressions as insincere or, on the other hand, may view them as signs of love or sexual advances. Similarly, the therapist's excessive disclosure of his own problems may feed the pessimism of the depressed patient: "He is too weak to help me."

There is no standard set of behaviors that will induce a sense of rapport with the patient. Some sorts of therapist responses are helpful for one patient (e.g., a serious, detached therapist style) while for others an opposite style (e.g., friendly, warm, outgoing) is most conducive to rapport.

The therapist will have a feeling that his remarks and comments are getting to or registering with the patient if there is a sense of rapport. The patient will appear relaxed, open, talkative, will be nodding his head or verbally agreeing, and will appear interested in, curious about, and reflective in response to the therapist's statements.

Rapport not only reflects but also influences the therapist–patient collaboration. For example, rapport can be used to reinforce specific adaptive behaviors on the patient's part. With a high degree of rapport, the patient will tend to be more influenced by the therapist's own behavior (therefore, will tend to identify with or model himself after the therapist). A feeling of rapport will keep the patient motivated for treatment and will motivate him to undertake specific treatment procedures (for example, doing the homework). Rapport stimulates a free expression of ideas and feelings. The patient's negative ideas or feelings which might induce him to leave treatment will more likely surface if the patient feels a strong sense of rapport.

How can the therapist establish or develop a sense of rapport? Many of the relevant behaviors "come naturally" to some therapists. Some specific techniques are useful to cultivate and use. A good base for building of rapport involves simple courtesy: not keeping the patient waiting, remembering important facts about him, and giving a sincerely warm (but not effusive) greeting. Maintaining eye contact, following the content of the patient's talk, trying to infer and reflect the patient's feelings, and phrasing questions and comments diplomatically help to build rapport.

Other factors which influence rapport include the therapist's appearance, mannerisms, and facial expressions. An attitude of warm neutrality and professionalism may be best. The therapist must carefully time when to talk and when to listen. If the therapist interrupts too frequently or in a tactless or curt manner, the patient may feel cut off, and rapport will suffer. If the therapist allows long silences or simply allows the patient to ramble without apparent purpose, the patient may become excessively anxious and rapport will diminish. The therapist's use of a mellow, soft, nonintrusive tone of voice also helps. The choice of words and labels is important (for example, "unproductive ideas" is preferable to "neurotic," "sick," or "irrational" thinking).

The therapist's own cognitive set or attitude toward the patient and treatment is important. Some therapists become frustrated and angry at depressed patients when they perceive the patient as passive or "resistant." In such cases, the therapist's attitude directly generates negative feelings and undermines rapport.

Initially, rapport can be facilitated by eliciting the patient's expectations for therapy and by informing him what to expect during the treatment process. For instance, we advise the therapist to discuss the length of treatment, frequency and length of the sessions, the objectives of each step of treatment, and the probability of "bad days" after improvement.

The therapist can also increase rapport by reflecting the patient's feelings back to him in the form of a sensitive summary, analogy, or metaphor. For example, one patient who had done quite well returned after a relapse and expressed suicidal thoughts. The therapist recalled to her a phrase she had used in a previous session, "I may feel like a mouse but I have the heart of a lion." At the moment, this phrase recaptured the feelings and attitude she needed to continue her struggle, while subtly giving her credit for persisting.

THE THERAPEUTIC COLLABORATION

Eliciting "Raw Data"

Initially, the therapist tries to engage the patient in a therapeutic alliance of collaboration. In contrast to "supportive" or "relationship" therapy, the therapeutic relationship is used not simply as the instrument to alleviate suffering but as a vehicle to facilitate a common effort in carrying out specific goals. In this sense, the therapist and patient form a "team." The initial focus of the collaboration is a common interest in the patient's thoughts, feelings, wishes, and behavior. Specifically, the therapist and patient work together to determine how and what the patient thinks, the basis for such thinking, and the practical benefits or losses which result from such thinking. The patient's unique contribution to this collaborative effort is to provide the raw data for this inquiry—namely, to report his thoughts, feelings, and wishes. The therapist's special contribution is to guide the patient about what data to collect and how to utilize these data therapeutically.

Each step in the progression of treatment is used to develop and deepen the collaborative aspects of the relationship. Initially, with the guidance and encouragement of the therapist, the patient learns to recognize and record his automatic negative interpretations of his experiences. Then, the therapist–patient team begins to analyze these data and looks for specific patterns in the automatic thinking. What sort of environmental events stimulate negative thoughts? How certain is the patient that these thoughts accurately describe the actual event? What sort of logical errors does the patient make in viewing himself, the future, and the world around him? For example, is he overgeneralizing from negative events while selectively failing to attend to positive events? Are there recurrent themes in the content of these cognitions (for example, is the patient continually assessing whether or not he is competent or approved of by others)? The manner in which the patient's thoughts and beliefs are elicited and validated or refuted is critical to fostering rapport and collaboration.

Authenticating Introspective Data

The therapist encourages the patient to identify, observe, and evaluate his thoughts in an objective manner. The patient's thoughts (or cognitions) are regarded as psychological events which may reflect the actual circumstance or situation to a greater or lesser degree. The therapist and patient collaborate to determine to what degree the patient's inferences and conclusions correspond to the observations and conclusions of other objective persons. In this way, the therapist and patient try to test the patient's inferences and conclusions. The therapist questions whether the patient is attributing the idiosyncratic meanings to certain events or whether he is making reasonable inferences.

Often these idiosyncratic depressive cognitions are stereotyped and contain recurrent themes, such as "I am incompetent," or "Nothing ever goes right." As the therapist identifies these themes, he tactfully brings them to the attention of the patient. Together, the therapist and patient begin to hypothesize what sort of assumptions underly these themes (for example, "Unless I do everything perfectly, I am a total failure."). In this way, the patient learns to identify these assumptions and to consider whether they are valid or logical.

Investigating Underlying Assumptions

Investigating the validity of underlying assumptions requires joint effort. The therapist asks the patient to provide evidence (usually from recent experience) for and against each assumption and belief. Alternatively, the therapist may ask the patient to contemplate applying these assumptions to other people to determine whether he is applying a special set of rules to himself that he would not apply to others. It is important in discussing these beliefs that the therapist not aggressively label or prematurely dismiss one or another of these beliefs as "obviously illogical" or "clearly ridiculous." Rather, a tactful, gentle, empathetic yet objective and logical viewpoint is indicated.

Setting Up Experiments

A powerful method with which to investigate the validity of a specific assumption consists of designing an experiment or task to test the assumption empirically. How is this experiment developed? The patient and therapist begin much as two detectives who have a hunch they want to explore. First, they specify the hunch or assumption they want to test. One example might be "If I assert myself with another person, he will reject me." The therapist derives a specific hypothesis from this general rule. The hypothesis is stated in specific operational terms, and the therapist and patient may formulate an experiment to test the prediction made from the general rule.

An illustrative specific hypothesis derived from the general rule stated above is, "If I tell my supervisor that I would like to take a day off because I need a rest, she will retaliate by telling me that I am lazy, shirking my responsibilities, and complaining." The therapist and patient may conclude that a test of this specific hypothesis would consist of the patient's actually talking to the supervisor. If so, the patient records the results of this experiment both in terms of precisely what was said and in terms of what ideas or inferences the patient develops from what happened. The therapist and patient use these data to evaluate the results of the experiment. They consider various interpretations of the results. Finally, the team compares the *actual* results with the patient's *predictions* based on the original hypothesis.

Homework Assignments

The manner in which the therapist goes about each step in therapy (for example, recording of automatic thoughts, assigning homework, testing the validity of thoughts and assumptions), will directly determine whether collaboration and rapport are increased or decreased. Conversely, the degree of collaboration and rapport will influence how well the patient will participate in each of the steps or tasks in the therapy program. The therapist can strengthen the therapeutic collaboration by engaging the patient in the formulation of the homework task itself. Each assignment is presented as an experiment—an opportunity to discover something new about the issues the patient is currently facing. The therapist can increase therapeutic collaboration by explaining the goal and rationale for each homework assignment. If patients understand both how to attempt the homework and why trying to do the homework might help, they are much more likely to be motivated to undertake the assignment.

The assignment of homework critically influences the therapeutic collaboration. Patients often regard the homework as a test of personal worth, personal skill, or motivation, or they may believe they must do the homework perfectly. The therapist tries to sense or directly inquire about such attitudes since they are distortions and antitherapeutic. He actively encourages the patients to share their thoughts and feelings about the homework task, both *before* and *after* attempting it. For instance, the patient who completes a small task successfully may regard this success as a failure "because anybody could do that." These sorts of cognitive distortions are actively identified and corrected. As with other cognitions, these thoughts are examined and, where appropriate, are corrected. The therapist might directly say, "Attempting the homework task is the assignment, not doing it as well as you could before you were depressed."

"Noncollaborative" Therapeutic Techniques

There are many techniques, for example, "paradoxical intention," that may have clinical relevance to depression. However, we generally eschew such methods if they do not fit into our conceptual and therapeutic framework. In addition, we believe that changing the patient's misinterpretations and dysfunctional behavior should be a collaborative enterprise between the patient and the therapist. In addition, we assume that lasting changes in the patient's thinking and behavior are more likely induced with the patient's understanding, awareness, and effort. The goal of the collaborative enterprise further contraindicates conveying to the patient that the therapist is manipulative or practicing "thought control." Thus, we avoid techniques which do not allow for the patient's conscious awareness and full understanding of the purpose of the methods as well as his voluntary participation in these procedures.

"TRANSFERENCE" AND "COUNTERTRANSFERENCE" REACTIONS

Too often, therapists view depressed patients as "willfully" passive, indecisive, and manipulative. The therapist becomes frustrated, and the patient feels criticized; his condition may deteriorate or he may drop out of treatment. These interactions are described in the analytic literature in the context of transference and countertransference reactions. The kind of therapeutic collaboration we have described tends to decrease these sorts of problems and frustrations.

The therapist should confront negative therapeutic reactions head on. By trying to identify and correct the patient's cognitive distortions which contribute to his passivity, lack of initiative, and "oppositionalism," the therapist and the patient collaborate in trying to solve the very problems which contribute to their mutual frustrations. In fact, the dysfunctional thinking which leads to passivity, indecisiveness, lack of motivation, etc., constitutes a specific target of treatment (see Chapter 7). As with other cognitive distortions, the therapist applies logic and the empirical method to correct the errors in such thinking.

Positive transference reactions may also impede the course of therapy. The patient may regard the therapist as a saviour and exaggerate his positive attributes. Such high evaluation and expectations have to be discussed and the positive distortions pointed out. The therapist needs to emphasize working together as a means of solving the patient's problems rather than as an end in itself. The therapeutic handling of "transference problems," such as the patient's infatuation with the therapist, have been described in Chapter 2.

There are a few aspects of structured, active therapy that can produce "negative" therapeutic reactions. Depending on the situation, any of the techniques described in this chapter could be construed by some patients as hostile, controlling, or coercive. However, some actions are particularly likely to be experienced as abrasive by depressed (and indeed many other) patients. These behaviors include preaching, demanding, threatening, arguing, blaming, moralizing, and cross-examining. If the therapist without explanation diverts or shifts the conversation away from topics which the patient wishes to pursue, or if he uses humor to poke fun at the patient (not at his *thinking*), the patient may feel manipulated and belittled.

A number of other difficulties may weaken the collaborative nature of the patient–therapist relationship; two of these are particularly common with depressed patients. First, the therapist may begin to believe the patient's persistent negative view of himself and his life situation. By stepping out of the role of the scientific observer, the therapist may "buy into" the patient's distorted construction of reality. Instead of regarding the patient's negative interpretations as *hypotheses that require empirical testing*, the therapist may begin to assume that these negative cognitions are accurate statements of fact which can be accepted at their face value. When this problem arises, the therapist may begin to regard the patient as a "born loser" or as inextricably caught in an impossible reality situation, rather than realizing that the patient may be so overwhelmed by his pessimistic outlook and self-critical view that he reports only negative observations and erroneous generalizations.* In order to maintain an objective but empathic view, the therapist should remind himself that the patient's negative views are only cognitions and beliefs; i.e., they should be tested and either confirmed or disconfirmed.

A source of disruption of the therapeutic collaboration may occur in the later stages of therapy if the patient should relinquish his objectivity toward his negative cognitions. For example, the patient may experience new disappointments or frustrations due to traumatic environmental events. If this should occur, he may be flooded with a stream of negative cognitions which he automatically regards as valid without subjecting them to further considerations. Consequently, he is likely to experience increasing depression and hopelessness. This symptomatic exacerbation may lead him to decide that cognitive therapy is ineffective and/or that he is incurable. He may also feel disillusioned with his therapist. Any of these views may lead the patient to stop cooperating with the therapist, resist carrying out assignments, miss appointments, or drop out of therapy. This reaction may lead to a *folie à deux* if the therapist unquestioningly accepts the patient's construction of the therapeutic relationship and his own progress in therapy. If the patient begins to miss appointments, the

---

* A number of patients, who had been referred to our clinic with the diagnosis of "realistic depression," were found to have misled the referring physician into accepting their accounts of their reality situations at face value.

therapist is advised to contact the patient and clarify the notions which are disrupting the therapeutic collaboration.

In actual practice, we find that symptomatic relapses during treatment are common. The therapist should inform the patient early in treatment to expect to have negative fluctuations. Such exacerbations provide a valuable opportunity for the patient to apply the techniques and skills he has learned in therapy. Further, they "keep him in practice" to deal with the problems that inevitably occur after termination of treatment.

Chapter 4

STRUCTURE OF THE THERAPEUTIC INTERVIEW

Specific Guidelines for the Therapist

Acknowledge the Patient's "Personal Paradigm"

The therapist should keep several specific principles in mind during treatment.* The depressed patient's personal world view, his negative ideas and beliefs, seem reasonable and plausible to him even though they appear far-fetched to the therapist. He seriously believes and is quite consistent in his beliefs that he is deprived, defective, useless, unlovable, etc. In fact, this internal consistency is often maintained in the face of repeated and dramatic external evidence contradictory to these beliefs. The beliefs are generally organized into a system similar to that Kuhn (1962) described as a scientific "paradigm." The patient's observations and interpretations of reality are molded by this conceptual framework. As in the case of change of scientific beliefs, a personal paradigm may be shaken and modified when the individual is prepared to recognize an anomaly that the existing paradigm cannot accommodate or evidence that disconfirms the paradigm.

The patient, however, generally does not pay attention to or does not assimilate the meaning of events which could disconfirm his depressing view. By accepting the patient's ideas as subjectively valid for him in his current state, the ideas actually have *objective validity*, a problem that can be explored at a later point. The patient often presents his negative ideas early in treatment. As the therapist begins to elicit the reasons why the patient holds these ideas, two sources of

---

* A comprehensive form outlining the general and specific procedures for cognitive therapy of depression is contained in the Appendix. This form, which includes sections on the personal and professional attitudes of the therapist, may be used as a guide for conducting as well as a scale for evaluating interviews.

data are usually discovered. First, the patient presents his views of specific *past* events which he believes substantiate his negative ideas. Secondly, he may construe one or more *present* events as evidence supporting these ideas. Therapy focuses more on current events because the patient can collect fresh data about the events and record his interpretations of current events (his cognitions). Misinterpretations of current events are more readily corrected since empirical evidence can be derived from more recent and, therefore, more reliable observations and recall than can cognitive correction of past events. However, some patients seem impermeable to fresh information that is contradictory to their preconceptions.

The following example illustrates how a patient enters treatment with a firmly held negative self-concept reflected in her interpretation of both current and past events. Evidence which disconfirmed this negative view was presented in the first treatment session. The patient found reasons to discount this evidence. After several sessions, the patient began to doubt this self-view and to volunteer new evidence which argued against her negative self-image. Subsequent testing of this view (for example, going to social gatherings) provided further data which the patient used to make her self-image more realistic.

A depressed mother of five children described herself as incompetent and stupid. She believed the following evidence strongly supported the notion of being stupid: her fear of taking a final exam, which had resulted in her receiving an incomplete grade while in college; the fact that she didn't have a professional career like her physician husband; and recent school problems with two of her teenage children (which led her to regard herself as an incompetent mother).

In the first therapy session, the therapist prematurely attempted to counter her negative self-view. He informed her that her intelligence quotient based on recent psychological testing was 135. She immediately gave several reasons why the test score was invalidly high.

Several sessions later she spontaneously reported several aspects of her life that she had not previously mentioned: she had been a straight-A high school student; she was a certified model; her husband considered her smarter than he was; she had taken flying lessons, had acting and modeling experience, was an amateur photographer, and at several recent social occasions she had heard that others (college deans, physicians, etc.) had found her charming and very interesting, rather than boring and dull as she had assumed.

Thus, although this patient's conceptualization of herself as stupid had no *external validity*, the concept had significant *internal consistency* (for the patient) until well into treatment; the internal "validity" of her beliefs was consistent with other notions about herself, her observations, her salient memories. Initially, the therapist tried to understand the basis for these apparent misconceptualizations; he accepted the patient's belief in her views and did not attempt to reject or dismiss her ideas as foolish. (In fact, an attack on her personal paradigm would have possibly resulted in confusion and possible disruption of the patient's methods for organizing and interpreting reality.) The objective validity of her negative beliefs was tested by gathering additional past-history data previously not recalled and reported and by "running an experiment" to gather data about her erroneous self-evaluation.

If disconfirming data are presented too early (for example, premature reporting of the I.Q. in this case), the patient may dismiss or distort these data. The therapist will find himself in an *adversary role* rather than a collaborator or guide. It seems that only after patients feel they have had a chance to "present their case" and be understood, will they be ready to consider disconfirming data and to run tests on the external validity of their beliefs.

Avoid "Labeling" the Patient and Making Value Judgments

We recommend that the therapist view his patient as a person who has problems and specific deficits or who holds some irrational beliefs, rather than as a person who is irrational or who has a defective character. In this context, it is wise to avoid the use of professional jargon in labeling the patient (for example, passive–aggressive, masochistic, neurotic, hysterical). Such pejorative labeling affects the therapist's and patient's attitude toward the patient. It also implies that the patient is relatively unchangeable and intrinsically defective. Furthermore, such global negative attitudes impede concentration on and delineation of specific problems and prescriptions of specific solutions. Actually, depressed patients generally are competent in many areas of functioning and in a wide variety of situations; their problem-solving skills tend to fail in highly specific conditions.

Depressed patients' chronic negative thinking may easily become a source of irritation to the therapist. The therapist may be tempted to blame patients for their "chronic symptom recitals" or "lack of will." These patients are often pigeonholed by others, including therapists, as chronic complainers, basically passive, overly dependent, and resistant. These negative constructions may lead the therapist to criticize the patient for not "cooperating in therapy" or for continuing to express pessimistic notions. When the therapist becomes frustrated, he is probably not sufficiently objective toward the patient's negative cognitions and beliefs to understand how the patient's behavior is completely consistent with his distorted thinking.

It is best to assume that given a free choice, the patient would prefer to be less helpless, more independent, and less passive (if he believed these choices were possible). When the patient does not attempt to carry out an assignment, misses an appointment, or derogates his ability, the skillful therapist will search for cognitions or attitudes which produce this regressive behavior. The therapist should regard the negative cognitions as a typical component of the depression, not as an inherent attribute of the patient.

Avoid Ascribing Self-Defeating Behavior to "Unconscious Wishes"

The therapist should avoid attempting to explain the patient's self-defeating behavior on the basis of "infantile wishes." In cognitive therapy the therapist assumes that the dominant factor in determining behavior is the patient's view of himself, his life situation, and his future expectations. Theories such as classical psychoanalysis assume that once the patient perceives the unconscious wishes presumed to underlie his oppositional and self-defeating behavior, he will choose more adaptive coping strategies. However, when depressed patients are confronted with a motivational interpretation of their behavior (for example, that they are seeking to satisfy desires for nurturance, revenge, sympathy, etc.), they generally use this "insight" to confirm their negative views of themselves as "bad" or "unworthy" and consequently feel more depressed.

Adjust Level of Activity and Structuring to the Patient's Needs

Most depressed patients have difficulty in concentrating and focusing their attention. Consequently, they are often unable to define problems, much less solve them. As a result, they feel helpless and overwhelmed by problems wherever they turn. Because of their negative cognitive set, they are likely to construe silences in therapy as rejections, or an open-ended time contract for therapy as evidence that they will never get better. They are prone to "find" evidence in the therapist's behavior or in his treatment that they are defective, unlikeable, and worthless. For these reasons, an unstructured interview provides full play to their negative fantasies.

The cognitive therapist is more active, and he exercises more initiative than does the therapist conducting traditional psychotherapy. The cognitive therapist takes the lead in guiding the patient into discussing those areas targeted for therapeutic work. This strategy contrasts with the more nondirective approaches in which the patient is left to select the agenda for the session while the therapist simply listens or reflects back what the patient is saying. The cognitive therapist functions as a fellow experimenter, a guide, an educator using a Socratic style. In this sense he tends to direct the flow of conversation and the patient's attention to specific targets.

The cognitive therapist tends to be most active during the earlier phases of therapy. He titrates his degree of activity according to the patient's apparent need for structure. Not infrequently, severely depressed persons are able to answer questions with only one or two words or a single sentence. The therapist is *very* active with these patients—as active as in crisis intervention—in order to energize the patient and to stir him out of his despondent state. Short, simple, direct, and concrete statements are most effective; moreover, the therapist tries to elicit specific, concrete responses to his questions.

When the depression lifts, the therapist is less active than at the outset. He expects and prompts the patient to take the lead in his treatment; for example, the patient might be expected to identify a theme in the cognitions he has reported, or he might try to identify the silent assumptions operative in a specific situation. However, in comparison to other therapies, the cognitive therapist remains quite active, often taking the initiative even in the later phases of treatment.

65

Naturally, even the most active cognitive therapist allows reasonable intervals after his questions or comments in order to allow the patient to organize his own thoughts and to formulate a response. The therapist must judge from experience with each patient whether each interval is too brief or too extended. Depressed patients may become confused and need further direction from the therapist in order to respond if the interval becomes too long. On the other hand, the retarded patient requires time to organize and articulate his responses to a question.

The degree of activity and structuring by the therapist requires an exquisite sensitivity to the patient's needs and reactions. No other aspect of cognitive therapy entails as many risks and requires as much skill. Being active and directive can be either underdone or overdone. Depressed patients usually feel reassured by a certain degree of structure and activity. For example, the depressed person may think, "The therapist talks to me so he must like me." In addition, structured and focused therapeutic interchanges tend to help the difficulties in concentration and attention experienced by more severely depressed patients. On the other hand, if the therapist is too active and directive, the patient may think the therapist is manipulative and not really interested in what *he* feels or wants; the patient may conclude that the therapist is more interested in trying out his techniques than in helping him.

Thus, cognitive distortions may influence how the patient interprets the therapeutic relationship. The experienced active therapist elicits the patient's view of therapy and tries to correct and clarify these views with the patient at frequent intervals.

Employ Questioning as a Major Therapeutic Device

We will see throughout this monograph that the preponderance of verbalizations by the therapist are framed in the form of questions. The utilization of questions serves a wide variety of functions intrinsic to cognitive therapy. In fact, a single question may simultaneously attempt to draw the patient's attention to a particular area, assess his responses to this new subject of inquiry, obtain direct information regarding this problem, generate methods for solving problems that had been regarded as insoluble, and, finally, raise doubts in the patient's mind regarding previously distorted conclusions.

The purposes of questioning may be summarized as follows:

1. To obtain important diagnostic, biographical, and background information.
2. To obtain a general idea of the nature of the patient's psychological problem.
3. To gain an overview of the patient's current life situation, specific stressors, and social support system.
4. To assess patient's coping mechanism, stress tolerance, functional level and capacity for introspection and self-objectivity.
5. To translate vague, abstract complaints into more concrete, discrete problems.

For example, a patient stated as her chief complaint, "I don't know where I am going." She had previously been diagnosed as having an "existential depression" because she talked in terms of not having a sense of identity and not being sure of her role. The therapist asked, "What specific problem have you been grappling with?" She replied, "My problem is that I can't decide whether to stay home and be a housewife or go back to school and start a career in law."

6. To initiate decision-making by inquiring into various alternative approaches to a problem.
7. To enable the patient to select a particular alternative. One approach is to weigh the pros and cons of each option and then begin to eliminate the least desirable.
8. To prompt the patient to examine the consequences of his maladaptive behavior: Asking, for instance, what do you have to gain by remaining in bed?
9. To assess the value of more adaptive behavior: What do you have to lose? What are the advantages of risking disapproval through asserting yourself? What are the disadvantages?
10. To elicit the patient's *specific cognitions* related to unpleasant affect or dysfunctional behavior.
11. To ascertain the *meaning* attached to a particular event or set of circumstances by the patient.
12. To induce the patient to examine the criteria for his negative self-appraisals (for example, worthless, weak, incompetent).

The therapist poses a series of questions such as the following: How do you define worthlessness? What characteristics or actions would I need to observe to recognize worthlessness in another person? Which of these apply to you? On what basis would you consider somebody else worthless? Is it possible that you apply one standard—a very harsh standard—to yourself and a more kindly standard to other people?

Similarly, the patient could be asked to list his criteria for "worthlessness," and then asked whether he meets any of these criteria.

Such questioning often enables the patient to recognize the arbitrary nature of his self-appraisals and their lack of congruence with any common sense definition of the negative terms he applies to himself.

13. To demonstrate the patient's selective abstraction of negative cues in forming his inferences. This kind of conceptual problem is illustrated in the following example: A depressed patient was disgusted with herself because she had broken a rule regarding eating candy when she was on a diet.

PATIENT: I don't have any self-control at all.
THERAPIST: On what basis do you say that?
P: Somebody offered me candy and I couldn't refuse it.
T: Were you eating candy every day?
P: No, I just ate it this once.
T: Did you do anything constructive during the past week to adhere to your diet?
P: Well, I didn't give in to the temptation to buy candy every time I saw it at the store. . . . Also, I did not eat any candy except that one time when it was offered to me and I felt I couldn't refuse it.
T: If you counted up the number of times you controlled yourself versus the number of times you gave in, what ratio would you get?
P: About 100 to 1.
T: So if you controlled yourself 100 times and did not control yourself just once, would that be a sign that you are weak through and through?
P: I guess not—not *through* and *through* (smiles).

14. To illustrate the patient's penchant for indiscriminately negating or disqualifying positive experiences:

PATIENT: I really haven't made any progress in therapy.
THERAPIST: Didn't you have to improve in order to leave the hospital and go back to college?
P: What's the big deal about going to college every day?
T: Why do you say that?
P: It's easy to attend these classes because all the people are healthy.
T: How about when you were in group therapy in the hospital? What did you feel then?
P: I guess I thought then that it was easy to be with the other people because they were all as crazy as I was.
T: Is it possible that whenever you accomplish you tend to discredit?

15. To open and explore certain problem areas that the patient had previously closed out.

The depressed person has a notorious tendency toward premature closure on certain topics. He often closes out a problem early because his conclusion, dictated by his dominant thought pattern, seems so plausible. On the other hand, he may think, "That's a stupid or neurotic idea, so I won't think about it anymore"; unfortunately, the erroneous belief persists and continues to influence his reactions.

Use Questioning Rather than Disputation and Indoctrination

A well-timed, carefully phrased series of questions can help the patient to isolate and carefully consider a specific issue, decision, or notion. A series of questions may open the patient's thinking around a specific issue, and thereby allow him to consider other information and experiences—either recent or past. The patient's curiosity can be raised by a series of questions. His apparently rigidly stated views become tentative hypotheses. In this way, questions are used to relieve depressed, constricted thinking.

It is important to try to elicit from the patient what *he* is thinking rather than telling the patient what the therapist believes he is thinking. Often, the patient's responses are quite different from what the therapist expected.

The following example illustrates how the therapist used a series of questions to open the patient's mind regarding a self-defeating behavior (staying in bed all day). The therapist emphasized the practical importance of feeling better and tried to help the patient to reflect realistically on the utility of returning to bed after the appointment.

THERAPIST: What is the probability that you will go back to bed when you leave the office?
PATIENT: About 100%.
T: Why are you going back to bed?
P: Because I want to.
T: What is the reason you want to?
P: Because I'll feel better.
T: For how long?
P: A few minutes.
T: And what will happen after that?
P: I suppose I'll feel worse again.
T: How do you know?
P: Because this happens every time.
T: Are you sure of that? . . . Have there been any times when lying in bed made you feel better for a period of time?
P: I don't think so.
T: Have you found that not giving in to the urge to return to bed has helped you at all?
P: I guess when I get active, I feel better.
T: Now to return to your wish to go to bed. What are the reasons for going to bed?
P: So I'll feel better.
T: What other reasons do you have for going to bed?
P: Well, I know theoretically that I will feel worse later.
T: So, are there reasons for not going to bed and doing something constructive?
P: I know that when I get involved in things I feel better.
T: Why is that?
P: Because it takes my mind off how bad I feel and I am able to concentrate on other things.

The therapist then asked the patient to rate his motivations. At this point, his wish to return to bed had dropped from 100% to 5% and his motivation to follow the preassigned activity on his schedule had increased from 0% to 50%.

Note that every verbal expression by the therapist was in the form of a question. Also observe that the therapist was persistent in getting the patient to express *both* sides of the argument and even to challenge the validity of the reasons for engaging in a constructive activity. Chapter 10 cites an example in which the therapist relied exclusively on questions to elicit the reasons for deciding to commit suicide and then to test the logic of this decision.

We have observed on many occasions that the patient tends to repeat the kind of conversation described above in a form of internal dialogue. Some patients do this spontaneously and even can "hear" the therapist's voice. In fact, some of these even have a visual image of the therapist talking to them. Other patients have to be trained to carry on the internal dialogue. They have to be "warmed up" through a cognitive rehearsal to ask themselves the kinds of questions listed in the previous extract. They also should be encouraged to write down the internal dialogue or dictate into a tape recorder so that they can listen to it later.

Questions constitute an important and powerful tool for identifying, considering, and correcting cognitions and beliefs. As with other powerful tools, they can be misused or artlessly applied. The patient may feel he is being cross-examined or that he is being attacked if questions are used to "trap" him into contradicting himself. In addition, open-ended questioning sometimes leaves the patient in the defensive position of trying to guess what the therapist "expects" for an answer. Questions must be carefully timed and phrased so as to help the patient recognize and consider his notions reflectively—to weigh his thoughts with objectivity.

Use Humor Judiciously

Humor and hyperbole can be useful tools for some cognitive therapists. Recently, a number of writers have emphasized the importance of humor in other forms of psychotherapy (Greenwald, 1973).

Humor is particularly useful if it is spontaneous, if it allows the patient to observe his notions or ideas with objectivity, and if the humor is presented in such a way that the patient doesn't think he is being belittled or ridiculed.

The therapist can often use a hypothetical example to exaggerate

71

a particular position the patient is taking. Exaggeration will often dramatize how unreasonable or inappropriate his thinking is. He may be able to laugh constructively at the incongruous aspects of his beliefs.

Humor also allows the therapist to shake up or loosen the patient's belief systems without directly attacking the specific belief. The therapist can indirectly raise doubts about the patient's actual statements without having to argue away at each specific piece of evidence for or against a given notion. In this way, the therapist can use humor to produce cognitive dissonance and, as a consequence, to set the patient searching for potential alternative explanations or ideas which may be more adaptive.

Again, a word of caution is in order. First of all, some therapists simply don't have a spontaneous sense of humor. As with many other therapy techniques, not all therapists are prepared to use humor. Secondly, even if the patient apparently laughs or smiles it is important to determine whether the patient construed the humorous sally in a negative way. Thus, potential misinterpretation should be sought for and corrected. Thirdly, the therapist must be clear that the target of his humor is the patient's thoughts or ideas—not the patient himself. Furthermore, substantial judgment is needed in order to choose which thoughts are appropriate targets for such therapeutic levity. Some patients are so convinced of the validity of certain ideas that poking fun at these thoughts may be disturbing and the therapeutic relationship will be weakened.

FORMAL STRUCTURE OF COGNITIVE THERAPY

Prepare the Patient for Cognitive Therapy

Two elements are important in the conduct of cognitive therapy. (1) The patient should understand the nature and rationale of cognitive treatment. (2) The patient should be prepared to deal with fluctuations in his level of depression during treatment.

Rationale: The therapist prepares each patient for cognitive therapy during most of the first and much of the second therapy session. The therapist carefully presents the general plan and rationale for cognitive treatment. The therapist then discusses the definitions and examples of cognitions or "automatic thoughts." For instance, during the first session, the therapist will describe the relationship between thoughts and feelings. Often, the patient can understand this relationship if the therapist uses an example. In the section following, a therapist describes how he illustrated to one patient the idea that thinking influences feeling:

THERAPIST: How persons interpret events determines how they feel about things. For instance, recently one of my patients who successfully completed treatment told me about the thoughts she had before each appointment while in the waiting room. She would carefully watch when I would begin each session. When I was late, even by a few minutes, she would think to herself, "He doesn't want to see me," and would feel sad. When I was early, she would think to herself, "I really must be doing poorly, since he is spending extra time to help," and would feel anxious. If I was right on time, she would tell herself, "He's really got a factory going. I'm just a number to him." And she would feel irritated. As you can see, no matter when I would begin the session (whether early, right on time, or late) this patient would be thinking negatively about the therapy and would feel bad about herself or the treatment. She could see the *connection* between her negative thought and her unpleasant feeling. After she learned to pinpoint and report her thoughts, she realized these negative thoughts were unrealistic. The next time she was thinking these sorts of thoughts and having unpleasant feelings in the waiting room, she began to correct these negative interpretations. As she corrected her arbitrary interpretations, her negative feelings disappeared.

The therapist may explain the cognitive approach to the sophisticated patient in the following way:

When depressed persons consider their experiences, they are generally drawn to the most negative meanings that can conceivably be attributed to those events. When this occurs, the negative thinking feels realistic to the patient. The more believable this negative thinking is, the more upset the patient will feel.

Throughout treatment, the therapist repeatedly focuses on the connection between feeling and thinking. If the patient says "I feel terrible," the cognitive therapist will ask, "What are you thinking about?" If the patient reports a recent event in his homework and records associated feelings such as "terrible" or "depressed," the therapist asks the patient about what thinking has occurred just prior to the unpleasant feelings. Alternatively, the therapist will ask about what the event means to the patient. Again, if a patient, feeling desperate and painfully sad, makes a phone call to the therapist, the therapist can use this phone conversation to help the patient identify upsetting automatic thoughts: "What are your thoughts right now?" Preparing the patient for the cognitive approach during the first interview is discussed more fully in the next chapter.

In our research study of the cognitive therapy of depression, we followed this procedure: After the therapist discusses the rationale for cognitive therapy, and after he explains the treatment processes, he gives the patient a booklet, *Coping with Depression* (Beck and Greenberg, 1974) which presents similar material in printed form. The therapist asks the patient to read this booklet, to underline sections about which he or she has questions or which are particularly pertinent to him, and to make notes in this booklet. This suggestion may constitute the first homework assignment. The patient's responses to this booklet are then reviewed in the second therapy session.

This general approach of providing clear explanations for each step in the treatment and each homework task is maintained throughout therapy. The therapist attempts to make treatment as comprehensible and credible as possible, so the patient can participate actively in identifying his problems and can help to develop strategies to approach each of these problems. As a consequence, the patient learns general principles in identifying and solving problems.

Recently, we have begun to pilot test a videotape designed to explain to patients the rationale and basis for cognitive treatment. This technique of "socialization for therapy" has been found to decrease premature discontinuation of treatment and to increase response to therapy in psychologically naïve or lower socioeconomic class patients (for a review, see Rush and Watkins, 1977). Patients also benefit from observing videotapes of their interviews. They are able to recognize the connections between their verbalized ideas and their subsequent emotional reactions.

Fluctuations in Symptoms and Relapses. It is important during the first few interviews for the therapist to elicit the patient's expectancies regarding treatment. Some patients expect a miracle cure and are likely to experience severe disappointment when this does not occur. Other depressed patients, as a result of the combination of their pathological pessimism and previous unsuccessful attempts at therapy, may believe that the therapy cannot produce any kind of enduring treatment. As a result of such expectations, these individuals are disposed to interpret any intensification of their symptoms or problems in a negative way.

For these reasons, it is important for the therapist to indicate that the natural course of depression has its ups and downs. A patient may experience a severe drop in his mood level after he has had several "good days." Moreover, many patients do not experience any substantial relief of their symptomatology for many weeks. It is important for the therapist to inform the patient that, although there is a reasonable expectation for improvement, they both must be prepared for the exacerbation of symptoms and intensification of problems.

As will be explained in Chapter 15, the therapist should indicate to the patient that an increase in symptomatology or external problems or relapse during or after treatment can afford an excellent opportunity for the therapist and patient to pinpoint the specific factors leading to such setbacks. We have frequently found that an apparent setback of this nature is actually an advantage in that it provides a very powerful learning experience for the patient in applying coping strategies to the entire experience. It is desirable, therefore, to prepare the patient to expect such fluctuations and to motivate the patient to try to utilize such occurrences in the service of strengthening himself.

Formulate a Therapy Plan for Each Session

The major objectives of cognitive therapy include (a) reasonably prompt relief of symptoms of the depressive syndrome and (b) prevention of recurrence. The aims are implemented by training the patient to (a) learn to identify and modify his faulty thinking and dysfunctional behavior and (b) recognize and change the cognitive patterns leading to dysfunctional ideation and behavior. The therapist outlines and explains these goals in the first treatment session. The relief of the symptoms of depression also includes increase in feelings of well-being and satisfaction. When this goal is presented to depressed patients, they may counter this notion with such arguments as, "I can't feel happy till my boyfriend comes back." In these cases, the therapist responds directly to this type of thinking: "Whether or not your boyfriend returns, you surely don't want to continue feeling as badly as you do," or "You may be better able to get him back if you set the goal to get over your depression."

This focus on techniques to solve problems deserves special emphasis. Although the overall initial goal is symptom relief, the steps to obtain this relief consist of definition and solving of problems. In this way, the patient learns to assess problems logically and to consistently apply one of several techniques to resolve the problems. Therefore, the emphasis is on learning or practicing a technique or skill rather than on neutralizing pain. An analogue to this formulation is found in the behavioral treatment of obesity in which the overall goal is weight loss. The therapist focuses on those *behaviors* and *attitudes* which decrease food intake rather than on weight loss itself. These constructive behaviors are concrete skills which eventually result not only in weight reduction but also enduring weight control.

In the same sense, the short-range goal of the relief of the depressive symptoms is achieved by a series of sessions or steps aimed at defining target problems and designed to impart concretely defined skills. Development of these skills consists of learning: (a) to assess personally relevant situations realistically, (b) to attend to all (not just biased) selections of the available data about these specific situations, (c) to generate alternative explanations about the outcome of interactions, and (d) to test maladaptive assumptions by behaving differently and thereby providing opportunities for a wider repertoire in relating to other people and solving problems.

The long-range goal of cognitive therapy depends on facilitating maturation, which includes refining skills in correcting cognitive distortions (and, therefore, in reality-testing) and incorporating more reasonable and adaptive attitudes. Furthermore, maturation includes developing more effective methods to master or adjust to difficult or complex environmental circumstances and to cope with unpleasant feelings, and the refinement of interpersonal skills.

Establish Agenda at Beginning of Session

The therapist functions as an expert guide, providing a plan, a map, and tools. However, he must insure that the patient is ready for and wants to follow the plan. Thus, the therapist and patient propose topics for the agenda of each therapy session near the beginning of each meeting. It is important that the agenda include a brief resume of the patient's experiences since the last session and feedback on his various assignments. Then they should agree on the specific goals for the session. The specific topics should be stated in concrete and precise terms so as to focus the patient's attention on the task at hand. For example, the therapist might say, "The first item we have listed is to review the automatic thoughts you collected and demonstrate how to reason with them."

The specific agenda for the interview depends on several factors. Obviously, one factor depends on the stage of therapy and the patient's progress to date. For example, has the patient learned to monitor and record maladaptive cognitions, to make reasonable responses, to identify and correct the specific logical errors in his thinking, etc.?

A second important factor influencing the items on the agenda relates to those problems that are most troubling for the patient at the present time. A third factor consists of the general severity of the depression. We tend to use more behaviorally oriented tasks and assignments with more severely depressed persons. As the depression lifts, more cognitively oriented tasks requiring more abstract reasoning are utilized.

Another factor is concerned with items which remain on the agenda from the previous therapy session. Alternatively, the patient may have had a delayed reaction to the previous meeting. The therapist should ask the patient whether additional feelings or concerns had followed the previous session, and if so, this material forms part of the current session's agenda.

Finally, the therapist should be alert to the patient's "hidden agenda," which may consist of topics he is reluctant to discuss and, indeed, may bring up voluntarily only at the very end of the session when it is too late to discuss these matters.

It is of critical importance that the therapist not be so bound by a predetermined sequence of defining and attacking problems or setting goals that he ignore *important current events.* Obviously, an acute crisis would supersede other topics on the agenda. The therapist can often determine the important topics by looking through the Daily Record of Dysfunctional Thoughts or the daily summary of activities recorded by the patient in his notebook. Is there a recurrent theme which ties these thoughts together (for example, assuming responsibility for everyone else's well-being)? Is suicidal preoccupation or hopelessness a dominant issue?

After considering these various factors, the therapist helps the patient develop an agenda for the meeting. Initially, the therapist attempts to sort out and define the various topics. Subsequently, they arrive at a consensus regarding the priority of the topics. Then the therapist can begin to reflect on which strategies should be used in approaching the specific problems, and he should discuss these proposed strategies with the patient. Because of the need to adapt the technique to the patient, it is generally desirable for the patient to make the final decision regarding which technique to use (for example, role playing, induced imagery, or refuting automatic thoughts).

In summary, the formulation of therapy consists of preparing an agenda *with the patient* for each session, usually at the beginning of the session. Items left over from the previous session are placed on the agenda for the subsequent session. The goals of each therapy session are stated explicitly at the beginning of each meeting: choosing the problems to be addressed (see Chapters 5–8) and selecting one or more techniques with which to approach the targets. Since cognitive therapy is time-limited, the therapist must judiciously use the time allotted for each therapy session. Formulating an agenda for each session helps the therapist and patient to distribute time in a rational fashion.

Formulate and Test Concrete Hypotheses

It is critical to construct a model—blueprint—that fits the particular patient. Based on the patient's responses to specific questions, the therapist can set up several hypotheses. Data are elicited by a logical sequence of questions (a) to test hypotheses, (b) to modify hypotheses, (c) to discard previous hypotheses, or (d) to derive new hypotheses. When the therapist feels reasonably confident about his hypothesis, he should "try it on" the patient. He elicits the patient's opinon on the "fit" of the hypothesis in question and he works with the patient to modify the hypothesis to improve its applicability to the patient's individual circumstance. These hypotheses are subsequently tested by the patient in his everyday life as though he were carrying out a specific experiment.

When the therapist poses a question or makes a comment, it should be based on a *definite rationale* derived from the framework of cognitive therapy; it should be phrased to elicit concrete information. We have found that specific questions most clearly help to delineate the patient's problem area. General, abstract, vague questions often produce similarly vague responses removed from the "hard" data of cognitions. In addition, vague phrases tend to confuse or unsettle the patient and are more easily interpreted in a negative manner by the patient. For example, if the therapist wants to know about the patient's ideation, he would ask questions such as, "What are you thinking right now?" or "How do you feel?" Specific direct questions facilitate specific direct responses. A comment such as, "I wonder what you have been thinking," is less likely to elicit specific cognitions than a more concrete question such as, "Try to recall just what words or pictures went through your mind right at the time of that event."

Based on the patient's report of his thinking, the therapist tends to develop specific notations about how the patient's misinterpretations, logical errors, and basic assumptions fit together. To identify logical inconsistencies *and* underlying assumptions, the therapist develops hypotheses based on recurrent themes which are identified in the patient's thinking. At an appropriate point, he checks out those hypotheses by sharing them with the patient.

For example, the patient might report continual automatic thoughts regarding whether other people like him or dislike him. The therapist might present hypotheses such as:

> You spend a lot of time guessing how each person you meet feels about you. Most of your attention to environmental events appears to be concentrated on whether or not you are a likable person. Even events that have little or no relation to that question—such as the way the checker acts at the supermarket—are interpreted by you to be relevant to the question of whether you are likable or not. Does this observation seem to fit the facts?

Such an inquiry is essential in order to prime the patient to consider the hypotheses formulated by the therapist. In this way, collaboration between the therapist and patient is strengthened. In addition, as the therapist formulates such hypotheses, he also helps the patient to regard his thoughts as a series of psychological events which consist of his own personal construction of reality and are not necessarily a true representation of reality.

In this illustration, the therapist might frame the hypotheses and the tests of the hypotheses as follows:

Hypothesis 1: "Your automatic response to any encounter with another person is 'He likes me, he likes me not.'" *Test:* "Observe how frequently you wonder about other people's reactions to you."

Hypothesis 2: "Since you are depressed, most of your expectations and interpretations will be negative." *Test:* "Click off on your wrist counter the number of negative expectations and interpretations."

Hypothesis 3: "You are prone to read evaluative responses (especially negative ones) into other people's reactions when there is no information at all for making a judgment, or when there is no reason for them to have any reaction to you at all." *Test:* "After each encounter, ask yourself, '(a) Did I feel hurt or rejected with the encounter?' (b) 'Is there any evidence the other person even noticed me?' (c) 'If he/she did notice me, is there any evidence that his/her reaction was anything but neutral?'"

Note: It is essential that the therapist bear in mind that his hypotheses are simply formalized conjectures and not *facts* or *data.* The data consist of the patient's introspective observations and reports plus the results of the "experimental" tests.

If these hypotheses are confirmed, the groundwork is laid for the formulation of the patient's underlying ("silent") assumptions, which will be discussed in later stages of therapy. Some of the underlying assumptions in the illustrative case might be: (1) "It is crucial to my happiness to be well-liked by everybody." (2) My self-worth as a person depends on how other people regard me." These postulated "assumptions" require testing as do any other inferred psychological constructs.

Elicit Feedback from the Patient

The therapist–patient collaboration normally involves a joint effort of identifying and evaluating cognitions, developing hypotheses, and conducting "experiments." Throughout these verbal exchanges, the therapist must actively observe the patient's reactions to his verbal and nonverbal behavior. Such feedback is particularly important in therapy with depressed persons—it is a crucial ingredient in enhancing the therapeutic alliance. Moreover, the feedback mechanism should encourage the patient to express in the sessions his perceptions and feelings about therapy, homework, or the therapist. The therapist initiates this procedure early in therapy by asking for the patient's feelings and evaluations of the present session, the previous session, homework assignments, etc. Depressed patients often are reluctant to "talk straight" to the therapist for fear of being rejected or criticized or of making a mistake. Thus they may agree with a formulation simply out of compliance. Thus, the therapist must make an extra effort to elicit feelings or wishes relevant to compliance (anxiety about rejection, wish to please) from the patient.

Feedback is particularly important since many patients often misconstrue therapists' statements and questions. For example, following the explanations about her negative self-evaluations, one patient—near tears—said, "I came in feeling depressed. Now you're telling me *my thinking is bad, too.*" Only with such feedback can the therapist ascertain whether he and the patient are on the same "wavelength" and correct his or her misconstructions of his behavior or techniques.

The pattern of eliciting this kind of feedback from the patient should be established in the first session. Following the introductory explanation of the methods of cognitive therapy, the therapist inquires how the patient reacts to what he said. He should encourage the patient to continue to report discordant reactions through all treatment sessions.

In the first session, the therapist may say:

> Now that we've discussed your negative emotions and thoughts, it's important to be aware that the same sort of negative reactions may

81

occur in therapy itself. That is, I may say or do something which you feel is hurtful, rejecting, or insulting. Your perception may be accurate or it might not be accurate. The only way to find out is to check out your perception with me. I have no way of knowing you have such a thought or feeling so you'll need to tell me. As you will see, such *reports are extremely valuable* in giving us information that will help the therapy. In fact, these reports are often the most valuable material that we obtain in treatment. Near the end of each session, we will check out your reactions to the interview and it is important to tell me anything that disturbed or confused you or any negative or unpleasant feelings that you experienced.

Many depressed persons are especially reluctant to express their negative perceptions of the therapist. They may think, "If I complain he won't like me or he may give up on my case." For that reason, it is initially the responsibility of the therapist to request feedback. After a while, the patient may begin to volunteer his discordant reactions without questioning or prodding from the therapist. By and large, the kinds of misunderstandings, exaggerated responses, or distortions reported by the patient in relation to other people are paralleled in his reactions to the therapist.

Typical cognitive responses to the therapist expressed by patients include:

1. "You don't like me."
2. "I am your worst patient."
3. "You can't get me well."
4. "You want to get rid of me."
5. "You don't want to hear my problems."
6. "You're going to hospitalize me, give me shock therapy, etc."
7. "I am boring you."
8. "You don't understand me."
9. "You are more interested in trying out your techniques than you are in me."
10. "You act as though you know more about what I am feeling than I do."
11. "You are always trying to put words in my mouth."

It is useful to ask for feedback at the beginning of the session about the last homework assignment *and* about the previous therapy session. For example, "Do you have any thoughts about the homework assignment?" or "You probably gave some thought to the last session we had. What reactions did you have?" In addition, it is important to elicit feedback near the end of each session about the session itself. For example, "Do you have any thoughts or feelings about this session, so far?", "Are you feeling any better or worse than when we started?"

The therapist should attend carefully to nonverbal behavior (for example, a sharp change in the facial expression, tears welling up, a change in voice modulation, etc.) as forms of feedback. If the therapist observes such nonverbal reactions, he can tactfully ask, "What was going through your mind just then?" When negative automatic thoughts are elicited during the therapy session, they are treated like cognitions collected as homework. The therapist gently asks for the stimuli evoking these responses and, possibly, for evidence or observations which support the cognitions reported. If specific cognitive errors (for example, arbitrary inference, over-generalization, selective inattention, etc.) are noted, these errors may become the focus of discussion. The therapist is cautioned not to reassure or correct the patient prematurely. It is often therapeutic for him to guide the patient in reconstructing how he arrived at his cognitive distortion.

At times, patients make sharp observations regarding the therapist's antitherapeutic behavior. A patient, for example, may say, "I feel that you talk too much and you don't give me a chance to say what's on my mind." The therapist should be prepared to acknowledge that he is fallible like any other human being and could respond in a fashion such as, "Other patients have made this observation. If you feel I am talking too much, I would appreciate it if you would interrupt me or use a signal such as waving your hand at me." Such an arrangement not only facilitates the working relationship but is a spur to the patient to assert himself—an effective antidote to depression.

Provide and Encourage Capsule Summaries

We have found that it is enormously useful for the therapist to make summary statements at appropriate times throughout the interview. Similarly, it is desirable to ask the patient for a brief resume of what he believes the therapist has been attempting to communicate to him. If applied systematically throughout the interview, these procedures help to insure that patient and therapist are on the same "wavelength" and aid the patient in focusing on concrete problems.

In the initial interview, for instance, the therapist summarizes the various themes he has extracted from the patient's descriptions of his problems and symptoms and inquires whether his recapitulation is accurate and complete. At times during the later therapeutic interviews, the therapist may paraphrase or briefly review the patient's verbalizations with prefatory remarks such as, "What I hear you say is . . .", or "You seem to be telling me . . ." If uncertain about the precise content of the verbal material, he may ask, "Am I correct in assuming that. . . ?" In each case, the therapist waits for the patient's confirmation, revision, or rejection of his resume before proceding further.

We also attempt to determine how well the patient understands the therapist's explanations or suggestions. At specific places during the interview the therapist may raise questions such as, "To make sure that we understand each other, I wonder if you would tell me in your own words what I have been saying." As the therapy progresses, the patient should assume more of the responsibility for summarizing the content of the discussion. The patient's version of what has been discussed often differs markedly from that of the therapist!

In actual practice, the therapist uses capsule summaries at least three times during the standard therapeutic interview: (1) In preparing the agenda, he reviews the main points that he and the patient believe should be discussed during the interview; (2) midway during the interview he recapitulates the material covered up to that point; (3) near the end of the session, he presents a final capsule summary of the main points of the interview—or he may ask the patient to do so.

We have found that the patients generally respond favorably to the elicitation of feedback and presentation of capsule summaries. Many of them have remarked that these procedures make them feel closer to the therapist. In analysis of videotaped interviews, we have concrete evidence that the development of empathy and warmth is facilitated by these techniques.

Utilize Significant Others

There is considerable evidence that the engagement of a relative or a friend can enhance the therapeutic impact of an interview. The therapist has to judge at what point it would be useful to involve another person such as a spouse or close friend. Unless there is some obvious contraindication, the significant other should be interviewed immediately after the initial interview with the patient. This procedure enables the therapist to obtain additional vital information regarding the patient's symptoms, level of functioning, suicidal threats, etc. It also provides an opportunity to explain the rationale of the therapeutic procedures and the homework assignments so that the significant other can reinforce the therapeutic regimen. Moreover, by securing the alliance of the relative or friend, the therapist can help to neutralize some of their antitherapeutic behaviors (for example, oversolicitousness, counterproductive suggestions, scolding, etc.). Finally, the interview with the significant other provides data regarding how stresses between that person and the patient may have contributed to the onset or the continuation of the depression. This information may suggest the value of doing "couples therapy."

In some instances, for example, with elderly or adolescent patients, a trained paraprofessional may be utilized to help to implement the total therapeutic program. Such an auxiliary therapist can assist not only in carrying out behavioral assignments but also in assisting the patient in identifying negative cognitions and formulating reasonable responses to them.

Utilize Ancillary Techniques

The therapist can draw on a variety of aids to reinforce and extend the impact of the therapeutic interview. It is often useful for a patient to listen to an audiotape of an interview immediately following the session. Unless there is some contraindication, the patient should be encouraged to listen to the taped interviews between sessions. Many patients find that watching videotaped recordings of their sessions is useful in correcting some of their distorted perceptions of themselves and also in dramatizing some of their maladaptive behaviors.

We have also used audiotapes and videotapes that have been specially designed to illustrate the therapeutic techniques and to demonstrate to the patient how he can learn some of these techniques; for example, recognizing and responding to negative "automatic thoughts."

Chapter 5

THE INITIAL INTERVIEW

STARTING THE INITIAL INTERVIEW

We have found in our experience that the therapy starts with the very first contact with the patient—whether it is over the telephone or in the therapist's office. As outlined in Chapters 2 and 3, the therapist attempts to form a relaxed personal relationship with the patient without, at the same time, artificially obscuring the obvious differences in their roles: the fact that the patient is a suffering individual who is seeking help from an expert. The formation of the working relationship, the gathering of important information, and the application of specific cognitive techniques can all be smoothly woven into the fabric of the intitial interview.

Many therapists find it helpful to start the interview with a question such as, "How do you feel about seeing a therapist?" or "How did you feel about coming here today?" Many patients respond with expressions of anxiety or pessimism. If so, the therapist can gently elicit some of the automatic thoughts behind these unpleasant feelings with questions such as, "Do you recall what you were thinking while you were waiting for me or traveling to my office?" or "What did you expect would happen when you came here?" Simply by sharing these expectations with the therapist, the patient can ease himself into a collaborative relationship.

The following interchange illustrates one way of opening the initial interview.

> THERAPIST: How did you feel about coming here today?
> PATIENT: I felt pretty nervous.
> T: Did you have any particular thoughts about me or the therapy before you came in?

P: I was nervous because I thought you would think that I was not suitable for this kind of therapy.

T: Did you have any other feelings or thoughts?

P: Well, to tell you the truth I was feeling kind of hopeless—I've been to so many therapists and my depressions keep coming back.

T: Now that we have had a chance to talk, do you still think that I am going to reject you as a patient?

P: I don't know . . . Are you?

T: No, of course not, but I want you to see that this is an example of how your expectations caused you anxiety . . . Now that you know that your expectation is wrong, how do you feel?

P: Well, I don't feel as nervous, but I still have this terrible feeling that you are not going to be able to help me.

T: Well, perhaps we can come back to this pessimistic feeling later on and see whether you still believe that. In any event, I think you have already brought out something very valuable and that is that your negative ideas lead to unpleasant feelings—in your case, anxiety and sadness . . . How do you feel now?

P: (more relaxed): Better, I guess.

T: Okay . . . Now, could you tell me in a few words what you would like help with?

This kind of interchange serves several purposes: (a) It helps to put the patient at ease, fosters a relatively informal therapeutic relationship, and facilitates therapeutic work. (b) It provides information to the therapist regarding the patient's expectations of another failure in therapy. (c) It presents an opportunity to point out the relationship between cognition and affect. (d) The prompt amelioration of the patient's unpleasant feelings will serve as an incentive for him to identify and correct his cognitive distortions.

ELICITING ESSENTIAL INFORMATION

It is important to note that skillful interviewing not only elicits essential information regarding the patient's (a) diagnosis, (b) past history, (c) present life situation, (d) psychological problems, (e) attitudes about treatment, and (f) motivation for treatment, but also serves to give the patient some objectivity regarding the particular disorder. This objectivity in itself is often quite reassuring. *

In our own research group, we attempt to obtain as much self-report information as possible *prior* to the interview so as to reduce the amount of time necessary for a clinical evaluation. The questionnaires provide demographic and biographic data and information regarding symptoms, previous illnesses, previous contacts with health professionals and agencies, and previous treatment. One of the useful therapeutic tools is the Depression Inventory (Beck, 1967; Beck, 1978), which not only gives a rapid assessment of the severity of the disorder but also may highlight certain symptoms (such as suicidal wishes) which would require prompt intervention. In addition, the various items on the Depression Inventory provide important information regarding the individual's negative thinking, which provides a natural lead into some of the patient's central problems (for example, the patient's expectations that everything will go wrong, his view of himself as a failure, his belief that he is unable to do anything without help, or his suicidal wishes). Similarly, the Hopelessness Scale (Beck, Weissman, Lester, and Trexler, 1974) contains many items that can serve as entry points into the patient's negative view of his future.

Most responses to the therapeutic questioning provide a blend of essential information about the patient's ideation and the connection between his negative thinking and his unpleasant emotions. The "socialization for therapy" is important and has already been described in the previous chapter. Although many patients are fully cognizant of the conceptual framework of cognitive therapy, almost all patients require demonstrations and illustrations relevant to their own problems in order to get a good grasp of this approach.

In some cases, particularly those in which the patient has great difficulty in expressing himself or is unaware of the basic format of cognitive therapy, it is often useful to present some introductory instructions and informational material regarding cognitive therapy and depression. This material helps to shape the expectations of the patients and to provide a general outline of the treatment. The

---

* A videotaped interview (with a transcript), specially designed to demonstrate the cognitive techniques of the initial interview, may be helpful in illustrating these points. See Appendix for details regarding obtaining a copy of this videotape or audio cassette.

following specific rationale for cognitive therapy is generally sufficient for these purposes. In fact, it may not be necessary to go into as much detail.

> Initially in our sessions we are going to pinpoint some of the difficulties or problems that you are having and use techniques which, hopefully, will resolve those difficulties. It will be important for us to find out how you react to specific situations in your life and what effect those reactions have on your feelings. By looking carefully at your reactions, we will have a better idea of how best to help you. We can then examine other ways of coping with stress, particularly those ways that could be used to prevent future depressions. Most of the procedures will become clearer after we get into them. Do you have any questions before we continue?

In our research studies of the cognitive therapy of depression, we have followed this procedure: After the therapist discusses the rationale for cognitive therapy, and after he explains the treatment processes, he gives the patient the booklet *Coping with Depression,* which presents similar material in printed form. The therapist asks the patient to read this booklet, to underline sections about which he has questions or which are particularly pertinent to him, and to make notes in this booklet. This suggestion may constitute the first homework assignment. The patient's responses to this booklet are then reviewed in the second therapy session.*

This general approach—providing clear explanations for each step in the treatment and each homework task—is retained throughout the therapy. The therapist attempts to make treatment as comprehensible and credible as possible, so the patient can participate actively in identifying his problems and help to develop strategies to approach each of these problems. As a consequence, the patient learns general principles in identifying and solving problems.

Recently, we have begun to pilot test a videotape designed to explain to patients the rationale and basis for cognitive treatment. This technique of socialization for therapy has been found to decrease

---

*As in other therapeutic procedures, we encourage the patient to express disagreement with the information or suggestions provided by the therapist. Such negative expressions provide useful information in correcting therapists' misunderstandings and patients' distortions, in counteracting automatic compliance, encouraging self-assertion, and in general promoting a collaborative effort.

premature discontinuation of treatment and to increase response to therapy in psychologically naive or lower-socioeconomic-class patients.

Note: The amount of information that can be gained from the patient is practically infinite but *the amount of time and the number of questions that can be asked is finite.* Because of practical constraints, the therapist is forced to make maximum use of limited information. Therefore, it is essential that the therapist try to make every question count. This means that the total background picture may not emerge for several interviews. However, it is essential that the crucial problems, particularly when the patient is severely disturbed, should be delineated fairly early in the first session and a tentative plan of treatment presented to the patient. Furthermore, through the careful blend of information-seeking questions and therapeutic sallies by the therapist, *it is to be hoped that the patient should feel better by the end of the first session.* This is particularly important in the case of suicidal patients who may decide to commit suicide before the next scheduled session if he feels discouraged at the end of the interview. In any event, it is advisable to allow at least one and one-half hours for the initial interview.

Diagnostic Information

It is obvious that the therapist should conduct a complete diagnostic evaluation of the patient unless a very thorough diagnostic workup has been conducted prior to the referral to the therapist. Even in that case, however, the therapist should ask pointed questions to confirm the diagnosis and should be alert to the nonverbal signs indicative of a particular diagnosis or type of psychopathology. In treating depressions, the therapist should have a strong grounding of knowledge and experience in recognizing the many "faces" of depression. He should be alert, for instance, to the "smiling depression," organic diseases masquerading as depression, and depressions masquerading as organic diseases (Beck, 1967). Many of these data can emerge from skillful history-taking.

Questions should not be framed in the kind of staccato rapid-fire interrogation used in psychiatric mental-status examinations in many institutions. Questions related to particular forms of symptomatology can also involve allusions to particular environmental stresses so that the therapist obtains information regarding the patient's life situation and the social context of his psychological disorder. For example, the following interchange yields a great deal of information regarding the type of symptoms, the kind of participating factors, and also the patient's life situation.

> THERAPIST: Can you tell me about some of the emotions that seem to trouble you?
> PATIENT: I am really depressed . . . I have to write a paper at school . . . I wake up early and I drag around all day and can't get to work . . .

The therapist pauses until he has obtained the optimum amount of information from his question before he goes on to the next question.

> T: What level paper is this?
> P: It's in my graduate course in archeology.
> T: What other painful symptoms do you get?
> P: I get upset whenever I have to call a girl for a date . . . That's a big problem.
> T: Have you ever been married?
> P: No, but I was living with a girl . . . We broke off three months ago.
> T: Was there any connection between the breakoff and the development of your depression?
> P: I guess so. I got so upset that I went back to living with my parents . . . Actually, I hate living with them.

As can be noted, a good deal of information was gathered regarding the patient's symptoms, level of education, stresses, and home situation. Also, notice that by pausing after the initial response to a question, the therapist was able to obtain additional information. The patient sensed from the therapist's silence that further elaboration was desired.

Note: The optimum duration of the silences requires a good deal of judgment; generally long pauses are counterproductive in that the patient may misinterpret silence as a rejection or he may lapse into obsessional self-criticisms.

Mental Status Examination

It is crucial that the therapist make his own evaluation as to whether or not the patient is psychotic. Also, it is critical that the therapist be able to determine rapidly whether the patient is suicidal. Suicidal clues may be provided by the patient's expression of hopelessness. For a further discussion of how suicidal wishes may be elicited in the interview, see Chapter 10 on the treatment of the suicidal patient.

The therapist also must be alert to various other "organic" problems such as brain damage, physical illness simulating depression, mental deficiency, etc. The Depression Inventory is a useful tool in covering the various facets of depression. However, since a wide variety of other symptoms may occur in conjunction with depression and in view of the fact that depression might be only a minor aspect of a more serious disorder, such as schizophrenia, the therapist needs to have a strong grounding in psychiatric evaluation and diagnosis and a reasonable knowledge of medical disorders.

Note: The course of the first interview and the patient's responses to some of the probes by the therapist can often yield very important information regarding the patient's capacity for introspection, his ability to view his ideas and his life situation objectively, his capacity to concentrate on a single subject, and his ability to reason and to apply some of the principles outlined by the therapist in a therapeutic way. Moreover, the interview can reveal information regarding the patient's capacity for rapport, his sense of humor, and his motivation for therapy. Thus, the therapeutic interview should not be geared as a stress-tolerance test but should be designed to elicit and mobilize the patient's assets (his "ego strength") so that the therapist will have a rational basis for formulating a treatment plan.

TRANSLATING "CHIEF COMPLAINT" INTO "TARGET SYMPTOM"

We have generally found that each depressed patient reports a particular set of symptoms or problems that represent the most troublesome aspect of the disorder to him. For this reason, it is generally useful for the therapist to try to pin the patient down to his chief complaints or his chief problems.

Often, these chief complaints will not be recognized as symptoms of the depression if the therapist takes the chief complaint at its face value. Some examples of chief complaints which were telltale signs of depression are as follows:

1. "My brain is deteriorating. That's why I want to die." The actual problem turned out to be that the patient was having difficulty in concentrating, a symptom which the patient misinterpreted as progressive brain disease.

2. "I want to divorce my husband." The underlying problem was that the patient was seeing all her relationships and interactions in absolutistic, black-and-white terms. She could only see the negative features in her spouse—and in fact, exaggerated these features. Another component of her depression was that she could no longer respond with affection to any of the individuals near her but specifically interpreted the loss of feeling toward her husband as a sign that her love for him was irreversibly lost. In fact, when not depressed, she had a happy, fulfilling relationship with her husband.

3. "I have no feeling." As indicated above, depressed patients frequently experience a reduction of the "positive" feelings such as love, pleasure, feelings of joy, humor, etc. Some patients interpret this lack of affective response as a sign that they have undergone a permanent transformation. Some patients have described this state as being a "zombie" or as being "subhuman." They do not see these symptoms as aspects of depression but rather as signs of some irreversible change in their personality.

4. "I cannot handle my problems." In this case, the patient greatly exaggerated some of her interpersonal difficulties and at the same time underestimated her coping abilities. As a result of such negative evaluations of herself, her confidence eroded further. Indeed, a vicious cycle was established that progressively undermined her capacity to master situations.

5. "I am a terrible person." The patient interpreted other symptoms of depression (such as slowing down, difficulty in concentrating, loss of affection for her family) in the typical negative, moralistic way seen among depressed patients. She viewed these symptoms as indicating that "I am lazy and self-centered; I don't care about anybody but myself."

6. "Life has no meaning" often is an indicator of suicidal wishes. (See Chapter 10.)

Note: Even though these "chief complaints" are manifestations of depression, they constitute serious problems that contribute to the *maintenance* and *aggravation* of depression. For this reason, they have to be defined and dealt with early in the course of therapy—preferably in the first interview. We include them among the "target symptoms" of depression and have developed a variety of strategies for dealing with them (Chapter 9).

THERAPEUTIC GOALS OF THE INITIAL INTERVIEW

A main therapeutic goal of the first interview is to produce at least some relief of symptoms. This obviously serves the patient's needs in terms of reducing his suffering and satisfies the therapist's desire to help another person in a meaningful way. Beyond this, the symptom relief helps to increase rapport, therapeutic collaboration, and confidence in the efficacy of the therapy. The relief of symptoms, in itself, is likely to make the patient more optimistic and the reinforcing effect of having "worked through" a particular problem usually stimulates the patient to do his homework between sessions.

In order to facilitate the therapeutic process, it is desirable that the symptom relief be based on more than simply rapport, a kindly sympathetic attitude, or implied promises of a "quick cure." Reassurance should be used judiciously since it has only a transient effect on the illogical cognitive processes, distortions of reality, and repetitive negative predictions. In fact, reassurance based on authoritative pronouncements by the therapist often backfires when the patient experiences fluctuations in his symptoms.

The most effective way to reach the immediate therapeutic goal and provide a *rational basis* for reassurance is to attempt to define a set of problems and, in the course of the interview, demonstrate to the patient some strategies for dealing with these problems. The technical application of the strategies should (ideally) begin during the interview and, of course, be carried out by the patient after the interview is completed. Any "success experience" by the patient— even achievement of the task of isolating a problem and viewing it objectively during the interview—is likely to give him an increased sense of mastery. In a sense, the therapeutic interview may be regarded as consisting of a series of "mini-confrontations": The therapist poses a "problem" (asks a question, proposes a possible project); the patient then offers a solution (answers the question; accepts, rejects, or modifies the proposed project). If there is a consensus that the patient's response is satisfactory or at least adequate, the procedure constitutes a successful experience for the patient. Seeing for himself that his response is adequate and receiving positive feedback from the therapist thus disconfirms the patient's notion that he cannot perform adequately or that interactions with other people are nonproductive. Continuous repetition of such "success" or "mastery" experiences throughout the interview is bound to counteract the patient's negative cognitive set. The therapist, of course, must be skillful in posing problems (questions) to which the patient can respond with "correct" solutions (answers). For instance, using the problem-solving model, the therapist should ask specific, concrete rather than abstract, open-ended questions since the patient can focus on and respond to concrete questions more readily.

SELECTING TARGET SYMPTOMS

It is difficult to stipulate in advance which problems should be selected during the first interview and at what level these problems should be approached. In general, however, in the moderately to severely depressed patient, the focus of the therapeutic intervention should be at the target symptom level.* The target symptom may be defined as any of the components of the depressive disorder that involves suffering or functional disability. These target symptoms may be broken down into the following categories (for a more complete description of these symptom categories, see Beck, 1967, pp. 10–43):

1. Affective symptoms: sadness, loss of gratification, apathy, loss of feelings and affection toward others, loss of mirth response, anxiety.

Contrast with Rational–Emotive Therapy, which focuses more on the general "Irrational Ideas" presumed to underlie all neurotic disorders. A complete discussion of typical target symptoms and their management is presented in Chapter 9.

2. Motivational: wish to escape from life (usually via suicide); wish to avoid "problems" or even usual everyday activities.
3. Cognitive: difficulty in concentrating, problems in attention span, difficulties in memory. The cognitive distortions—which are more on a conceptual or information-processing level—will be discussed in the next section.
4. Behavioral: often a reflection of the other previously mentioned symptoms; includes passivity (for example, lying in bed or sitting in a chair for hours on end), withdrawal from other people, retardation, agitation.
5. Physiological or vegetative: includes sleep disturbance (either increased or diminished sleeping); appetite disturbance (either increased or decreased eating).

The therapist (with the assistance of the patient) makes a determination as to which of the *target symptoms* should be addressed on the basis of many factors:

a. Which are the most distressing to the patient?
b. Which are most amenable to therapeutic intervention?

The specific *techniques* to be used will not be discussed at length here since they will be the focus of the next five chapters. In general, the techniques may be classified as (a) predominantly behavioral—which generally consists of engaging the patient in specific activities or projects which, in themselves, help to ameliorate some of his suffering and will have a spreading effect onto the other symptoms; (b) predominantly cognitive—in which the major focus is on the patient's thinking.

When the patient's depression is less severe, the therapeutic focus is often on external problems that are related to the precipitation or aggravation of the depression. These problems may include stresses or difficulties at home, school, or work. They frequently have a component of loss, such as a disruption of a close personal relationship, a failure to achieve a desired goal, or the deprivation of some pleasurable activity. Thus, the therapist and patient may work on helping the patient to make an important life decision regarding a problem contributing to his depression, discuss specialized techniques to help him cope better with a difficult life situation, or consider ways of relieving stresses or external demands. This type of approach (concentration on external problems) is also used after the patient's acute or severe symptoms have been relieved. The therapist should bear in mind that situational problems and depression may aggravate each other. This reciprocal interaction may be modified to improve both the external stresses and the depressive symptomatology.

COUNTERACTING THE TARGET SYMPTOMS

In this approach, we attempt to delineate the configuration of cognitive problems which contribute to the maintenance and aggravation of the symptoms of depression previously listed. The paradigm (and the supporting experimental evidence) that explains how resolving the conceptual problems leads to an alleviation of depressive symptoms has been described in detail elsewhere. (In order to pursue this therapeutic approach, the therapist should read Beck, 1967; Beck and Greenberg, 1974; and Beck, 1976, Chapters 5 and 11). The techniques are described in detail in later chapters in this book but will be briefly sketched here for purposes of illustration.

Briefly stated, this treatment approach attempts to identify and correct the specific cognitive distortions, deficits, or disturbances that feed into a patient's symptoms. To illustrate this approach, we can focus on the relations between cognitive problem and symptom as follows: If the patient feels sad, likely focal problems are his indiscriminate misreading of situations or internal stimuli as representing losses, deprivations, or disease, and his belief that his life situation will continue to get worse.

If the target symptom is "suicidal wishes," we look for (a) a desire to escape from an "intolerable" life situation, (b) an exaggeration of the actual reality problems, (c) an underestimation of the patient's coping abilities, (d) a lack of consideration or an unreasonable exclusion of potentially effective options for solving the "reality problems," and (e) an intolerance for dysphoria or for waiting until the problem can be resolved.

If the patient's major difficulty is in concentration, focusing, and recall, a step-wise progression of cognitive tasks can be given to help him gradually increase the duration of concentration on relevant details. We generally find that such deficits in concentration and recall are related to the continual intrusion of depressing cognitions.

Thus, the therapeutic strategy consists of specific techniques of "walling off" the peremptory cognitions, practice in focusing, distraction, "time-outs," etc.

If the major symptoms are passivity and retardation, behavioral tasks such as the Graded Task Assignment can be employed. When the target symptom is the patient's lack of gratification from activities that ordinarily would bring him pleasure, then a scheduling of potentially pleasurable activities may be employed. This strategy is designed to make the patient more "cognitively aware" of potentially satisfying events and also to make him more conscious of feelings of pleasure. Because of his all-or-nothing thinking, the patient tends to consider totally unpleasurable any activity that elicits less than his normal amount of satisfaction. Thus, we might ask him to rate the degree of pleasure on a 0–5 scale. This strategy also involves special tactics for enabling the patient to recall pleasant events.

When the main problem is functional impairment in the patient's capacity to carry out normal activities such as vocational tasks, housework, academic work, or even problems of physical hygiene, specific projects such as the Graded Task Assignment may be devised.

FOCUSING ON FAULTY INFORMATION-PROCESSING

In some respects, the depressed patient's cognitive problems are involved with faulty information processing. He tends to perceive his present, his future, and the outside world (the cognitive triad) in a negative way and consequently shows a biased interpretation of his experiences, negative expectancies as to the probable success of anything he undertakes, and a massive amount of self-criticism. Thus, one approach is to focus on the stream of cognitive distortions having to do with such content areas as a sense of loss; perceiving the self as either ugly, diseased, undesirable, or deficient; and regarding external problems as overwhelming and insoluble.

Concomitantly, the therapist may focus on the stylistic and logical errors that provide the matrix of the patient's negative thinking. The formal "thought disorder" shown by depressed patients included characteristics such as overgeneralization, selective abstraction, obliviousness to positive information ("tunnel vision"), arbitrary inference, etc. The patient also shows a tendency to think in extremes or absolutistic terms (black-and-white thinking) and shows a tendency to overpersonalize events. Moreover, he has a penchant to make continual moralistic value judgments ("worthless," "lazy," "irresponsible," "hateful") in reference to himself. Further, he castigates himself for his presumed moral deficiencies.

Feedback in the Initial Interview

In the previous chapter, we discussed the importance of receiving feedback from the patient. This is of the utmost importance in the first interview. Such feedback consists not only of the observation of the patient's overt emotional responses during the interview but also explicit statements by the patient of his reaction to the therapist and the therapy process itself.

Reciprocal feedback is important in establishing (a) whether the therapist understands the patient's problem and (b) whether the patient understands what the therapist is saying. The feedback may be obtained in a number of ways. Typical interchanges between patient and therapist might proceed as follows:

1. The therapist summarizes the patient's narrative or extracts the major problems. For example, one-third of the way through an initial interview, the therapist capsulizes the patient's problem in a fashion similar to this.

> Now, boiling down the various problems that seem to be troubling you, we see three main areas. First, you are disturbed about your son's problems in school; you have felt so upset and guilty about his alleged misbehavior that you have not really been able to pinpoint the precise problem and possibly help him with it. The second major area seems to have to do with your husband. You are concerned that since he seems to be coming home late more frequently, he may have a girlfriend. You are afraid to broach the subject with him because he may confirm your suspicion. You also are concerned that if you ask him to come home early, he is going to take this as more nagging on your part . . . Do I seem to be on the right track so far? . . . Okay, . . . Then the third problem is that you are disgusted with yourself because you don't seem to be taking very good care of yourself. You've let yourself go. You have

been gaining weight and you generally seem to be out of control. Does that seem to summarize the problems?

The patient then has the opportunity to modify or add to the capsule summary. If the summary is accurate, the patient is often pleased that he is understood and that his seemingly enormous problems can be reduced to manageable proportions. If the summary is incorrect, then the therapist can get on to the right track before he loses contact with the patient's problems.

2. To make sure that the patient is really "tuned in" to the therapist's summary of conceptualizations, he should ask the patient what he or she abstracts from the therapist's statements. The following is an illustration from the first interview with the same case. About two-thirds of the way through the interview, the therapist inquires as to how the patient perceives the therapist's analysis of the problems. The patient replies,

> I can see that I have been looking only at the bad points of Johnny's behavior and I have been so obsessed with his being a bad boy and I have been so furious at him, that I haven't even attempted to find out what the true facts are in the case. What I should do is speak to the teacher and then to Johnny . . . I guess you are suggesting that I stop nagging my husband and blaming him when he comes in late. When I feel up to it, I guess I can try to inquire as to whether there is another woman. In the meantime, I can work on my depression and make myself more attractive so that I'll be in a better position to work on the problem with my husband later on.

This summary demonstrates not only that the patient accepts the therapist's analysis of her problems but shows that she is capable of volunteering constructive solutions to her problems.

3. The third type of feedback has been alluded to previously. The therapist tries to elicit covert reactions to the interview that may be counterproductive. If there is any sign of "static" in the interview, it is desirable for the therapist to inquire as to what the patient is thinking.

In any event, as a good general rule, it is valuable for the therapist to inquire before the end of the interview into the patient's reactions so as to forestall any delayed negative reactions following the interview. This can be accomplished by the therapist's posing a question such as, "We've covered a lot of territory so far in this interview. Is there anything I said that troubled you? Or would you like further explanation? Do you think we left out anything important?" Often the therapist learns that the patient actually has misconstrued or failed to understand something that he has said. Such unclarities in communication are inevitable and, of course, are accentuated when one is dealing with a person who is already in a state of turmoil and has a tendency to distort other persons' statements.

4. Similarly, after proposing a homework assignment, the therapist can say to the patient, "How do you feel about this assignment? Do you feel that it is something that you would like to tackle, or does it seem onerous to you. Or would you prefer to think about it?" By giving the patient a multiple choice, as it were, the therapist is more likely to get a genuine response from the patient.

5. Finally, it is important for the therapist to get some feedback sometime during the first part of a subsequent interview regarding the patient's reactions to the previous interviews; that is, reactions that had occurred following the termination of the interview. This would also be a good time to get the patient's possible negative reactions to the homework assignments. As we have found that the patients are generally more likely to volunteer positive reactions regarding their homework assignments from the previous interviews, it is not so necessary to explore for positive reactions as it is to try to uncover negative reactions.

SUMMARY

1. The therapist treating depressed patients requires a solid background in psychopathology and diagnosis.
2. Interviews should be geared to establish:
    a. A therapeutic working relationship, including rapport
    b. Consensus on goals and treatment procedures
    c. Collaboration in defining and "solving" problems
    d. Appropriate interchange to provide optimum feedback to both patient and therapist regarding reciprocal understanding, stumbling blocks in therapy, progress toward goals, etc.
3. The therapist should attempt to utilize technical procedures

to provide some symptom of relief in the first session as well as in subsequent sessions. A mechanism for maintaining symptom relief needs to be set up to utilize the time between sessions optimally (for example, homework assignments, listening to a tape recording of the previous therapy session, etc.).

4. The ideal way to motivate the patient to work on his problems is to produce prompt lessening of symptoms through working together on particular problems. Thus, "education" or "re-education" is preferable to prestige suggestion or authoritarian reassurance.

5. The therapist should work within the arbitrary time constraints of the interview to achieve several concomitant technical goals:

    a. Establish a diagnostic profile

    b. Assess the degree of psychopathology

    c. Estimate the patient's assets for therapy and his social support system

    d. Obtain a solid data base in order to formulate the patient's problems. This involves setting up and testing a hierarchy of hypotheses.

    e. Improvise and test out a variety of treatment strategies appropriate for the particular stage of therapy.

6. Utilizing time optimally may involve diplomatically interrupting the patient when he rambles and guiding him back to focusing on his problem.

Chapter 6

SESSION BY SESSION TREATMENT:
A TYPICAL COURSE OF THERAPY

OVERVIEW OF THE SESSIONS

This chapter illustrates the course in treatment of a patient receiving cognitive therapy for depression. The practical "mechanics" of cognitive therapy were extracted by reviewing treatment case notes. This specific case was selected because it reflects a typical response to cognitive psychotherapy, including "setbacks" and therapeutic "roadblocks." While our intent is to provide the relevant treatment details, it is only possible to present the therapist's interpretations of critical data.

Initially, therapy focused on developing a common conceptualization; that is, the therapist presented a rationale for cognitive therapy and discussed the patient's reaction to the model. Prior to the first treatment session, the therapist sent the patient the booklet, *Coping with Depression,* with a request that she read it to assist with this aspect of treatment. The therapy then centered on the patient's symptoms with initial attention to behavioral and motivational difficulties. Once the patient showed some significant changes in these areas, the emphasis was directed to the content and pattern of her thinking; namely, recognizing, recording, and testing specific cognitions. In the later sessions, the therapist and patient discussed her basic assumptions that were viewed as resulting in her vulnerability to depression.

Note: Our experience indicates that the moderately–severely depressed to the severely depressed patients require twice-weekly sessions initially. In the study reported by Rush *et al.* (1977), the protocol called for a maximum of 20 sessions over a 15-week period. In implementation of this research plan, we found that the patients in this group (mean Beck Depression Inventory score = 30.2) averaged

15 therapy sessions over an 11-week period. Thus, on the average, the patients received cognitive therapy twice a week for 4 weeks and then once a week for 7 weeks. If not bound by the constraints of a research design, the therapist should be flexible in "tapering off" therapy (for example, to bi-weekly, monthly, etc.).

It is obvious that the frequency and duration of therapy has to be adjusted to the needs of the individual case. The severely depressed patient described in this chapter had 22 sessions of cognitive therapy over a period of 14 weeks (twice a week for 8 weeks; once a week for 6 weeks).

In this case report, the Beck Depression Inventory scores will be specified following the session heading (for example, Session 3, BDI = 37) as an indicator of the severity of the patient's depression. The treatment plan (agenda items) for the therapy session will be listed in point form followed by a narrative of the important therapeutic interchanges.

CASE HISTORY

Personal Data

The patient was a 36-year-old married homemaker, the mother of 2 boys (ages 14 and 9) and a girl (age 7). Her husband of 15 years was sales manager of an automotive supply company, age 37, who was described by the patient as a "confident, loving person." The patient described herself as a "nobody who can't do anything right, a failure as a wife and mother." She questioned whether she loved her husband or her children and, on several occasions, considered suicide as a way of "unburdening" her family.

Assessment

The patient was initially assessed by a psychiatrist (other than the therapist) who determined she had a "severe depression and personality problems." She was referred for cognitive therapy because of her tendency toward self-criticism and hopelessness. Two previous therapeutic approaches (marital therapy for 6 sessions and pharmacotherapy with two antidepressant preparations over 17 weeks) resulted in slight but transient symptomatic improvement in the previous 19 months. The therapist interviewed the patient and confirmed the diagnosis of primary depression. The Beck Depression Inventory score was 41, and the Hamilton Rating Scale for Depression was 23, both measures indicative of severe depression.

Session 1 (BDI = 41)

Plan (Agenda):

- Review symptoms of depression.
- Assess suicidal ideation and hopelessness.
- Discuss influence of thinking on behavior with specific reference to booklet, *Coping with Depression.*
- Review activity level, if indicated.

The patient came to the first session indicating that she felt at the "end of the rope." She was particularly concerned about her loss of affection for her family members. She had considered suicide but had obtained some hope when she recognized the description "of myself" in the *Coping with Depression* booklet. She criticized herself for being "selfish" and "thinking as a child." She believed that her work around the home was "unimportant" and she feared "total rejection" from her husband. She acknowledged that her self-criticisms made her feel worse but noted, "The truth hurts." The therapist clarified that she was depressed and that her negative reactions could be signs of her depression.

Assigned Homework:

- Keep activity schedule: to ascertain how active the patient is and to obtain "objective" data about her present level of functioning.
- Complete Minnesota Multiphasic Personality Inventory (to evaluate degree of psychopathology as well as obtaining research data).
- Complete Life History Questionnaire (Lazarus, 1972) to obtain relevant past history.

Session 2 (BDI = 43)

Plan:

- Review symptoms of depression.
- Review activity schedule checking for possible *omissions* and *distortions.*
- Begin to demonstrate relationship between thinking, behavior and affect by using specific experiences of patient.

In this session, the patient presented herself in tearful state and reported that her marriage was certain "to end in divorce." She described an event in which her husband responded to a slight, positive change in her mood by inviting her out to a movie. The patient responded that she "didn't deserve to go out" and then berated her husband for proposing an activity that would "waste money."

She said that she couldn't understand why her husband didn't "sense" her irritability toward the children and him. She concluded that his "insensitivity" was indicative of his uncaring attitude ("and I don't blame him"), an attitude that would lead to divorce. The therapist pointed out her selective inattention to his offer of an evening out and indicated how this was contradictory to her conclusion. This comment appeared to have little effect on the patient.

Homework:

- Continue with activity schedule with patient's agreeing to attempt mastery and/or pleasure activities.
- Define problems that patient sees as contributing to her depression.

Session 3 (BDI = 38)

Plan:

- Review "Mastery and Pleasure" activities.
- Continue to elicit thoughts related to sadness.

The patient brought in her activity schedule: her mornings had been filled with routine housecleaning jobs; her afternoons consisted of "watching the soaps and crying." She criticized herself for "not doing what I should be doing." She referred to her inability to control her children; she specifically described the problems she faced getting her oldest boy out of bed in the morning. This latter problem quite simply resulted from the patient's failure to give her son sufficient responsibility for his own behavior. She was in the habit of repeatedly calling him every morning and thereby reinforcing his reliance on her. She agreed to change this behavior by telling her son about a "new rule" of personal responsibility, for getting oneself up.

Other problems that were listed included a lack of communication with her husband and a lack of fulfillment in her activities. In general, the patient remained relatively active during the day: this indicated a reasonable level of motivation and activity, and, thus, treatment focused more directly on her cognitions.

Homework:

- Record cognitions during periods of sadness, anxiety, and anger and during periods of "apathy," in order to elicit the relationship between thinking, behavior, and affect.

Session 4 (BDI = 31)

Plan:

- Discuss specific cognitions leading to unpleasant affect.

The patient brought a list of 12 situations in the previous three days that led to depression, anger, or guilt. Most of the situations involved interactions with her children which had resulted in the conclusion that she was an "incompetent mother." She tended to punish her children for any misbehavior in an attempt to change their behavior so that others (her husband, family, friends) would not criticize her. On the other hand, she spent most of her time catering to her children's needs and demands.

Her cognitions included many references to activities she "should" do around the home. She tried to maintain a high level of activity (housework and cooking) in order to please her husband even though she believed she "deserved to be rejected."

108

The therapist was able to break through the patient's self-criticisms of "incompetence" by pointing out that instead of labeling herself as incompetent, she could perhaps correct the "misbehavior" of her children by different training techniques. She demonstrated an interest in learning new methods of child rearing but maintained skeptical attitude.

Homework:

- Continue recording cognitions—if possible, record alternative explanations; avoid labels such as "incompetent" and "selfish" since these pejorative terms serve to disguise problems.
- Rate on a scale of 0–10 the degree to which she *"wanted* to complete the activities" as opposed to meeting the therapist's or her husband's expectations.

Session 5 (BDI = 36)

Plan:

- Discuss cognitions and identify recurrent or common themes.

The main theme of the patient's cognitions was her belief that she was failing in her duties as wife. These "duties" ranged from doing housecleaning to responding sexually. She believed that her husband would eventually leave her unless she "snapped out" of her depression. The therapist informed her that she would not suddenly "snap out" of the depression but by examining her thinking she would gradually learn to cope with her depression and eventually to understand herself better. It was interesting that the therapist's negation of her self-demand to "eliminate" her depression was received by the patient with considerable relief. She "knew" that her feelings would not change overnight and in fact recognized she was mimicking her husband's directives to improve. She also complained of a sleep disturbance (getting to sleep at night). This reaction appeared to result from self-criticisms about her loss of libido and "loss of love."

Homework:

- "Beds are for sleeping." If not asleep in 15 minutes, get up and do something to distract thinking.
- Continue to record thoughts and list responsibilities to husband and vice versa.

Session 6 (BDI = 29); Session 7 (BDI = 26); Session 8 (BDI = 26)

Plan:

- Review cognitions, particularly her expectations for herself and her "shoulds" rather than "wants."
- Discuss her thoughts regarding her marital responsibilities.

In these three sessions the therapist attempted to pinpoint the patient's expectations. In past sessions, she had been able to recognize how her self-criticisms and hopelessness were clearly related to comparing herself with an *ideal* mother, wife, person, etc.

She ruminated about past mistakes and selectively ignored the realities of her accomplishments. For example, at one point her husband was interviewed and, with the exception of acknowledging frustration with her "negative attitudes," he expressed a caring, concerned attitude. He indicated that he tried to express his affection toward his wife to counter her notion of his "rejection" of her, but that these actions resulted in further periods of crying and guilt. The patient started to understand that her own ideas did not mirror reality but rather were her misinterpretations of reality and thus, subject to reevaluation.

The patient had great difficulty *defining* a reasonable set of goals. She tended to speak in global terms about being a "better mother," "better wife," etc., without realistically defining what she meant. When she was guided toward specific behavior change such as asserting herself with her husband about her desire for more shared activities, or setting limits on her oldest son's behavior, her initial reaction was "I can't do it." With specific directions, role-playing, and cognitive rehearsal, however, she surprised herself with a series of successes. As would be expected at this stage, her reaction was, at best, transient pleasure since she continually downgraded her accomplishments (she viewed her achievements as "*normal* reactions, what I *should* do, nothing special"). After a success, she would think of the "overwhelming" series of problems that she still had to face.

The therapist pointed out the patient's "no win" cognitive set and spent considerable therapeutic time discussing the self-defeating nature of her thought pattern. She recognized, for instance, that initially she castigated herself for being ineffective but after she tested and disconfirmed this idea, she devalued herself for not trying hard enough. Once she became aware of her cognitive errors and was able to practice more reasonable responses to her "automatic thoughts," she observed a significant decrease in her depressive symptoms. Interestingly, the patient's sisters-in-law commented on her increased confidence, a change the patient had not recognized; this feedback supported her therapeutic efforts. On the other hand, she began to experience an increase in anxiety when she received favorable comments from her husband. This anxiety was not readily understandable at this point in therapy.

Homework:

- Continue to recognize cognitive errors and review alternative explanations for her negative "automatic thoughts."

Session 9 (BDI = 23); Session 10 (BDI = 22); Session 11 (BDI = 30)

Plan:

- Focus on self-criticisms and work on coping responses (that is, *realistic* evaluations of problem areas rather than self-criticisms).
- Pursue responding to her "wants" rather than her "shoulds."

The patient recognized a variety of situations in which she would criticize herself. Some of these situations involved her husband and family and concerned her family duties. For example, she found it particularly difficult to cook the main meal and on some occasions, she used frozen dinners. In the past she had criticized herself for her "uncaring" behavior in this regard. With considerable effort she began to cook basic meals and gradually increased her accomplishments in this area until she was almost "back to normal."

One focus was on the patient's self-critical reactions to her meals; during her meals she made comments that indicated that the food was poorly presented. Her family would usually disagree ("They're trying to make me feel better") but they would on occasion make critical or nonsupportive comments themselves. As a result, the patient found mealtime to be particularly upsetting. These were essentially "no-win" situations. During this period of treatment, the patient learned to refrain from stating her criticisms but rather rated her *effort* in making the meal. As a result, she received "honest" reactions from her family and made changes in her own unrealistic reactions.

A second focus was on her "wants." The treatment goals included assertiveness discussions ("If I express my feelings, I'll get rejected"), time management ("I have to look after the needs of others and no one should have to help"), and future planning ("I used to enjoy working in a store but couldn't do it now"). As indicated by the above thoughts, considerable work on the patient's dysfunctional ideas was required. Interestingly, her reaction to an inquiry about what it would mean if someone didn't agree with her distorted ideas, she stated, "It means I'm no good, I'm not worth anything, my opinion doesn't count."

Session 12 (BDI = 15); Session 13 (BDI = 20); Session 14 (BDI = 17); Session 15 (BDI = 17)

Plan:

- Continue to attend to self-criticisms with focus on underlying assumptions. (At this point the patient was ready to assess the basis for her unrealistic self-criticisms and other depressive reactions. The therapist decided to investigate the patient's attitudes and beliefs that contributed to her depression.)

The patient began to believe that her depression could be controlled if she managed her tendency to criticize herself. When she was able to evaluate situations objectively, she learned that her husband had, indeed, been highly critical of her if she did not keep a "spotless" house and prepare his favorite foods. The patient would often act on her expectations of criticism by criticizing herself before her husband had an opportunity to do so.

The patient had never communicated with her husband about *her* "wants" and "needs." She eventually stopped criticizing herself for being "a burden" and a "terrible mother"—with the knowledge that these labels served no purpose except to make her feel sad and/or guilty. Labeling herself had no effect on the reality-based problems in her life. Initially, when she managed to meet her own expectations that involved perfectionistic standards she received little gratification. As therapy continued to focus on her expectations and their consequences she gradually recognized that she did not like many of the household tasks and, thus, deserved self-praise when she was successful. She deserved this praise for doing a job she didn't like rather than one that she "should" accomplish. Her basic assumption had often been, "People will dislike and even reject me unless I meet their expectations." Thus, the patient tended to do what she should do, criticized herself in reaction to perceived criticisms from others, and continued to restrict her own activities in order to meet the needs of others.

In this stage of therapy, the patient began to recognize her self-abnegating pattern of thinking and behavior and to question why she didn't act on what she "wanted" to do rather than what she "should" do. Her level of anxiety increased at this time and she required considerable reassurance that she was taking a reasonable approach. For instance, she worried that she would become a selfish, egocentric person, always demanding that others do what she wanted. She learned that the important factor was that she think about what she wanted. In fact, there were occasions when she put her own "wants" aside and did what her husband wanted. This kind of compromise was particularly gratifying to her.

Homework:

- List "wants," particularly future goals. This assignment was designed to focus the patient on her own needs and expectations.

Session 16 (BDI = 22); Session 17 (BDI = 18); Session 18 (BDI = 12); Session 19 (BDI = 14)

The patient indicated a desire to return to a part-time job but immediately began to devalue the idea, a pattern that had not occurred for four sessions. When the therapist pointed out this reaction to her, she registered surprise.

She noted that she had been feeling depressed again and had initially believed her depression came "out of the blue." One incident appeared to add further to her uncertainty about herself. Her parents visited and her mother was observed to be very critical of her father. The patient had the idea that she (the patient) was responsible for her father's happiness. She also had the notion that her mother might suffer a heart attack because she was a "worrier" and thereby leave her father in a helpless position. Thus, the visit of the parents started a series of doubts about her parents. The patient concluded that she had to keep her own family happy and this would require being at their beck and call.

This reaction again involved meeting the expectations of others and for a while the patient became very concerned that she was making a mistake by following her own judgments about her family. For instance, she ruminated about whether it was a good idea to take a job even though she wanted it and received pleasure from working. She worried that her husband might respond by leaving her or criticizing her to her family.

This period of therapy was critical because *there appeared to be a possibility of a relapse.* The patient had been strongly affected by her parents' interaction, and from a clinical theory point of view, it seemed that she was again flooded with her previous dysfunctional cognitions and maladaptive methods, namely, "Do what is expected of you, otherwise you'll screw things up." This belief then led her to approach her problem in the old way by acting on what she thought others expected of her.

Two key interventions were made at this point. First, the therapist reviewed the similarities between her present reaction and her past pattern of thinking. The therapist reviewed the events with the patient and she proposed that she was "following the old pattern." Second, her husband commented that he liked her "new

114

self" better than her "old self." These interchanges were highly significant and the patient at that point regained her motivation to pursue a reasonable course of action.

Soon after this session the patient obtained a part-time position in a store. She noted that she was not particularly happy or pleased ("It feels different") but her reaction was understandable, given her conflict about her decisions.

Homework:

• Discuss goals with husband in greater detail with particular reference to homemaking responsibilities.

Session 20 (BDI = 8); Session 21 (BDI = 6); Session 22 (BDI = 7)

The final sessions attempted to consolidate the gains made in therapy. The patient provided one anecdote that perhaps best illustrated the result of her cognitive and behavior changes.

When she initially went to her job she returned home and complained to her husband that she derived no pleasure from working. Her husband, who had encouraged the patient previously (but with some unspoken reservations), reacted by stating, "If you're not happy, then quit." Thus, the patient was faced with a crisis and thought she should resign her position. She had learned to list the "pros and cons" prior to any decision and to pay specific attention to her problem of automatically responding to the expectations of others. After this analysis the patient concluded that her displeasure in the job resulted from her own unrealistically high expectations (that is, the job had to be perfect in order to justify the time away from her home responsibilities).

Her statements of displeasure, in fact, uncovered her husband's doubts and she decided to discuss these doubts rather than simply act on them. As a result, her husband admitted his own uncertainty and boredom when she wasn't at home. He agreed to pursue activities at home that *he* enjoyed and surprised himself with a new "freedom." As a final consequence, the patient reacted positively to this change in her husband's behavior and began to enjoy her job.

Follow Up: 1 month (BDI = 9); 2 months (BDI = 5); 6 months (BDI = 2)

During the follow-up period the patient remained nondepressed and noted with considerable pleasure that she was more confident. She and her husband enrolled in a child management course with the purpose of becoming "more effective parents." She still was faced with problems, particularly when significant others (husband, children, parents) became emotional or demanding. The patient recognized that her "old automatic thoughts" would still be elicited but she remained convinced that the best approach to this ideation was a careful reappraisal of the situation.

With the exception of long-term followup, treatment was terminated at this point.

Chapter 7

APPLICATION OF BEHAVIORAL TECHNIQUES

COGNITIVE CHANGE THROUGH BEHAVIORAL CHANGE

The cognitive *therapy* of depression is based on the cognitive *theory* of depression. By working within the framework of the cognitive model, the therapist formulates his therapeutic approach according to the specific needs of a given patient at a particular time. Thus, the therapist may be conducting cognitive therapy even though he is utilizing predominantly behavioral or abreactive (emotion releasing) techniques.

In the early stages of cognitive therapy and particularly with the more severely depressed patients, it is often necessary for the therapist to concentrate on restoring the patient's functioning to the premorbid level. Specifically, engaging the patient's attention and interest the therapist attempts to induce the patient to counteract his withdrawal and to become involved in more constructive activities. The rationale for this approach is based on the clinical observation that the severely depressed patient, and often the important people in his life ("significant others"), believe that he is no longer capable of carrying out the typical functions expected in his role as a student, wage earner, homemaker, spouse, parent, etc. Furthermore, the patient can see no hope of gaining satisfaction from those activities that had previously brought him pleasure.

The severely depressed patient is caught in a vicious cycle in which his reduced level of activity leads to labeling himself as ineffectual. This labeling, in turn, leads to further discouragement and ultimately to a drift into a state of immobility. He finds it difficult to carry out intellectual functions (such as reasoning and planning motor activities — even walking and talking spontaneously as well as performing complicated acts requiring specialized skill and training.

These forms of behavior are generally instruments for achieving satisfaction and maintaining one's self-esteem and the esteem of others. The disruption of these functions as a result of diminished concentration, fatigability, and low mood produces dissatisfaction and a reduction of self-esteem.

The role of the therapist is clear. There is no easy way to "talk the patient out" of his conclusions that he is weak, inept, or vacuous. He can see for himself that he simply is not doing those things that once were relatively easy and important to him. By helping the patient change certain behaviors, the therapist may *demonstrate* to the patient that his negative, overgeneralized conclusions were incorrect. Following specific behavior changes, the therapist may show the patient that he has, in fact, not lost the ability to function at his previous level, but that his discouragement and pessimism make it difficult to mobilize his resources to make the necessary effort. The patient thereby comes to recognize that the source of his problem is a cognitive error: He *thinks* (incorrectly) that he is inept, weak, and helpless, and those beliefs seriously restrict his motivation and behavior.

The term *behavioral techniques* may suggest that the immediate therapeutic attention is solely on the patient's overt behavior; that is, the therapist prescribes some kind of goal-directed activity. In actuality, the reporting of the patient's thoughts, feelings, and wishes remains critical for the successful application of the behavioral techniques. The ultimate aim of these techniques in cognitive therapy is to produce change in the negative attitudes so that the patient's performance will continue to improve. Actually, the behavioral methods can be regarded as a series of small experiments designed to test the validity of the patient's hypotheses or ideas about himself. As the negative ideas are contradicted by these "experiments," the patient gradually becomes less certain of their validity and he is motivated to attempt more difficult assignments.

Many of the techniques described in this chapter are also part of the repertoire of the behavior therapist. The impact of the therapeutic techniques derived from a strictly behavioral or conditioning model is limited because of the restriction to observable behavior and selective exclusion of information regarding the patient's attitudes, beliefs, and thoughts—his cognitions. Hence, even though the behavior therapist induces the patient to become more active, his pessimism, self-disparagement, and suicidal impulses may remain unchanged. For the behavior therapist, the modification of behavior is an end in itself; for the cognitive therapist it is a means to an end—namely, cognitive change.

It is important to note that cognitive changes *do not necessarily* follow changes in behavior. In contrast to the typical findings in the social-psychological studies of normal subjects, we find that depressed individuals do not readily alter their hypervalent, negative cognitions despite distinct behavior changes. This point is illustrated in the following example.

A 36-year-old depressed woman had withdrawn from participating in the tennis games she had previously enjoyed. Instead, her daily behavior pattern consisted of "sleeping and trying to do the housework I've neglected." The patient firmly believed that she was unable to engage in activities as "strenuous" as tennis. Her husband arranged for a private tennis lesson in an attempt to help his wife to overcome her depression. The patient reluctantly attended the lesson and appeared to be "a different person" in the eyes of her husband. She stroked the ball well and was agile in following instructions. Despite her good performance during the lesson, the patient concluded that her skills had "deteriorated" beyond the point at which lessons would do any good. She misinterpreted her husband's positive response to her lesson as an indication of how bad her game had become—because *in her view*, "He thinks I'm so hopeless that the only time I can hit the ball is when I'm taking a lesson." In essence she rejected the obvious reason for her husband's enthusiasm in favor of an explanation derived from her negative image of herself. She also stated that she didn't enjoy the tennis session because she wasn't "deserving" of any recreation time.

This vignette illustrates the importance of placing the behavioral changes into perspective for the patient. The negatively biased cognitions are not necessarily altered simply by a change in behavior. Rather the change in behavior allows the identification of such negative appraisals. Behavior change is important insofar as it provides an opportunity for the patient to evaluate empirically his ideas of inadequacy and incompetence. The therapist has to base the rationale for his therapeutic procedure on an understanding of the patient's frame of reference. In this case, although the husband initiated an appropriate plan of action (a tennis lesson), his ignorance

119

of his wife's belief system prevented him from helping her to solve her cognitive problem. In fact, his effort backfired in that she misinterpreted the entire experience. Later in the chapter we will describe the therapeutic strategies of defining and dealing with the cognitions related to mutually agreeable behavioral goals and behavior change.

SCHEDULING ACTIVITIES

Many depressed patients report an overwhelming number of self-debasing and pessimistic cognitions at times when they are physically and socially inactive. They criticize themselves for being "vegetables" and for withdrawing from other people. Paradoxically, they may justify their withdrawal and avoidance on the basis that activity and social interaction are meaningless or that they are a burden to others. Thus, they sink into increasing passivity and social isolation. Furthermore, it is not unusual for the depressed patient to interpret his inactivity and withdrawal as evidence of inadequacy and helplessness and thereby complete a vicious cycle.

The prescription of special projects is based on the clinical observation that depressed patients find it difficult to undertake or complete jobs which they accomplished with relative ease prior to the depressive episode. They are prone to avoid complex tasks, or, if they do attempt such tasks, they are likely to have considerable difficulty achieving their objective. Typically, the depressed patient avoids the project or stops trying soon after he encounters some difficulty. His negative beliefs and attitudes appear to underlie his tendency to give up. Patients often report, "It's useless to try," for they are convinced they will fail. When they engage in goal-directed activities they tend to magnify the difficulties and minimize their ability to overcome them.

The use of activity schedules serves to counteract the patient's loss of motivation, inactivity, and his preoccupation with depressive ideas. The specific technique of scheduling the patient's time on an hour-by-hour basis is likely to maintain a certain momentum and prevent slipping back into immobility. Furthermore, focusing on specific goal-oriented tasks provides the patient and therapist with concrete data on which to base realistic evaluations of the patient's functional capacity.

As with other cognitive techniques, the therapist should present the patient with a rationale. Often the patient is aware that inactivity is associated with an increase in his painful feelings. The patient can generally accept the idea that inactivity increases his negative ruminations and dysphoria. At the very least, the therapist can request the patient to engage in an "experiment" to determine whether activity diminishes his preoccupations and possibly improves his mood. The therapist and patient determine specific activities and the patient agrees to monitor his thoughts and feelings while engaged in each task. In every difficult cases, the therapist may seriously question the patient, "What have you got to lose by trying?"

The therapist may choose to provide the patient with a schedule to plan his activities in advance and/or to record the actual activities during the day. A "graded task" hierarchy should be incorporated into the daily plan.

Planning specific activities in collaboration with the patient may be an important step in demonstrating to him that he is capable of controlling his time. Severely depressed patients often report a sense of "going through the motions" with the sense that there is little purpose in their activities. By planning the day with the therapist, they are often able to set meaningful goals. Later, the patient's record of the actual activities (compared to what he planned for the day) provides the therapist and patient with objective feedback about his achievements. The record also provides a reference to self-ratings of mastery and satisfaction for successful goal-attainment (see Figures 1 and 2).

It may tax the therapist's ingenuity to get the patient sufficiently involved in the idea of carrying out a program of activities or even filling his activity schedule retrospectively. Thus, the therapist explains the rationale (for example, that people generally function better when they have a schedule), elicits the patient's objections, and then proposes making a schedule as an interesting experiment. It should be emphasized to the patient that the immediate objective is attempting to follow the schedule rather than seeking symptomatic relief: Improved functioning frequently comes before subjective relief is apparent.

It is important for the therapist to stress the following principles to the patient prior to using a schedule to plan daily activities.

1. "No one accomplishes everything he plans, so don't feel bad if you don't realize all of your plans."

WEEKLY ACTIVITY SCHEDULE
NOTE: Grade activities *M* for Mastery and *P* for Pleasure

	M	T	W	Th	F	S	S
9-10		Go to grocery store	Go to Museum	Get ready to go out			
10-11		Go to grocery store	Go to Museum	Drive to Dr.'s appointment			
11-12	Doctor's Appointment	Call friend	Go to Museum	Doctor's Appointment			
12-1	LUNCH	LUNCH	Lunch at Museum				
1-2	Drive home	Clean front room	Drive home				
2-3	Read novel	Clean front room	Washing				
3-4	Clean bedroom	Read novel	Washing				
4-5	Watch T.V.	Watch T.V.	Watch T.V.				
5-6	Fix dinner	Fix dinner	Fix dinner				
6-7	Eat with Family	Eat with Family	Eat with Family				
7-8	Clean kitchen	Clean kitchen	Clean kitchen				
8-12	Watch T.V., Read novel, Sleep	Call sister, Watch T.V., read novel, sleep	Work on rug, Read novel, sleep				

FIGURE 1. Assigned Activity Schedule for Patient A.

WEEKLY ACTIVITY SCHEDULE
NOTE: Grade activities *M* for Mastery and *P* for Pleasure

	M		T		W		Th		F	S	S
9-10			Went to grocery store	M3 P0	Back to bed	M0 P0	Ready to go out	M2 P0			
10-11			Went to grocery store	M3 P0	Back to bed	M0 P0	Drove to town				
11-12			Went to grocery store	M3 P0	Called repair-man for dishwasher	M3 P0	Appointment				
12-1	LUNCH	M0 P1	LUNCH	M0 P0	LUNCH	M0 P1					
1-2	Drove home	M0 P0	Called friend	M0 P3	Washing	M4 P0					
2-3	Read	P3	Watched T.V.	M0 P1	Washing	M4 P0					
3-4	Cleaned Room	M5 P2	Watched T.V.	M0 P1	Washing	M4 P0					
4-5	Cleaned Room	M5 P2	Watched T.V.	M0 P1	Watched T.V.	M0 P2					
5-6	Fixed Dinner	M4 P2	Fixed Dinner	M3 P0	Fixed Dinner	M2 P0					
6-7	Cleaned kitchen	M4 P0	T.V.	M0 P0	T.V.	M0 P1					
7-8	Watched T.V.	M0 P1	T.V.	M0 P0	T.V.	M0 P1					
8-12	Watched T.V. Sleep	M0 P1	T.V. Clean kitchen Sleep	M0,P0 M3,P0	T.V. Sleep	M0 P1					

FIGURE 2. Completed Activity Schedule for Patient A.

2. "In planning, state what kind of activity you will undertake, not *how much* you will accomplish. What you accomplish often depends on external factors you can't plan, such as interruptions, mechanical failures, and weather, as well as subjective factors such as fatigue, concentration, and motivation. For example, you say that you wish the house was cleaner. Plan to do housework for one specific hour each day, say 10–11:00 a.m. The actual number of hours you will need to finish cleaning the house can be predicted after you have followed the schedule for several days."

3. "Even if you don't succeed, be sure to remind yourself that *trying* to carry out plans is the most important step. This step provides useful information for setting the next goal."

4. "Set aside time each evening to plan for the next day; write your plans for each hour of the next day on the schedule."

These principles are important since they are designed to counter negative ideas about attempting the scheduling task.

The activity schedule serves to structure the day and it provides information to assess the patient's daily activities. In making this assignment, the therapist clearly states that the initial purpose of the program is to *observe* and not to *evaluate* how well or how much the patient does each day.

The following table is taken from the schedule reported by a depressed 40-year-old male. The patient was asked to rate on a scale from 0 to 5 the degree of mastery (M) and pleasure (P) associated with each activity.

Monday		M	P
6–7 a.m.	Woke up, stayed in bed	0	0
7–8 a.m.	Dressed, washed	0	0
8–8:30 a.m.	Read paper, drank coffee	0	0
8:30–10 a.m.	Back to bed—couldn't sleep	0	0
10–12 a.m.	Watched TV	0	1
12–1 p.m.	Paid bills	0	0
3 p.m.	Friends visited	0	3
3–4 p.m.	Watched TV	0	0
4–5 p.m.	Tried to wash car	0	0
5–6 p.m.	Ate dinner with family	0	1
6–7 p.m.	Did dishes with wife	0	0

The daily record activity provided the basis for testing the recurrent idea expressed by the patient that "I don't do *anything.*" Without such specific evidence, the therapist cannot realistically and constructively refute the patient's belief that he did things and wasn't capable of doing anything.

The daily activity schedule also induces the patient to become aware of the activities which provided even slight relief from the feelings of depression. In this case, the therapist asked, "Did you feel better or worse when you were in bed and not sleeping compared to when you visited friends?" To his surprise, the patient realized that the social interactions had relieved his dysphoria. Thus, with an activity schedule and the associated therapist questions, the patient learned that his depression does fluctuate depending on his behavior and on external circumstances. Ideas such as, "Nothing makes any difference" or "I feel equally terrible all day" can be altered to the more reasonable view that "Sometimes I can do something which will provide relief for me." Even the most depressed, retarded patients seem to feel better when involved in an activity—if for no other reason than the distraction it provides. Furthermore, by rating the degree of satisfaction associated with each activity, the patient becomes "sensitized" to feelings of satisfaction and thus is more likely to experience and recall pleasurable sensations. Such experiences counteract his belief that he is incapable of experiencing any gratifications. (For further elaboration, see the section on Mastery and Pleasure techniques.)

If the patient is unable to decide what to plan, the therapist suggests various possible projects which the patient wishes he could carry out (for example, housework, shopping, paying bills, etc.). Once a job has been selected, a time slot is picked and the scheduled plans are recorded on the Activity Schedule form at the appropriate times (for example, cleaning the house 10–11 a.m. Monday and Wednesday; one hour of shopping Tuesday 10–11 a.m.). The actual details of carrying out the plans are discussed in a step-by-step manner and may be facilitated by the Cognitive Rehearsal technique discussed later in this chapter. The patient should be encouraged to observe and report any negative ideas that occur while trying to carry out the plan. These ideas should be dealt with in the same way as any other dysfunctional cognitions.

The flexible application of the principle of scheduling activities is illustrated in the following example.

A 42-year-old unemployed depressed male complained of inertia which he defined as "an inability to do anything." In the session, the patient indicated particular difficulty in deciding what task to start since, as he described it, he was overwhelmed with jobs around the house. The therapist decided to use an activity schedule and set out with the patient to plan a "reasonable" day using the graded task concept in addition to outlining an hour-to-hour schedule. The therapist emphasized the value of the patient's planning his day so he would have a concrete set of guidelines. The guidelines were formulated so that the patient would not view the schedule as something which "must" be followed. As with all behavioral assignments, the therapist elicited the patient's reactions to the proposed schedule. In this case, the patient was relieved that he was not expected to follow the schedule rigidly and agreed to *attempt* each item.

The items on the agenda included getting up, washing, etc., making breakfast, scanning the newspaper for job opportunities, beginning to mow the lawn (the emphasis being on initiating the activity, not completing it), preparing a resume for a job, and watching television. The patient reported the schedule to be extremely useful as it helped to break his day into discrete units. He continued the scheduling throughout therapy and established a system of planning his day in the prior evening since the mornings were the most difficult decision-making times for him.

The next example demonstrates how the therapist elicited a general sense of hopelessness about a specific task—shopping. Then, each of the problems raised about the task was specified, assessed, and answered. Finally, the therapist and patient constructed a schedule to accomplish an aspect of the goal, recognizing that "everything" could not be accomplished in one trial.

A 48-year-old severely depressed mother of five reported, "I can't do the shopping. I can't plan one meal to the next." Her reasons for not being able to shop included these: (1) "My five children are all on weird diets and I can't keep them all in mind," (2) "I can't tell when my husband's coming home so I don't know what to buy," (3) "I forget what I wanted to buy when I get to the store."

THERAPIST: If you shop for the next day's menus, would you consider that useful?

PATIENT: Yes, but I used to shop for a month at a time.

T: Shopping for one day is not as "efficient" as you used to be—I understand. But by comparing yourself to your best performance, you overlook the value of accomplishing at least one day's shopping now.

P: That's true. I see that.

T: Let's plan one hour a day for shopping. Which hour is best?

P: Eleven to twelve.

T: Okay. Let's mark "shopping" into the 11–12 block for the three problems you know about shopping: (1) forgetting, (2) many individual menus, and (3) an unpredictable number of people for dinner. First, how would you solve the problem of forgetting?

P: I try to make a shopping list.

T: So one thing you'll need to do is make a list during the 11–12 period each day.

P: Right.

T: Next. Are there any foods which all the various diets have in common?

P: Yes, hamburgers, cottage cheese, and salads. But I am tired of fixing and eating those foods.

T: Changing the diets is one issue. Shopping is another. Let's stick to shopping for now. We'll get onto other issues when we're ready. (Note: The therapist did not bring up the patient's probable assumption that she must please everyone in order to be a good mother. When her depression was reduced, the idea was discussed.)

P: Okay. I could plan on hamburger and salads each day.

T: Next, since you're buying the same things for each meal, it doesn't matter how many are present at dinner each night. You can save any extra food for the next day.

P: (smiles): That's true.

T: Do you have enough ideas to plan on working on shopping each day for the one hour? Be sure to record exactly what you do in that hour when it comes and to record any negative thoughts you have while you're trying to shop.

MASTERY AND PLEASURE TECHNIQUES

Some depressed patients engage in activities but derive little pleasure from them. This failure to derive gratification often results from either (a) an attempt to engage in activities which were not plesurable even prior to the depressive episode, (b) the dominance of negative cognitions which override any potential sense of pleasure, or (c) selective inattention to sensations of pleasure.

In the first instance, patients undertake generally unexciting activities, such as housework, with the result that they do not find that successful completion is gratifying. The patient may hold back from participating in pleasurable activities or he may not readily recall past activities which were pleasurable. The therapist's first objective is to elicit the patient's reasons for not engaging in pleasant activities. A reason such as "I don't deserve to have fun because I have not accomplished anything" is commonly heard from depressives. To counteract this type of thinking, the therapist could describe one purpose of increasing pleasurable activities, namely, to improve the patient's mood even if temporarily.

Activities which are likely to be pleasurable may be assessed with the Reinforcement Survey Schedule (Cautela and Kastenbaum, 1967) or the Pleasant Events Schedule (MacPhillamy and Lewinsohn, 1971). The therapist may assign the task of undertaking a particular pleasurable activity for a specified number of minutes each day and request that the patient note changes in mood or reduction of depressive ruminations associated with the activity. When the patient engages in various activities, it is useful to have him record the degree of Mastery (M) and Pleasure (P) associated with a prescribed activity (see section on Scheduling Activities). The term Mastery refers to a sense of accomplishment when performing a specific task. Pleasure refers to pleasant feelings associated with the activity. Mastery and Pleasure can be rated on a 5-point scale with 0 representing no mastery (pleasure) and 5 representing maximum mastery (pleasure). By using a rating scale, the patient is induced to recognize *partial successes* and *small degrees* of pleasure. This technique tends to counteract his all-or-nothing thinking.

It is often valuable to explain the concepts of Mastery and Pleasure to the patient. "Mastery" may not be directly related to the completion nor to the magnitude of the task. Patients tend to compare how well they complete the task to their predepression level of achievement. He or she may say, "What's the big deal about calling up a friend? I used to be able to make a dozen calls without thinking about it." Or, "So what if I did some housework. I *should* be able to do that. It's what's expected of me." The therapist explains to the patient that judgment of current performance (degree of mastery) is logically based on the difficulty of the task in his *present* state and not his ideal state: Because of his depression, he is "carrying a 100-lb. weight on his shoulders" or is "dragging a heavy anchor"; in this context, reaching even a minimal goal can be judged a major achievement.

Pleasure refers to feelings of enjoyment, amusement, or fun from an activity. Sometimes even a mild satisfaction that patient attributes to his own actions may help to restore his morale and produce a sense of optimism.

Thus, Mastery and Pleasure may be totally independent. A patient should be encouraged to regard any Mastery as a forward step even though he may not experience any Pleasure. The failure to score either Mastery or Pleasure after successfully engaging in a prescribed activity is likely to be related to a negative interpretation of the event. For example, a patient reported that reading the newspaper had been pleasurable in the past and yet he obtained no pleasure from it when depressed. An inquiry about the loss of pleasure produced responses such as, "I thought of how I lost my job" and "The world seems to be falling apart from the newspaper reports." Similarly, he did not have any sense of mastery from washing the car. He reported, "I couldn't get the whitewalls clean" or "I did not have enough energy to clean the upholstery." By focusing on what he did not accomplish, the patient misses what he *did* accomplish. The therapist points out how this all-or-nothing thinking prevents the patient from having any perspective regarding his present capacity and achievements.

Thus, scheduling activities and rating each for mastery and pleasure provides data with which to identify and correct cognitive distortions. Furthermore, activities which are no longer sources of pleasure can be isolated and, with further experimentation, replaced. The following clinical example demonstrates how an activity schedule is used to identify and correct negative thoughts. Assignments often elicit absolutistic or perfectionistic standards. Thus, further assignments are designed to elicit and "work through" these thinking problems.

While severely depressed, a 38-year-old executive returned his Activity Schedule with the following ratings of Mastery and Pleasure on a 0–5 scale.

Saturday		M	P
8–9 a.m.	Awoke, dressed, ate breakfast	1	1
9–12 noon	Wallpaper kitchen	0	0
12–1 p.m.	Lunch	0	0
1–3 p.m.	Watched TV	0	0

The report indicates that although breakfast provided some pleasure and just getting up was rated as achievement, the remainder of the day provided no sense of pleasure or mastery. Yet the patient did wallpaper a kitchen while very depressed. How did he discredit this apparent achievement?

> THERAPIST: Why didn't you rate wallpapering the kitchen as a mastery experience?
> PATIENT: Because the flowers didn't line up.
> T: You did in fact complete the job?
> P: Yes.
> T: Your kitchen?
> P: No. I helped a neighbor do his kitchen.
> T: Did he do most of the work? (Note that the therapist inquires about any other reasons for a sense of failure which might not be offered spontaneously.)
> P: No. I really did almost all of it. He hadn't wallpapered before.
> T: Did anything else go wrong? Did you spill the paste all over? Ruin a lot of wallpaper? Leave a big mess?
> P: No, no, the only problem was that the flowers did not line up.
> T: So, since it was not perfect, you get no credit at all.
> P: Well . . . yes.

[Note that the irrational belief "If I don't do everything perfectly, I am useless, inadequate, and a failure," is implied by this reasoning. However, the correction of this assumption will be left to a later phase of therapy when the patient is less depressed. For now, the correction of the cognitive distortion is the objective.]

T: Just how far off was the alignment of the flowers?

P: (holds out fingers about ⅛ of an inch apart): About that much.

T: On each strip of paper?

P: No . . . on two or three pieces.

T: Out of how many?

P: About 20–25.

T: Did anyone else notice it?

P: No. In fact, my neighbor thought it was great.

T: Did your wife see it?

P: Yeh, she admired the job.

T: Could you see the defect when you stood back and looked at the whole wall?

P: Well . . . not really.

T: So you've selectively attended to a real but very small flaw in your effort to wallpaper. Is it logical that such a small defect should entirely cancel the credit you deserve?

P: Well, it wasn't as good as it should have been.

T: If your neighbor had done the same quality job in your kitchen, what would you say?

P: . . . pretty good job!

The therapist initially reviewed the reported activities and tried to identify apparent discrepancies between what was accomplished (the activity) and what was felt (feelings of mastery and pleasure). Next, by careful inquiry, the therapist sought the reasons for the discrepancy. Then, he elicited the data for the cognition, "The flowers didn't line up." The data were examined objectively by (1) putting the patient's evaluation into perspective with other data (the patient did the bulk of the work, others didn't notice the flaws, etc.) and (2) asking the patient to assess the data from an objective point of view ("What would you say if someone else wallpapered your kitchen in that way?"). Thus, the patient began to see his selective attention to minimal flaws and to reassess the actual facts of the situation.

GRADED TASK ASSIGNMENT

After successful completion of a series of tasks, depressed patients generally experience some (even though transient) improvement in their mood. They then feel motivated to tackle more difficult tasks, provided the therapist is vigilant to detect and rebut the patient's inclination to disparage his achievement.

An example of the Graded Task Assignment was described by Goldfried (personal communication, 1974), who independently arrived at this technique. Interestingly, his technique and rationale were similar to those used by our group. While treating a depressed outpatient, Dr. Goldfried reported:

> Working from the assumption that the depression might be construed as a perceived inability of the patient to control her environment, I assigned her a number of specific tasks such as making the beds, getting dressed in the morning, and straightening out rooms around the house, to demonstrate to her that she could, indeed, control the world around her. As she became more adept at these lower level tasks, she was assigned more complex ones. As a significant part of the treatment, I had her continually stand back to evaluate her performance and particularly note that the changes occurring in her life resulted from her own efforts.

The key features of the Graded Task Assignment are:

1. Problem definition—for example, the patient's belief that he is not capable of attaining goals that are important to him.
2. Formulation of a project. Stepwise assignment of tasks (or activities) from simpler to more complex.
3. Immediate and direct observation by the patient that he is successful in reaching a specific objective (carrying out an assigned task). The continual concrete feedback provides the patient with new corrective information regarding his functional capacity.
4. Ventilation of the patient's doubts, cynical reactions, and belittling of his achievement.
5. Encouragement of realistic evaluation by the patient of his actual performance.
6. Emphasis on the fact that the patient reached the goal as a result of his own effort and skill.
7. Devising new, more complex assignments in collaboration with the patient.

The use of graded assignments is illustrated in the following case:

The therapist visited a 40-year-old woman patient on the first day of her hospitalization. Instead of following rather loose instructions by the ward personnel to be involved in ward activities, she was lying in her bed and was ruminating about her problems and "feeling miserable." She did not believe she could get satisfaction from anything.

The therapist was able to determine that in the past, she had enjoyed reading. She stated, however, "I haven't even been able to read a headline in a newspaper for the past couple of months." Despite her doubts regarding whether she would be able to concentrate, she was willing to make an effort to read a few lines. The therapist selected the shortest story in a collection from the library and urged her to read it while he was with her. She said, "I know I won't be able to read it." He replied, "Well, try reading the first paragraph *out loud.*" She responded, "I may be able to mouth the words but I won't be able to concentrate." He then suggested, "See whether you can read the first sentence."

She read the first sentence aloud and continued until she had completed the paragraph. He asked her to read some more but to try reading to herself. She gradually became engrossed in the short story and spontaneously continued onto the next page. He told her to keep reading and that he would return later. About an hour later, the therapist received a call from the psychiatric resident who said, "I just saw the patient whom you *claim* is depressed." When he returned to the ward, the therapist observed that her depression had indeed lifted (temporarily). He encouraged her to undertake a regimen of reading progressively longer short stories; by the end of the week, she was reading a long novel. Within ten days after admission and with continued treatment, she was well enough to return home.

As illustrated in this case, the therapist should elicit the patient's reactions to undertaking a simple project. Most often, the patient's ideas center around a belief that he can't do anything or can't do the specific task. It is important for the therapist to divide a large task into small parts or steps and then to start with a relatively easy first step that he is reasonably certain the patient can complete. As the patient finishes each step, he goes on to the next part. After successful completion of a few tasks during the therapy session, the therapist suggests "homework assignments." The assignments proceed step by step, for example, from boiling an egg to the eventual goal of preparing a meal.

The therapist is careful to set modest goals to avoid the patient's strong tendency to give up because of his automatic thought, "I can't do it." After a successful attempt the therapist discusses the achievement with the patient and tries to provide an opportunity for the patient to assimilate the success. After the successful experience, the patient usually feels motivated for the next step, but still has to work against the resistance caused by self-doubt and cynicism. Repeated successes generally undermine the patient's belief that "I can't do it." As the patient continues to master each problem, his attitudes such as, 'I can't do anything" or "It is all meaningless" are gradually eroded.

A poorly designed Graded Task Assignment is likely to result in failure. The patient is likely to magnify a failure and use it to confirm his attitude of "I can't do anything." For this reason, a preliminary exercise in carrying out graded tasks may be used in the therapy session and subsequently graded tasks may be assigned as homework. The therapist should formulate the assignment in such a way as to avoid the appearance of failure. For instance, if the therapist suspects that the patient is likely to fail at a task, he should break it into smaller, more easily accomplished steps. The therapist should initially suggest they attempt to determine *how much* the patient can do; "Even if you don't get very far, it will give us important information." In this way, even a "failure" may be construed in a positive way by the therapist; namely, as a source of data for devising other projects.

An important source of error in the application of the Graded Task Assignment is the therapist's failure to check with the patient about his evaluation; that is, how well he *thought* he did in carrying out an assignment. Although depressed patients are likely to do better than they expected, they are also prone to disqualify an accomplishment after the task is completed. A patient may think, for example, "I would have done this in half the time before I was depressed." "Of course I accomplished this, but I am still depressed."

It is crucial to elicit such disclaimers and qualifications from the patient and to provide reasonable answers to them. For example, in response to the first objection, the therapist may respond, "The question we tested with the task was whether you could do it at all. You predicted you couldn't. Yet you did *in fact do it*. You lost sight of the original purpose of the project by noting you didn't do it at top efficiency. That's a completely separate question." The therapist may respond to the other objection with the explanation, "The project wasn't designed to relieve your depression. It was to see whether your prediction about your inability to do it was accurate. Do you now believe that your prediction was right? . . . We don't expect relief of your depression until we have finished a number of steps. However, your mood does change depending on whether you think you can influence your feelings of depression by carrying out an assignment and then evaluating your success accurately.'

COGNITIVE REHEARSAL

One of the difficulties in treating depressed patients is the fact that, once depressed, they have problems in carrying out well-learned tasks. A number of psychological factors may interfere with their normal behavioral repertoire. Difficulty in concentration may impede the formulation or execution of normally automatic, habitual behaviors. A housewife may wander into the kitchen to get a glass of water and then forget what she came for. Her problem was not amnesia, but obsessive ruminations; she simply failed to focus on the purpose of the trip to the kitchen. Such an unpleasant experience intensifies her belief that something is seriously wrong with her mind.

"Cognitive rehearsal" refers to the technique of asking the patient to imagine each successive step in the sequence leading to the completion of the task. This procedure forces the patient to pay attention to the essential details of the activities and counteracts the tendency of his mind to wander. Further, by rehearsing the sequence of steps, the patient has a preprogrammed system to carry out the assignment.

Another aim of cognitive rehearsal is to identify potential "roadblocks" (cognitive, behavioral, or environmental) which might impede the achievement of the assignment. The central plan of the therapist is to identify and develop solutions for such problems before they produce an unwanted failure experience. Interestingly, some patients report that they feel better simply as a result of the completion of the assigned task in imagery.

Identification of the psychological barriers by using cognitive rehearsal is illustrated in the following example.

The patient was a 24-year-old single unemployed female who after some discussion agreed to attempt to attend her neglected exercise classes.

> THERAPIST: So you agree that it would be a good idea to go to an exercise class.
>
> PATIENT: Yes, I always feel good after them.
>
> T: Okay, well I'd like you to use your imagination and go through each step involved in getting to the class.
>
> P: Well, I'll just have to go the way I've always gone.
>
> T: I think we need to be more specific. We know that you've decided to go to class before but everytime you've run into some roadblocks. Let's go over each step and see what might interfere with getting to class. I'd like you to go through all the steps needed to get to your class. Go over each step in your imagination and tell me what they are.
>
> P: Okay. I know what you mean.
>
> T: The class starts at 9 a.m. What time should we start?
>
> P: About 7:30. I'll wake up to the alarm and probably be feeling lousy. I always hate starting the day.
>
> T: How can you handle that problem?
>
> P: Well, that's why I'll give myself extra time. I'll start by getting dressed and having breakfast. Then, I'll pick up my equipment . . . (pause) . . . Oh, oh, wait, I don't have a pair of shorts to wear. That's one roadblock.
>
> T: What can you do to solve that problem?
>
> P: Well, I can go out and buy some.
>
> T: Can you visualize that? What comes next?
>
> P: I picture myself all ready to go and the car isn't there.
>
> T: What can you do about it?
>
> P: I'll ask my husband to bring the car early.
>
> T: What do you picture next?
>
> P: I'm driving to the class and I decide to turn round and go back.
>
> T: Why?
>
> P: Because I think I'll look foolish.
>
> T: What's the answer to that?
>
> P: Well, actually, the other people are just interested in the exercise, not in how anybody looks.

[By preparing herself with coping techniques for each of those "obstacles" the patient was able to get to the class—in fantasy. She was then asked to rehearse the entire sequence again and this time was able to imagine the various steps without any interfering cognitions. Subsequently, she indeed drove to the class and did not experience any difficulties. In the event that unexpected problems did arise, she had been instructed to write them down, attempt to master them on the spot, and discuss them at the next session.]

ASSERTIVE TRAINING AND ROLE-PLAYING

The procedures which form the basis of the assertive training have been well documented. In general, the training focuses on specific skills and includes techniques such as modeling, coaching, and behavior rehearsal. The efficacy of the treatment package and the relative contribution of its components have been reported elsewhere (McFall and Twentyman, 1973).

Role-playing simply involves the adoption of a role by the therapist, the patient, or both, and the subsequent social interaction based on the assigned role. Assertive training and role-playing can be effectively employed in the treatment of depressed patients. As with other techniques with a behavioral focus the therapist attempts to clarify self-defeating or interfering cognitions. Role-playing may also be employed to demonstrate an alternative viewpoint to the patient or to further elucidate the factors which interfere with appropriate emotional expression. (For a list of such cognitive factors see Wolfe and Fodor, 1975.)

A 20-year-old female patient reported a "humiliating experience" in which she became flustered while buying some clothes in a large department store. She was preoccupied with thoughts that her purchase may not have been suitable and that she gave the clerk less money than was requested. When the clerk asked for more money, the patient concluded, "She must think I'm a fool. I'm so clumsy and inept." The therapist asked the patient to take the role of the clerk and to draw some conclusions from her observations.

> PATIENT: (in role of clerk) Well, I see a woman who is obviously flustered and embarassed to have given me the incorrect change. I would try to console her by saying, "Everyone makes mistakes."

THERAPIST: Do you think it's possible the clerk also came to a similar conclusion with the exception that she did not console you?

P: Well, if she had tried to console me, I would have been shocked. No, she couldn't have been so understanding . . . I know what it's like to be a klutz, so I can put myself in the other person's shoes.

T: And what evidence do you have that the clerk didn't understand your mistake? Did she make any comments? Did she act disgusted?

P: No, actually she was quite patient. She even smiled but that made me feel more like a fool.

T: Well, without much data it's difficult to draw definite conclusions about her reactions. So let's work on your tendency to view yourself as a fool when you make mistakes. Later we can rehearse how you could have responded if she had acted critically to you.

Role-playing may be used in similar manner to elicit a "self-sympathy" response from the patient. The therapist may take the role of the patient in an attempt to change the patient's cognitive set from self-critical to sympathetic. It is common for depressed patients to be more demanding and critical of themselves than of others in the same situation.

One of the essential aspects of cognitive therapy is the evaluation of cognitions which may interfere with behavioral performance. Some depressed patients behave nonassertively because of the negative beliefs rather than as a result of a deficiency of behavioral skill.

A 29-year-old depressed male had returned to a university after a 10-year period during which he worked as a factory worker. He came to a therapy session particularly disturbed by the behavior of his 20-year-old chemistry laboratory partner. The younger student persistently left their shared equipment dirty and disarranged with the result that the patient spent time every week cleaning the equipment. The patient clearly outlined a way of discussing the problem with his lab partner but changed his mind each time he was about to confront him. The therapist pursued the patient's cognitions related to his attempts at self-assertion.

PATIENT: Well, even though I know what to say and when to say it, I always get the thought, "He'll think I am over-meticulous."

THERAPIST: And what would it mean to him if you were "over-meticulous."

P: He'd think I was a rigid, conservative type.

T: Are you a "rigid, conservative type."

P: No. You know what? I'm concerned that he might rebel and I'd be causing even more trouble.

From this point, it was apparent the patient was not behaving in an assertive manner because of his desire to avoid "causing trouble," particularly since he was "considerably older." His lack of assertiveness resulted in further concern about his decision to return to university. When the therapist and patient were able to list the "pros and cons" of his being assertive in this instance, the patient decided to speak to the other student and had no difficulty accomplishing his objective.

This example illustrates the vital importance of an individual's negative cognitions in interfering with assertive behavior.

BEHAVIORAL TECHNIQUES: RATIONALE AND TIMING

It is extremely important that patient understand the rationale for the various behavioral assignments. The therapist faces a considerable challenge with depressed patients since they are prone to distort the purpose of the tasks *post facto*. It is the therapist's responsibility to insure that the patient interprets the results of an assignment within the confines of the initial objective. The initial objective, therefore, must be made clear from the beginning.

One helpful strategy to evaluate the patient's understanding of a task is to use a role-reversal (the patient takes the role of the therapist). The patient can then review the reasons for the assignment (for example, recording daily activities) and the therapist can subsequently correct any misconceptions.

When outlining a behavioral assignment, the therapist needs to avoid making generalized statements which may imply that the completion of one task will make the patient feel better. The therapist should simply underscore that the patient is "moving in the right direction." Positive expectations of the patient are helpful, of course, but the patient should be guided away from the absolute ("all or nothing") evaluation of the results of any one assignment.

Note: The utilization of a "significant other" (spouse, other relative, or close friend) is often very helpful in setting and implementing behavioral assignments. In addition to encouraging the patient in initiating and completing projects, the significant other can provide valuable feedback to both patient and therapist.

Some patients respond to success in a behavioral assignment by dramatically increasing their activity. While this result is generally desirable, the patient may overextend himself to the point of failure or may experience anxiety from undertaking new projects before he is prepared for them. A reminder that the initial goals of therapy involve testing negative ideas and gradually increasing activity, rather than making tremendous accomplishments, may be indicated.

As previously noted, most of the behavioral techniques are employed in the initial therapy sessions. The appropriate targets include passivity, avoidance, lack of gratification, and an inability to express appropriate emotions (such as anger and sadness). While these symptoms may be evident across the range of depressed patients, the behavioral techniques are clearly indicated with severely depressed patients. An individual with severe depression commonly has considerable difficulty focusing on more abstract conceptualizations. His attention span may be limited to well-defined concrete suggestions. Research findings in the area suggest "success" experiences on concrete behavioral tasks are most effective in breaking the vicious cycle of demoralization, passivity and avoidance, and self-disparagement.

Homework assignments also need to be graded to the patient's level of understanding. In general, homework is not assigned in the initial stages of treatment until the patient completes a form of the assignment in the session. Obviously, it is impossible to comply absolutely with this rule since many assignments require the patient to be in his natural environment. Nevertheless, cognitive rehearsal and telephone conversations between patient and therapist will circumvent many problems. We have found that the agreement to call the therapist when the patient is "stuck" in carrying out an assignment is very helpful. This practice enables the patient to identify and master his problems in the "real life situation" and also motivates him to continue with his assignments. "Reporting in" to the therapist by telephone when the patient has completed a series of assignments also provides a powerful motivation to carry out the projects.

Once the patient understands the rationale and application of the behavioral techniques, therapy proceeds to more "purely" cognitive approaches. If behavioral symptoms or problems reappear, the patient may need a "refresher course" or may simply reinstitute the behavioral techniques. In times of stress, many former patients return to activity scheduling or recording. Since the techniques have already been mastered, they are easily used to prevent incipient regression.

In summary, behavioral techniques are useful insofar as they improve level of functioning, counteract obsessive thinking, change dysfunctional attitudes, and give a feeling of gratification. By observing changes in his own behavior, the patient may then be more amenable to examining his negative self-concept. An amelioration of the negative self-concept then leads to more spontaneous motivation and an improvement in mood.

Chapter 8

COGNITIVE TECHNIQUES

THE RATIONALE OF COGNITIVE TECHNIQUES

As pointed out previously, the novice therapist should be aware of the fact that many depressed patients are so preoccupied with negative thoughts that further introspection may aggravate the perseverating ideation. As the patient begins to engage in more constructive goal-directed activities and thereby changes the negative estimates of his capabilities, the therapist may focus directly on the cognitive components of his depression. Of course, if a patient seems accessible to exploration of his thoughts, wishes, and feelings at the beginning of treatment, these introspective techniques may be applied immediately and behavioral strategies may be deemphasized. These cognitive techniques should be utilized early in treating the suicidal patient. Many or most clinically depressed patients require a combination of behavioral and cognitive techniques.

The specific cognitive techniques are aimed at providing points of entry into the patient's cognitive organization. The techniques of questioning, of identifying illogical thinking, of ascertaining the rules according to which the patient organizes reality, are employed to help both the therapist and the patient to understand the patient's construction of reality. Since the therapist's questions and other verbal techniques are derived from his own theory, he must be especially vigilant regarding "putting ideas in the patient's head." The therapist should be aware of his leading questions, the patient's suggestibility, and his desire to please the therapist by providing the answers he believes the therapist is seeking.

Since there is more verbal interchange during the "cognitive phase" of treatment, this aspect of the therapy is likely to be much closer to a joint enterprise than the earlier phase, which emphasizes behavioral techniques. Although the therapist may initiate the spirit of collaboration during the behavioral phase, he frequently is impelled to take the reverse position because of the patient's inertia and indecisiveness during his more depressed phases.

In applying specific cognitive techniques in therapy, it is important that the therapist work within the framework of the cognitive model of depression. As pointed out in Chapter 1, the reductionist conception of cognitive therapy views this approach as a standard series of steps executed along the style of a waltz or tango. Actually, cognitive therapy is a broad system concerned with providing specific procedures to identify and modify the patient's "personal paradigm." A crucial part of the therapy, thus, consists of the therapist's obtaining adequate information, so that he can step into the patient's world and can experience the way in which the patient organizes reality. He needs to become involved with the patient's idiosyncratic concepts—the specific cognitive patterns that lead to or sustain his depression.

The joint exploration of the patient's inner life frequently engenders a spirit of adventure, and the discovery by the patient of his peculiar construction of reality generally motivates him to focus more directly on actual events and the meanings he attaches to them. By discovering the faulty meanings he has been ascribing to his experiences, life can take on a "new meaning"—geared to reality and open to the kinds of satisfactions and goals he seeks. He can sharply define the real obstacles to reaching his main objectives and sources of satisfaction and develop methods of surmounting or detouring around these blocks.

Explaining the Rationale to the Patient

The therapist first reviews the patient's attempt to define and solve his psychological problems. To alter the dysfunctional or distorted ideation associated with the problematic areas, the therapist briefly explains the cognitive model of depression. The explanations include the close relationship between the way a person thinks about himself, his environment, and his future (the cognitive triad) and his feelings, motivations, and behavior. The therapist outlines the negative effect that thinking in a self-defeating manner may have on the patient's feelings and behavior. However, telling the patient that he "thinks irrationally" may be detrimental. Depressed patients earnestly believe they are seeing things "as they really are." Instead, the therapist provides the patient with evidence that his way of thinking contributes to his depression and that his observations and conclusions may be "inaccurate" (rather than "irrational"). The therapist may point out, for example, that when many interpretations of an event are possible, the patient consistently selects the most negative. Specific methods for providing evidence for these tendencies will be described later in the chapter.

The main idea for the therapist to communicate is that they (the patient and the therapist) will act as scientific collaborators who will "investigate" the content of the patient's thinking. In their work together, the definition of the crucial information to be obtained and investigated by the collaborators is crucial. The central information required for cognitive therapy is the patient's understanding (or misunderstanding) and interpretation of the events in his life.

The investigation of the patient's thinking is based on two premises. First, depressed patients think in an idiosyncratic way (that is, they have a systematic negative bias in the way they regard themselves, their world, and their future). Second, the way the patient interprets events maintains his depression.

As previously stated, the typical strategy adopted by the cognitive therapist is to elicit the patient's ideas about the nature of his problems rather than providing the patient's interpretations or explanations. The therapist attempts to understand what the patient considers to be the most essential factors that are keeping him depressed.

A knowledge of the patient's expectations for treatment (for example, what will happen, what goals are reasonable, what outcome can be expected) is essential to treatment. To illustrate, one of us (B.F.S.) had a patient who indicated that she had been in treatment before and had been told that her depression was caused by biochemical abnormalities. Prior to her referral, she had been on trials of three different antidepressant preparations without a clinically significant effect. In this case, the patient was convinced that her depression was untreatable by any method. Consequently, she required specific information about "talking" (interview) therapy, how it differed from chemotherapy, its theoretical basis, and its implications and the probability of improvement.

Similarly, a patient who is convinced that he is depressed simply because of his childhood experiences and who believes it is necessary to recall, "relive," and analyze significant childhood events needs to be oriented regarding the rationale of cognitive therapy. Otherwise, he may conclude cognitive therapy with its focus on the here and now is simply a "first aid" approach. In such a case, it may be useful for the therapist to discuss the fact that one can change a pattern of thinking or behavior without identifying the cause and course of previous learning.

An analogy may be of some value to illustrate this point. For example, if a person learned to use short, slang-laden, and ungrammatical speech, it would not be necessary to review his past experiences with grammar. Instead, he would require specific training, including the correction of his errors and a specification of acceptable statements. At times, however, it may be useful to review previous learning experiences to demonstrate to the patient that he is interpreting life events inappropriately.

One method of assessing the patient's views about therapy while providing a conceptual model for cognitive therapy is to have him read an introduction to the approach, such as *Coping with Depression*, or *Cognitive Therapy and the Emotional Disorders*. He can direct the patient to outline the areas which he considers to be relevant to his case. The therapist, in particular, is vigilant to ascertain whether the patient understands the concepts of distorted thinking in depression, and the relationship between thinking and the other symptoms of depression.

An example of the exploration of the *meaning* of events is provided by the following interchange with a 26-year-old graduate student who had a history of a four-month recurrent depression.

PATIENT: I agree with the descriptions of me but I guess I don't agree that the way I think makes me depressed.

THERAPIST: How do you understand it?

P: I get depressed when things go wrong. Like when I fail a test.

T: How can failing a test make you depressed?

P: Well, if I fail I'll never get into law school.

T: So failing the test means a lot to you. But if failing a test could drive people into clinical depression, wouldn't you expect everyone who failed the test to have a depression? . . . Did everyone who failed get depressed enough to require treatment?

P: No, but it depends on how important the test was to the person.

T: Right, and who decides the importance?

P: I do.

T: And so, what we have to examine is your way of viewing the test (or the way that you *think* about the test) and how it affects your chances of getting into law school. Do you agree?

P: Right.

T: Do you agree that the way you interpret the results of the test will affect you? You might feel depressed, you might have trouble sleeping, not feel like eating, and you might even wonder if you should drop out of the course.

P: I have been thinking that I wasn't going to make it. Yes, I agree.

T: Now what did failing mean?

P: (tearful): That I couldn't get into law school.

T: And what does that mean to you?

P: That I'm just not smart enough.

T: Anything else?

P: That I can never be happy.

T: And how do these *thoughts* make you feel?

P: Very unhappy.

T: So it is the meaning of failing a test that makes you very unhappy. In fact, believing that you can never be happy is a powerful factor in producing unhappiness. So, you get yourself into a trap — by definition, failure to get into law school equals "I can never be happy."

The most critical stage of cognitive therapy involves training the patient to observe and record his cognitions. Obviously, without agreement on the relevant data to be studied, meaningful and therapeutic communication will be limited. The training in the observation and recording of cognitions makes the patient aware of the occurrence of images and self-verbalizations ("stream of thought"). The therapist trains the patient to identify distorted and dysfunctional cognitions. The patient may need to learn to discriminate between his own thoughts and the actual events. He will also need to understand the relationship between his cognitions, his affects, his behaviors, and environmental events.

Training the patient to observe and record his cognitions is best accomplished in several steps: (1) Define "automatic thought" (cognition); (2) demonstrate the relationship between cognition and affect (or behavior) using specific examples; (3) demonstrate the presence of cognitions from the patient's recent experience; (4) assign the patient homework to collect cognitions, and (5) review the patient's records and provide concrete feedback.

Defining "Cognition" for the Patient

The therapist can define a *cognition* as "either a thought or a visual image that you may not be very aware of unless you focus your attention on it." Characteristically, a cognition is an appraisal of events from any time perspective (past, present, or future). The typical cognitions observed in depression and other clinical disorders are often described as "automatic thoughts," part of a habitual pattern of thinking. Except in certain well-defined situations (such as the artist's or poet's attempt to extend the realm of reality), cognitions are generally viewed by the individual as factual representations of reality and hence, tend to be believed. Since his cognitions are automatic, habitual, and believable, the individual rarely assesses their validity. Thus, it is not uncommon for the depressed patient to be overwhelmed with rhetorical questions (for example, "Why am I so weak?" "Why am I such an incompetent person?") or with unpleasant visual images (for example, "seeing myself looking like an ugly pig"). He takes for granted that he is weak, inept, or ugly and wonders why he has been afflicted in this way.

The Influence of Cognitions on Affect and Behavior

There are a number of methods to demonstrate the relationship between thinking and feeling and behaving. Many patients can relate themselves to a specific vignette which does not involve them personally. A typical vignette is presented in the following interchange between a therapist and a 43-year-old depressed patient.

THERAPIST: The way a person thinks about or interprets events affects how he feels and behaves. For example, say he was home alone one night and heard a crash in another room. If he thinks, "There's a burglar in the room," how do you think he would feel?

147

PATIENT: Very anxious, terrified.

T: And how might he behave?

P: He might try to hide or if he was smart he would phone the police.

T: Okay, so in response to a thought that a burglar made the noise, the person would probably feel anxious and behave in such a way as to protect himself. Now, let's say he heard the same noise and thought, "The windows have been left open and the wind has caused something to fall over." How would he feel?

P: Well, he wouldn't be afraid. He might be sad if he thought something valuable was broken or he might be annoyed that one of the kids left the window open.

T: And would his behavior be different following this thought?

P: Sure, he would probably go and see what the problem was. He certainly wouldn't phone the police.

T: Okay. Now, what this example shows us is that there are usually a number of ways in which you can interpret a situation. Also, the way you interpret the situation affects your feelings and behavior.

This particular example is designed to provide the patient with a psychological distance from his own problems while at the same time providing the framework for examining his own thoughts and feelings. It is difficult to predict the difficulty (or ease) with which a particular patient will grasp these concepts. The therapist's major strategy is to try a few demonstrations but also to be prepared for the model to evolve as a result of the patient's experiences.

Another technique to demonstrate the relationship between thinking and affect involves an "induced imagery" technique. The therapist first asks the patient to imagine an unpleasant scene. If the patient indicates a negative emotional response, the therapist can inquire about the content of the patient's thoughts. The therapist then asks the patient to imagine a pleasant scene and to describe his feelings. Typically, a patient is able to recognize that by changing the content of his thought he is able to alter his feeling state. For some patients, this simple technique will clearly illustrate the impact of their own imagery and they are able to understand how modifications in their thinking may lead to a shift in their mood. This technique is indicated with the mildly depressed patient who is most likely to experience transient sad moods.

Cognition and Recent Experiences

Some patients may have difficulty identifying dysfunctional thoughts or images, or they may not see the connection between thoughts and feelings. Other patients may readily understand the nature of cognitions and may even spontaneously offer typical negative cognitions from their own experiences. In either case it is desirable to demonstrate to the patient the presence of cognitions in his sphere of awareness. In the first instance, it is essential for the patients to become aware of and to identify their negative cognitions. In the second case, it is worthwhile to scrutinize the cognitions with the patient to insure that he understands the importance of his thoughts. The latter approach also acts as a safeguard since automatic agreement with the therapist's formulations generally is more indicative of compliance than of genuine learning. Such patients require the same training as the patient who is uncertain of the role of cognitions in his depression.

An early method of demonstrating the presence of cognitions is to inquire about the patient's thoughts just prior to the first appointment. Most patients report having had thoughts about the therapist, the treatment, and the chances of receiving help. The therapist then labels these thoughts and images for the patient as "automatic thoughts" (cognitions). If the therapist believes the patient's vocabulary is limited he may use other terms to describe cognitive phenomena such as "the things you say to yourself" or "self-statements."

In addition to ascertaining the presence of such cognitions, the therapist is able to correct any incorrect conceptions or misinformation regarding treatment. For example, a 38-year-old married female who was the mother of two small children was asked to report any thoughts she experienced in the waiting room. She indicated a major concern that she was not going to survive the period of time during which she would require treatment. Although she had been informed of the general time span of cognitive therapy (weekly 1-hour sessions for approximately 12 weeks) she could not reconcile this information with another consultant's comment that she would require treatment for a 2-to-3-year period with 3 sessions per week. In fact, the patient had failed to understand that the previous consultant was referring to a different system of therapy (psychoanalytic therapy) *and* a different set of objectives ("complete personality reconstruction"). When she recognized that cognitive therapy would focus on her problems (and specifically, her depression), the dread she had experienced in the waiting room was reduced to the more relevant concerns, namely, "Will *this* therapy be successful?" and "What if I don't get better?"

Detection of Automatic Thoughts

Once the patient understands the definition of a cognition and recognizes the presence of automatic thoughts and images, the therapist assigns a specific project designed to delineate his dysfunctional cognitions.

The specific assignment depends on the particular problem under investigation. Typically, the patient is instructed to "catch" as many cognitions as he can and to record them in writing. Since a person is rarely, if ever, "completely blank," the patient can use changes in affect or the experience of dysphoria as a marker or cue to recognize or recall his cognitions. *

The most accurate identification of cognitions is accomplished right after they occur. However, for a variety of reasons, an individual may not be able to record his cognitions immediately. Therefore, a second method is to direct the patient to set aside a specific brief period of time, for example, 15 minutes each evening, to replay the events that led to his cognitions as well as the actual cognitions. The therapist instructs the patient to record any upsetting thoughts as precisely as possible. That is, rather than noting, "I had the feeling I was incompetent in my job," as he would be likely to report the thought in a conversation, the patient would write, "I'm incompetent in my job," a more precise reproduction of the thought. This training method of collecting cognitions outside of the therapy session is particularly useful with patients who have been instructed to keep busy to avoid depressive ruminations.

A third method of pinpointing cognitions depends on identifying the specific environmental events associated with the patient's depression. For example, a 31-year-old mother of three children

---

* The identification of automatic thoughts will be facilitated by reading the description of their characteristics in "Coping with Depression" (Beck & Greenberg, 1974).

150

indicated that the "worst time of the day" was between 7 a.m. and 9 a.m. in the morning. During this time period she habitually prepared her breakfast for her family. She could not explain why this period was so difficult until she began recording her cognitions at home. As a result, she discovered she consistently compared herself with her mother who she remembered was irritable and argumentative in the morning. When her children misbehaved or made unreasonable requests, the patient often thought, "Don't get angry or they'll resent you," with the result that she typically ignored them. With increasing frequency, however, she "exploded" at the children and then thought, "I'm worse than my mother ever was. I'm not fit to care for my children. They'd be better off if I were dead." She became even more depressed when she imagined her negative childhood experiences such as "my mother slapping me if I complained about anything." Once she identified these cognitions, the patient and her therapist entered into a successful discussion that involved a listing of the similarities and differences between her mother and herself, a review of her views of reasonable behavior for her children and a refutation of her belief that any display of anger by her would make her children permanently resent her.

Alternatively, the therapist may choose to confront the patient with one of the upsetting environmental events with the purpose of arousing and identifying depressive cognitions. For example, a 49-year-old woman had lost a son as a result of suicide 2 years prior to her treatment. The patient blamed herself for her son's death. She found that many objects and events (for example, guitars, music, art exhibits) reminded her of her son and triggered a torrent of negative cognitions, marked despondency, and guilt. In order to feel better she had been trying to avoid these reminders. The patient, thus, had difficulty in identifying clear-cut depressogenic cognitions. Consequently, the therapist suggested that the patient attend a local art gallery and focus on her cognitions. As a result, she observed specific self-accusatory automatic thoughts that centered on "her inability to listen to her son," her decision to remain in an unhappy marriage, and her "incompetence" as a mother. It was useful for the patient to recognize these cognitions since she was then able to ascertain their validity. When the patient and therapist discussed the specific aspects of her negative ideas, the patient concluded that her self-accusations were unfounded. The patient's extreme guilt feeling dissipated and she was then able to manage the sadness associated with her son's death.

A profitable tactic involves instructing the patient to record cognitions which have a common theme. A 21-year-old mildly depressed college student was in her sixth week of treatment when her therapist explained the necessity of canceling her next appointment.

> PATIENT: That's okay, I know you have to go to a meeting. (pause) You know, I think I should tell you, I got the thought that you were rejecting me. I don't know why. Because if I think about it, it's obvious you have to cancel the appointment.
>
> THERAPIST: Was there any evidence which supported your idea?
>
> P: Well, frankly, I wondered whether you could make an extra effort and see me. And I don't even know whether you'll be in the area.

In this case, the patient was asked to pay particular attention to similar kinds of thoughts which centered on the theme of rejection. She returned in the next session and stated her surprise that she had experienced 27 such thoughts in a one-week period. In addition, she felt more depressed if she believed that the "rejecter" did so purposely. As a result, the therapist and patient focused their attention on her definition of a "rejection" as well as her tendency to expect others ("the people who care") to act in her best interest all of the time. It was then clear that she had interpreted the cancellation of her appointment as a rejection since, according to her formula, the therapist's behavior indicated that he "did not care" about her.

Thus, there are a number of methods to help the patient specify the cognitions that maintain or aggravate his depression. Once the patient learns to specify these cognitions, the therapist and patient examine the source of his depression.

Examining and Reality Testing Automatic Thoughts and Images

The therapist engages the patient in the reality testing of his ideas not to induce a spurious optimism by inducing him to think that "things are really better than they are," but to encourage a more accurate description and analysis of the way things are. While the depressed person characteristically views his world in a negative light, the therapist should not fall into a trap of assuming that all of the patient's pessimistic or nihilistic statements are necessarily invalid. He should examine a sample of the patient's thoughts in collaboration with the patient. The basis or evidence for each thought should be subjected to the scrutiny of reality testing with the application of the kind of reasonable standards used by nondepressed people in making judgments.

For example, a depressed young student expressed the belief that she would not get into one of the colleges to which she had applied. When the therapist explored the reasons which led to her conclusion, he discovered there was little basis for it. The questioning went as follows:

THERAPIST: Why do you think you won't be able to get into the university of your choice?

PATIENT: Because my grades were really not so hot.

T: Well, what was your grade average?

P: Well, pretty good up until the last semester in high school.

T: What was your grade average in general?

P: A's and B's.

T: Well, how many of each?

P: Well, I guess, almost all of my grades were A's but I got terrible grades my last semester.

T: What were your grades then?

P: I got two A's and two B's.

T: Since your grade average would seem to me to come out to almost all A's, why do you think you won't be able to get into the university?

T: Because of competition being so tough.

T: Have you found out what the average grades are for admissions to the college?

P: Well, somebody told me that a B+ average would suffice.

T: Isn't your average better than that?

P: I guess so.

In this case, the patient was not deliberately trying to thwart the therapist but had, indeed, reached the negative (erroneous) conclusion regarding her chances for being admitted. Her logic can be seen as an example of "all-or-nothing" thinking in that any grade less than an A was viewed as a failure. The patient backed up this erroneous conclusion with another inaccurate conclusion regarding her class standing relative to other students. She ascertained that,

153

although she assumed she was an average student, she was closer to the top in her class rank. Only after the therapist was able to elicit the facts was the patient able to see how she had distorted reality.

In this case the therapist could have used two different approaches which might have had some positive influence on the patient but would probably not have actually taught her to examine and authenticate her ideas. For example, he could have reassured her that on the basis of her obvious intelligence she certainly should be able to get into college. Secondly, he could have used one approach advocated by Rational–Emotive therapists (Ellis, 1962) and challenged her belief that entrance into college was an index of her worth as a person. Using a different RET technique, the therapist could have explored with her what the catastrophe would be if she could not get into college.

If the therapist chose these approaches at this point in therapy, however, he would be in essence missing an essential point because (a) he would not have established a solid data base against which the patient's conclusions could be tested, and (2) he would not have provided the patient with the opportunity of applying evidence in order to test out her conclusions. Consequently, while she might temporarily feel better as a result of a rational–emotive approach, her negative cognitive set might continue to operate. Thus, she might misinterpret other situations or even return to the initial erroneous conclusions regarding admission to college. Once she learns to test her cognitions against the available reality-based evidence, she will have a chance to assess her assumptions. Depressed patients require reality testing prior to attempting to change their beliefs (if their beliefs are demonstrated to be erroneous). *

Of course, we all know that not every student who applies to

---

* In response to this statement, Ellis (personal communication, 1978) writes: "RET does *not* preclude getting what you call a 'solid data base' against which the patient's conclusions could be tested. Although RET therapists are not required to do this as you seem to do it, they can easily choose to do so. In many instances, I would proceed almost exactly as your therapists did in the dialogue given in this section of the manual; in other instances, I might possibly proceed to discussing the patient's worth or her catastrophizing—and in the course of doing so derive the 'solid data base' information. In a few other cases, I might help her to fully accept herself or to stop catastrophizing without the data base information brought out in your instance—but with various other kinds of information brought out. RET does *not* have one special way of questioning and disputing."

college has a high grade average, and a depressed student who predicts rejection may, indeed, be accurate. In that case, once the therapist has determined the accuracy of the person's recall of his school record and the plausibility of his predictions, he can then go on to explore the *meaning* of being rejected at college and the cluster of attitudes surrounding this meaning. For instance, suppose the therapist was able to determine that a college career was, indeed, uncertain or even unlikely, he would then ascertain the patient's attitudes regarding admission to college. For example, the student might say, "If I don't get into college, it really means I am stupid," or ". . . I can never be happy," or "My family and friends will be terribly disappointed." These attitudes themselves can be further explored in terms of whether they are realistic. If it is true that family and friends will be indeed disappointed, therapist and patient can then explore why the patient has to be controlled by what other people will think or feel. The therapist may point out that other people cannot *make* him disappointed but rather by incorporating their attitude, the patient *"makes"* himself feel disappointed. That is, his own thinking, not that of others, produces the unpleasant emotions.

The essence of reality testing is to enable the person to correct his distortions. An analysis of meaning and attitudes exposes the unreasonableness and self-defeating nature of the attitudes. However, we have found that as the individual continues to distort reality, the attempts by the therapist to bring the person's system of assignment of meanings and of attitudes into a more reasonable framework are ineffective.

A woman who complained of severe headache and other somatic disturbances was found to have a very high depression score. When asked about the cognitions that seemed to make her unhappy, she said, "My family doesn't appreciate me"; "Nobody appreciates me, they take me for granted"; "I am worthless."

As an example she stated that her adolescent children no longer wanted to do things with her. Although this particular statement could very well have been accurate, the therapist decided to determine its authenticity. He pursued the "evidence" for the statement in the following interchange:

PATIENT: My son doesn't like to go to the theatre or to the movies with me anymore.

Therapist: How do you know that he doesn't want to go with you?

P: Teenagers don't actually like to do things with their parents.

T: Have you actually asked him to go with you?

P: No, as a matter of fact, he did ask me a few times if I wanted him to take me . . . but I didn't think he really wanted to go.

T: How about testing it out by asking him to give you a straight answer?

P: I guess so.

T: The important thing is not whether or not he goes with you but whether you are deciding for him what he thinks instead of letting him tell you.

P: I guess you are right but he does seem to be inconsiderate. For example, he is always late for dinner.

T: How often has that happened?

P: Oh, once or twice . . . I guess that's really not all that often.

T: Is his coming late for dinner due to his being inconsiderate?

P: Well, come to think of it, he did say that he had been working late those two nights. Also, he has been considerate in a lot of other ways.

Actually as the patient later found out, her son was willing to go to the movies with her.

Thus, the therapist does not accept the patient's conclusions and inferences at their face value but pursues them to determine their validity. If indeed the patient's conclusions had been valid, then the therapist could explore the way she assigns meanings to her son's "rejection." The therapist could also encourage her to pursue other activities and relationships with other people.

One characteristic of depressed patients is their tendency to view their ideas as facts. Although this characteristic is typical of human beings in general, it is of particular importance in depression because of the degree of distortions that occur. Furthermore, the problem is increased when the patient behaves in a manner consistent with his thinking.

Once the patient has acquired the relevant observational and recording skills, he will recognize that certain cognitions are particularly frequent at times of painful affect. The specific structure and content of each cognition is related to the ensuing painful affect (Beck, 1976). For example, anxiety is associated with cognitions in which the patient sees himself in immediate danger (either by physical threat or social disgrace). Cognitions associated with depression often reflect the patient's belief of his lack of competency, unattractiveness, failure to "meet responsibilities," or his social isolation.

Generally, with the therapist's guidance, the patient can categorize his cognitions by the major themes (for example, self-blame, inferiority, deprivation). The therapist can help the patient to recognize the different interpretations and meanings that can be assigned to a specific life experience. He should point out the patient's systematic negative biases in his choice of interpretations and indicate how he indiscriminately makes negative inferences even in the face of contradictory evidence. Of course, the therapist should not expect the patient to change his views simply because he becomes aware of his biased selection of interpretations. Instead, the accuracy of each interpretation requires a careful examination so that the patient can improve both his observational skill and his ability to form realistic and logical inferences.

The therapist may use a variety of cognitive techniques to evaluate and validate specific conclusions. It is essential to alter the depressed patient's stereotyped negative responses since (1) they result in the experience of intense negative affect and (2) they divert the patient from focusing on his actual, reality-based problems. Two techniques designed to increase the patient's objectivity involve "reattribution" and "alternative conceptualization." One of the central advantages of these techniques is that the patient learns to "distance" himself from his thoughts; that is, he begins to view his thoughts as psychological events.

REATTRIBUTION TECHNIQUES

A common cognitive pattern in depression involves incorrectly assigning the blame or responsibility for adverse events to oneself. Depressed patients are particularly prone to self-blame resulting from the negative consequences of events beyond their control as well as those relative to their actions and judgments. The technique of "reattribution" is used when the patient unrealistically attributes adverse occurrences to a personal deficiency, such as a lack of ability or effort. The therapist and patient review the relevant events that apply the laws of logic to the available information to make an appropriate assignment of responsibility. The point is not to absolve the patient of all responsibility but to define the multitude of extraneous factors contributing to an adverse experience. By gaining objectivity, the patient not only lifts the weight of self-reproach but he may then search for ways of salvaging bad situations and also of preventing a recurrence.

The following case illustrates the usefulness of the appropriate attribution of responsibility in solving realistic problems.

The patient was a 51-year-old moderately depressed bank manager who complained primarily of "ineffectiveness in my job." By "ineffectiveness" the patient referred to a difficulty he experienced in making business decisions. The patient came to his fourth session in a state of deep depression.

> PATIENT: I can't tell you how much of a mess I've made of things. I've made another major error of judgment which should cost me my job.
> THERAPIST: Tell me what the error in judgment was.
> P: I approved a loan which fell through completely. I made a very poor decision.
> T: Can you recall the specifics about the decision?
> P: Yes, I remember that it looked good on paper, good collateral, good credit rating, but I should have known there was going to be a problem.
> T: Did you have all the pertinent information at the time of your decision?
> P: Not at the time, but I sure found out 6 weeks later. I'm paid to make profitable decisions, not to give the bank's money away.
> T: I understand your position, but I would like to review the information which you had at the time your decision was required, not 6 weeks after the decision had been made.

When the therapist and patient reviewed the pertinent information available at the time of his decision, the patient reasonably concluded that his initial decision was based on sound banking principles. He even recalled checking the client's financial background intensively. The patient was helped by the method of reattribution, that is, identifying the cause of the difficulty as residing outside of himself. Nevertheless, he was left with a significant problem with the account. As a result of his self-criticisms, he had avoided contacting the central office to begin the appropriate legal proceedings against the client. He was left with "a problem of my own making," but was encouraged that there was still time to "correct the damage." The patient and therapist worked out a step-by-step plan designed to amend his previous errors. Although the patient was criticized by his superiors for his tardiness, he found that he could accept their "constructive" criticism without castigating himself.

Reattribution is particularly useful with patients who are prone to excessive self-blame and/or with patients who assume responsibility for any adverse occurrence. The therapist may elect to counter the cognitions of the self-blaming patient by (a) reviewing the "facts" of the events which result in self-criticism (as in the case above); or (b) demonstrating the different criteria for assigning responsibility applied by the patient to his own behavior as compared to the behavior of others (double standard); or (c) challenging the belief that the patient is "100 percent" responsible for any negative consequences. The term "de-responsibilitizing" has also been applied to this technique.

The Search for Alternative Solutions

The depressed patient's closed system of logic and reasoning opens as he distances himself from his cognitions and identifies the rigid patterns and themes of his thinking. Problems which were previously perceived as insoluble may be reconceptualized. At this point, the "search for alternatives" may prove useful. This technique simply involves the active investigation of other interpretations or solutions of the patient's problems. This approach forms the cornerstone of effective problem-solving.

Through the careful definition of his difficulties, the patient may spontaneously arrive at solutions to problems that he considered insoluble. Also, with an understanding of the reality-based undistorted problems, options that he had previously discarded may now appear practical and useful. The therapist should not be diverted by the patient's claims that he has "tried everything." While depressed patients sincerely believe that they have explored every possible option, it is more likely that they automatically rejected several options and stopped the search for others because they had made a prejudgment that the problem was insoluble. As noted previously, the depressed patient's basis for his conclusion of hopelessness is derived from his sytematically biased selection of negative data. The following case example illustrates the tendency of depressed patients to view problems as insoluble on the basis of their negative cognitive set.

The patient was a 28-year-old moderately depressed woman whose husband had abandoned the patient and their three children one month previously. She continually referred to her idea that she couldn't survive without her husband. She "proved" her point by describing the difficulties she had experienced in the past with "independence." The patient had been phobic about being alone when she was a teenager. She "always had trouble coping" when her husband would go on business trips. She hadn't received any training in financial matters and was convinced that her children would suffer the consequences. She described her attempts to cope with the loss of her husband as "a nightmare."

Using the "alternatives" method, the therapist first listed the problems (for example, management of finances, discipline of children, loneliness). In each case, the patient concluded that she wouldn't be able to solve her problems because she hadn't been able to succeed in the past. She claimed, "I've never been good at math," "I've always left discipline to Jack," "I've always been afraid of being alone in case something goes wrong."

These statements may have been generally correct in the past but the crucial question was whether the patient could apply the specific skills or coping techniques with the appropriate guidance and training in the present. The therapist learned that she was a high school graduate and that she had, in fact, resented to a certain degree the dominance of her husband who had insisted on "taking care of everything." The alternative solutions generated by the patient revealed a well-developed problem-solving ability. For example, in the area of finances, she was aware of a number of assistance programs, knew the name of her bank manager, and had considered applying for a position as a secretary (her high school diploma was in business and commerce). The therapist, after underscoring a series of alternatives, then returned to the patient's original belief that she "couldn't survive without her husband." By this time the patient experienced a considerable improvement in her mood and she agreed to pursue one of the possible solutions (short-term financial assistance) to her financial problem. She was able to secure a loan and this successful venture disconfirmed her original notion of incompetence. As a result she was willing to actively pursue solutions to her other problem areas.

It is notable that the "pursuit of solutions" often leads to an affect shift in the depressed patient. The sudden recognition that his life situation may not be "hopeless" accounts for this change. The therapist's objective, however, cannot be achieved simply by the consideration of alternative approaches to problem-solving. The therapist also reviews the patient's conclusion ("I've never been good at anything") from an objective standpoint. Although it is highly unlikely that such a conclusion is valid, nevertheless, the depressed patient *believes* that it is and he may present "persuasive" evidence of failure or incompetency. The therapist, therefore, should be prepared to provide the patient with sufficient time to integrate his new conclusion ("I have some knowledge but also need some concrete advice in the area of finances, child-rearing, and coping with loneliness"). The search for alternative ways to deal with problems constitutes an important technique in the treatment of suicidal patients (see Chapter 10).

Searching for alternative explanations provides another approach to "insoluble problems." The depressed patient shows a systematic negative bias in his interpretations of events. By thinking of alternative interpretations, he is enabled to recognize and counter his bias and to substitute a more accurate conclusion. The result of this change in thinking is a positive change in his affect and behavior. The following example further illustrates the effect of correcting a negative cognitive set.

A 22-year-old depressed graduate student was convinced that her English professor thought she was "a reject." To prove her point, she provided a copy of a recent essay which had received a C grade along with two pages of critical comment. The student was distraught about the results. She had written the essay during a period of great distress precipitated by the belief that "she couldn't make it in school." She now had "proof she couldn't make it" and was prepared to drop out.

The therapist elicited two relevant points regarding the patient's conclusions. First, the patient had been depressed when she wrote the essay and it could be anticipated that her performance would not accurately reflect her abilities. In fact, when she reflected on her thinking at the time she handed in the essay, she was surprised that she had even completed it. Her actual grade and performance, therefore, needed to be placed in context with this information. Prior to pursuing this course of action, however, the therapist recognized that the grades and comments had to be construed accurately and his first priority was to help the patient investigate her idea that she was "a reject."

The therapist inquired about alternative explanations for the grade and professor's criticisms and these alternatives were discussed and rated by the patient. The rating simply consisted of the proportion of 100% that would represent the degree of "believability" of each explanation. The listing in decreasing order of "believability" went as follows:

1. "I'm a reject who doesn't have any ability in English." 90%
2. "The professor has a personal bias against female graduate students." 5%
3 "The grade was not very different from other students'." 3%
4. "The professor provided the comments to help with future essays and therefore thinks I have some ability." 2%

Fortunately, the therapist convinced the patient to get some more information before she withdrew from the course. He encouraged her to call her professor from the therapist's office ("There's no time like the present."). On the telephone she found out (1) that the average class grade was a C, and (2) the professor thought that although the style of the essay was "wanting" the content was "promising." He suggested that they have a further discussion to explain his criticisms. As a result of this new information the patient became more animated and cheerful. Instead of viewing herself as a "reject," she readily agreed that she required concrete instruction on her writing style. She decided to get some tutoring and to complete the term in preference to her decision to withdraw from the course.

This example demonstrates the affective and behavioral effects of the patient's negative interpretations. She experienced intense dysphoria not only because of the mediocre grade but also because it meant to her that she was a failure. In addition, however, she was prepared to *act* on her negative conclusion. Withdrawal from the course would have been a major mistake in light of the evidence. In fact, it would have convinced her of the validity of her negative judgment of her ability. When she had investigated the other possible interpretations, she was able to reach a more reasonable decision.

It was useful for the patient and therapist to list and rate the patients's beliefs for they were able to develop empirically testable hypotheses. The patient re-rated her interpretations at the end of the session and was able to see how she had overrated the "reject–no–ability" hypothesis because of the limited amount of evidence available. Interestingly, once the patient gained some perspective on her professor's comments, she focused her attention away from her idea that she was a failure (which no longer seemed plausible), to a reasonable accounting of the deficiencies in her creative writing. Unlike the therapist who practices "the power of positive thinking," the cognitive therapist did not attempt to deny or ignore these realistic deficits.

Of course, it is not always possible to have the patient collect relevant data in the office as in the present case. When feasible, however, the effort is worthwhile since progress in other areas will be impeded if the patient is overwhelmed with ideas of rejection. If data cannot be collected in the office, the patient should be assigned an "emergency homework assignment"; that is, obtain the information (for example, contact the professor) and recontact the therapist as soon as possible. In this way, there is less opportunity for the negative thinking and conclusions to spread to other aspects of the patient's life. Incidentally, we generally find that the greater the discrepancy between the original erroneous conclusion and the relevant data collected by the patient, the more that conclusion is undermined. At times, it may be useful to engage the help of a "significant other" or an auxiliary therapist to help the patient to obtain adequate data outside of the treatment session.

RECORDING DYSFUNCTIONAL THOUGHTS

Recording cognitions and responses in parallel columns is a way to begin examining, evaluating, and modifying the cognitions. The patient is instructed to write his cognitions in one column and then to write a "reasonable response" to the cognitions in the next column. The written assignment may also include additional columns for describing the patient's affect and behavior, and the specific description of the situation or event which preceded the cognition. Thus, depending on the number of columns used, the technique may be referred to as the double-column, the triple-column, or even the quadruple-column technique. A recording form is available to aid the patient in recognizing his dysfunctional thoughts and images. The columns of the form are labeled Date, Situation, Emotion(s), Automatic thoughts, Rational response, and Outcome.

The therapist should explain in detail the use of the form after the patient understands the notion of automatic thoughts (or cognitions). Is is useful to provide some examples of dysfunctional cognitions and reasonable responses in the therapy session. The therapist also teaches the patient to rate the degree of his emotional experiences and the degree to which he believes his automatic thought. The rationale for this approach is to teach the patient more precise discriminations of his emotions and to insure that the patient writes down even thoughts which are "foreign" (that is, have a low degree of belief) to him. The ratings, of course, also provide a method of quantifying changes in the patient's emotional responses and his thinking. The Daily Record of Dysfunctional Thoughts is a useful adjunct to cognitive therapy. Following treatment, many patients use their records as a reminder of the kinds of situations and errors in thinking that maintained or accentuated their depression.

The therapist's major task is to help the patient think of reasonable responses to his negative cognitions. The following case example demonstrates the use of the recording form. As situations and cognitions are recorded, the patient gains some distance from their effect. The therapist's goal is to increase the patient's objectivity about his cognitions, to demonstrate the relationship between negative cognitions, unpleasant affect, and unproductive behavior and, most important, to differentiate between a realistic accounting of events and an accounting distorted by idiosyncratic meanings.

The therapist may choose to label the columns according to specific needs of the patient. The following examples illustrate either an adaptation of the alternative technique or the use of an "objective third person" as the responder to cognitions.

A medical records librarian had a 6-yr history of depression.

Event	Feelings	Cognitions	Other possible interpretations
The charge nurse in the coronary care unit was curt and said "I hate medical records" when I went to collect charts for the record review committe	Sadness Slight anger Loneliness	She doesn't like me	The charge nurse is generally unhappy. Hating medical records is not the same as hating me; she actually hates paper work. She is under a lot of pressure for unknown reasons She is foolish to hate records; they are her only defense in a lawsuit.

A 24-year-old nurse recently discharged from the hospital for severe depression presented this record.

Event	Feelings	Cognitions	Other possible interpretations
While at a party Jim asked me "How are you feeling?" shortly after I was discharged from the hospital.	Anxious	Jim thinks I am a basket case. I must really look bad for him to be concerned.	He really cares about me. He noticed that I look better than before I went into the hospital and wants to know if feel better too.

Further descriptions regarding the use of the Daily Record of Dysfunctional Thoughts are contained in Chapter 13.

USE OF THE WRIST COUNTER

We have found that since most patients are unaware of the stereotyped, repetitive nature of their negative automatic thoughts, the use of a technical aid helps them to identify and monitor these cognitions.

A specially designed Response Counter adapted from a golf counter (resembling a wrist watch) may be used for this purpose. After the patient has been instructed by the therapist to recognize automatic thoughts and has read *Coping with Depression*, he is asked to write down his automatic thoughts. As soon as the therapist is satisfied that the patient correctly identifies these cognitions (and distinguishes them from "normal," adaptive, or neutral thoughts), he should demonstrate the use of the wrist counter.

It is essential that the therapist check regularly to insure that the patient is "checking" the kinds of cognitions of importance to the therapy. As described in *Cognitive Therapy and the Emotional Disorders* (Beck, 1976) and *Coping with Depression,* these negative cognitions have specific criterial attributes: (1) They are *automatic*—they occur as if by reflex, without prior reasoning; (2) they are *unreasonable* and *dysfunctional;* (3) they seem completely *plausible* and are uncritically accepted as valid even though they seem bizarre upon reflection; (4) they are *involuntary.* The patient may have great difficulty in "turning them off."

In the course of time, the therapist will discover that each patient has his own *idiosyncratic* kind of automatic thoughts. For some patients the thoughts may take the form of construing every interaction as a rejection; others may think continually of failure; others may characteristically make negative predictions as they move from one activity or interaction to another. Some patients may perseverate all day in thinking about how worthless, or defective, or diseased they are.

The use of the clicker is helpful in demonstrating to the patient how his thoughts produce, maintain, or intensify his unpleasant feelings and other symptoms of depression. However, in some cases the use of the clicker and recording automatic thoughts is *contraindicated:* When the patient is so immersed in his negative thinking that he cannot concentrate on anything else, he needs to be trained to *ignore* the cognition and concentrate on the task at hand.

Chapter 9

FOCUS ON TARGET SYMPTOMS

We have already discussed the importance of providing the patient with symptom relief by translating his major complaints into *solvable problems* (Chapter 5). Any of the components of depression that involve discomfort or immobility may be considered target symptoms, which may similarly be reformulated in terms of solvable problems. Chapters 7 and 8 provided general treatment procedures; in this chapter we will outline the range of interventions for specific target symptoms. Since the selection of a focal point takes into account not only what the patient perceives as his crucial realistic problems but also the feasibility of resolving these problems promptly, there are times when consideration of the patient's more general problems has to be postponed until his disabling symptoms are alleviated. For example, one patient was extremely depressed over not finding work. But before this crucial issue could be addressed directly, he first had to become active. It was only after the patient had become mobilized and had begun to feel better that he was then able to handle the social anxiety aroused by looking for work.

Because depression consists of affective, motivational, cognitive, behavioral, and physiological components, the therapist can concentrate on any one or a combination of these components to induce a change in the total syndrome of depression. Each of the components has a reciprocal relationship with the other components, and, therefore, improvement in one major problem area generally spreads into the others. In each case, the delineation of the specific problem to be treated and the special techniques to be used depend on a variety of factors. The therapist needs to discuss the goals with the patient in order to reach a consensus on which "target" problem to aim at and what methods to use. The cognitive therapist then formulates the patient's problems in terms of the thoughts and images underlying the patient's responses. Thus, the therapist's first task is to understand how the signs and symptoms of depression reflect a profound shift in the patient's cognitive organization.

As noted previously, the depressed person tends to regard himself, his experiences, and his future in a negative way. These negative concepts are evident in the way the patient systematically misconstrues his experiences in the content of his thinking. The patient's negative concepts contribute to the other symptoms of depression, such as sadness, passivity, self-blame, loss of pleasure response, and suicidal wishes. A vicious cycle is established: the negative thinking, unpleasant affects, self-defeating motivations, and general passivity reinforce each other. The cognitive therapist begins to break the vicious cycle by selecting one or more of the symptoms that appear to be most susceptible to therapeutic intervention. Thus the early focus may be directed to any one or a combination of affective, cognitive, motivational, or behavioral symptoms.* (For long-term results, the dysfunctional assumptions underlying the symptoms must be changed.)

Selection of Targets and Techniques

The choice of symptom-cluster and technique(s) can be made on the basis of several considerations.

1. The principle of the "therapeutic collaboration" often provides a good basis for making these decisions. The therapist can outline several areas that seem accessible to

---

* The Depression Inventory (Beck, 1967, 1978) may provide a useful tool for eliciting problems from patients who have difficulty in focusing on distressing symptoms or life situations. We have found that almost any of the items in the Inventory may provide a point of entry into the patient's distorted or dysfunctional constructs. For example, specific questions regarding high scores on items labeled Sense of Failure, Crying Spells, or Fatigability often yield a wealth of data regarding the patient's negative self-evaluations, fixation on imagined or actual deprivations, and negative expectations regarding any goal-directed activity, respectively.

intervention and also describe some of the therapeutic approaches that seem indicated. After discussion, he can make a joint decision with the patient (provided the patient is not too locked into inertia or indecisiveness to participate in decision-making).

2. Generally, in the earlier phases of treatment and in the treatment of the more severely depressed patients, the behavioral approaches are likely to be more useful than the strictly cognitive approaches. Thus, techniques such as scheduling activities, assigning graded tasks, and behavioral rehearsal would be given more attention than identifying and modifying dysfunctional cognitions.

3. The therapist should attempt to gear his approach to the patient's level of sophistication, personal style, and typical coping techniques.

4. The relative urgency and severity of the various problems and symptoms may dictate the priorities; that is, which problem(s) to deal with first.

5. A certain amount of "trial and error" is usually necessary. The patient should be told: "We have a number of approaches that have been shown to be successful for various problems. We may have to try out several before we find the one that really fits you. Thus, if one method is not particularly helpful, it will provide us with valuable information regarding which method is likely to succeed."

In summary, then, the problem-oriented approach consists of breaking up the complex phenomenon of depression into component problems, selecting the specific problems to be attacked in a given case, and then determining what types of therapeutic intervention would be appropriate for the patient. The following are major symptom targets.

AFFECTIVE SYMPTOMS

Sadness

Most depressed patients report some degree of sadness or unhappiness. Some patients experience fluctuating periods of feeling blue, while others are incapacitated by the severity of the affect. At times patients will describe these feelings in terms of body sensations; for example, "I have a sad feeling throughout my body." The patient is usually suffering this psychic pain at a time when his tolerance and ability to cope with any type of pain is at a low level. For this reason, providing the patient with some relief from his dysphoria is often an early target for intervention.

When working with the patient's affect, the therapist has to know precisely what the patient means when describing specific feelings.

Patients often intensify their dysphoria by such thoughts as, "I can't stand feeling this way," "I feel terrible all the time," and "I'll always be miserable." The therapist can use any of the previously described cognitive/behavioral methods to help the patient correct these distortions.

The patient's cognitions leading to sadness are not always apparent. He may be unable to pinpoint the thoughts which would cause feelings of sadness. In such an instance, the therapist has to provide the patient with other ways of relieving or reducing his dysphoria.

The therapist can provide the patient with some easing of his dysphoria by inducing the patient to "feel sorry for himself." Beck (1976) has written on this method:

> Encouraging a patient to express his unpleasant emotions through verbalizing them or crying sometimes reduces their intensity and makes the patient feel more alive, more like a "whole person." (Of course, some patients feel worse after emotional release: hence, such methods should be used with caution.) When a patient cries, he may feel sympathy for himself. Thus, his cognitive set toward himself changes from rejecting or derogatory to sympathetic. Sympathy with oneself is inconsistent with the cognitive set of self-blame. (p. 295)

The process can be accelerated by a number of other techniques. Telling the patient a story of another person with a similar problem and with whom the patient can identify frequently evokes sympathy in the patient. Feeling sympathy for another person in the same condition helps the patient to regard himself sympathetically. Dramatic techniques such as role-playing in which the therapist assumes

170

the role of his depressed patient, may also help the patient to change his cognitive set from self-critical to sympathetic.

Self-sympathy procedures are particularly helpful with patients who want to cry but are unable to. Traditionally, men in our society have trouble crying, but as sex roles change we are finding more and more females with the same problem. The therapist can also use selective self-disclosure to help the patient cry. One patient, for example, was unable to cry after his wife died. Her death followed a lengthy and painful hospitalization. The patient was able to cry and to feel self-sympathy after the therapist described his own painful feeling when his wife had been hospitalized for an accident.

Induced Anger

Experiencing anger often can counteract the patient's feelings of sadness. However, unless carefully controlled, the patient can blame himself for expressing anger and thus feel worse. In the office, the therapist can use techniques for inducing anger to help the patient alleviate sadness. However, the ultimate goal is to teach the patient to use these methods to combat feelings of sadness outside the office. After the patient has learned to use these methods in the office, he is instructed to practice them between sessions. To prevent the patient from becoming bogged down in anger, he is instructed to sharply limit the duration of the expression of angry feelings and follow them with some form of distraction.

Diversion

Patients can use diversion to reduce (temporarily) nearly all forms of painful affect. Diversion is particularly effective in relieving sadness. When teaching diversion as a coping skill, the therapist first asks the patient to rate his degree of sadness; the patient is then instructed to focus on some item in the office, such as the light switch plate or a piece of furniture and describe this in detail. After he has done this, the patient rerates his degree of sadness, which has usually diminished to some degree.

If the office "exercise" is successful, the patient is asked to practice diversion techniques between sessions. When the patient begins to feel sad, he is asked to use this dysphoria as a cue to begin diverting himself. The distraction can take the form of such activities as taking a walk, reading, engaging in conversation, talking on the telephone, and observing his environment. Quite often the patient is able to divert himself for only a few minutes in the beginning. As with other cognitive methods, the patient is instructed to start at his current level and usually finds he can gradually increase the duration of the procedure.

Sometimes a patient can learn to divert his attention from sadness by increasing his sensory awareness. In this procedure, while focusing on the environment, the patient uses as many of his sensory modalities as possible, including taste, hearing, sense of smell, body sensations, and heightened visual acuity. This procedure is often effective with negatively ruminating patients. A salesman, for example, with chronic dysphoria was able to control these feelings while working by increasing his awareness of environmental stimuli as he drove from call to call. The more sensory modalities he used, the fewer negative ruminations he experienced and the greater was his relief.

Some patients can use visual imagery as a diversion from dysphoria by imagining pleasant scenes, such as playing tennis in Florida or winning the lottery. The more details used in these images, the more effective they are likely to be. The patient can also mentally visualize those times in the past when he was happy, or he can try to picture a time in the future when he will no longer be sad. The use of visual imagery is usually detrimental in the more severely depressed patients, however, because of the encroachment of negative themes into the daydreams.

Use of Humor

Humor often succeeds in distracting a patient from his feelings of sadness. Many patients retain their sense of irony despite a general loss of mirth, and therapists adept at pointing out the ironic nature of a situation can divert the patient's attention, if only temporarily, with humor. When a depressed patient is able to appreciate the humor in a situation, it is usually a sign that he is developing or applying an important coping skill.

In this procedure, the patients are instructed to look for the humor or irony in a situation whenever they begin to feel sad. In one instance, a patient felt himself becoming sad as he was walking to his car in the morning. He stopped and realized he was sad because he had just seen the trashman carelessly throwing his trash can around, an act which had triggered thoughts about how the patient hated the neighborhood. Instead of giving in to the sadness, the patient looked for humor in the situation and observed that the name of the trash collection company was Vile and Sons. The amusement he found in this coincidence successfully counteracted his sadness.

The use of humor and other forms of diversion are not ideal solutions to a patient's problems. One would prefer long-term attitudinal changes. However, it is often necessary to get the patient feeling and functioning better before more basic solutions can be worked out. Just knowing he has adaptive ways of dealing with sadness often increases the patient's sense of control, which in turn increases his sense of security and well-being.

Limiting Excessive Expression of Dysphoria

Persons suffering from psychological pain, like those suffering from physical pain, often seek relief by telling others about this suffering. While attention of others is not, as many believe, the cause of sadness, prolonged discussion of these feelings can intensify them. When telling others of their suffering, patients become needlessly involved in focusing on these feelings. Furthermore, through excessive "ventilation" of feelings, patients often strain their relationships with friends and relatives. For these reasons, patients are encouraged to set strict limits to their discussion of their unhappiness.

After the therapist presents the rationale for limiting discussions of unhappiness, he may ask the patient to monitor the amount of time he spends talking about his feelings, for many patients are unaware of how much they do this. The patient can seek the aid of others in changing this behavior, and can tell those who are continually asking how he feels that he appreciates their concern but that he is presently trying to limit emotional "temperature-taking." If necessary, the therapist can talk about this issue to others of significance in the patient's life.

We have occasionally assigned a special time during the day for "feeling bad." For example, the therapist may suggest that the patient try to postpone the full experience of his feelings to a block of time late in the afternoon, say, from 4–5 p.m. Those patients seem to find that by knowing they will have a definite opportunity for "letting themselves go," they can be more oriented to achieve specific goals during the rest of the day.

"Building a Floor" under Sadness

Another helpful approach is to teach the patient to increase his tolerance for dysphoric feelings. This approach is useful in dealing with negative emotions, such as anxiety. In place of or in response to thinking, "I can't stand this," the patient is encouraged to tell himself, "I'm strong enough to take this" or "I will time how long I can stand this." With practice, people can learn to increase their tolerance for nearly all forms of discomfort.

A patient can be told that by increasing his tolerance for sadness, he is strengthening himself and "inoculating" himself against future bouts of dysphoria. By observing that he actually is able to tolerate high levels of dysphoria without becoming agitated, a patient frequently develops an increased sense of control that in itself can arrest the downward spiraling effects of sadness. In coping with sadness, patients often resort to maladaptive behavior mechanisms, such as oversleeping, overeating, or excessive drinking. The patient can increase his tolerance for sadness by increasing the time elapsed between feeling sad and resorting to such "antidotes." Similarly, postponing even the use of adaptive counteractive measures when he feels sad helps the patient to increase his level of tolerance.

Since it is expected that the patient will continue to feel varying degrees of sadness as long as his depression lasts, it is important for him to apply certain strategies that will *prevent him from aggravating his dysphoria.* The demonstration that he is capable of arresting the progress of his painful feelings serves as an antidote to the thought, "This pain will get so bad, it will be unbearable."

A simple technique applicable for patients who regularly experience their worst period at a particular time each day or week (e.g., in the early part of the morning) is to prepare a plan of diverting activities for that time interval. For example, an author instituted the program of outlining chapters and writing as many paragraphs as possible between 6 a.m. and 8 a.m.—her period of most intense dysphoria each day. A housewife used the same period to do cleaning and washing. On weekends, which had been particularly painful for her, she scheduled a number of social activities.

Such diversions not only diminish the degree of awareness of the dysphoria but are useful in channeling the patient's thought processes away from making interpretations regarding the significance or meaning of his dysphoria.

A specifically cognitive technique is often helpful in counteracting the patient's tendency to attach "catastrophic" meanings or self-condemnation to his low mood. We have found, for instance, that some individuals berate themselves for feeling sad and thus make themselves feel worse. One patient who had recently moved with her husband and children from a row house in the city to a new house in the suburbs condemned herself for feeling bad. Her thoughts were "I have plenty of room—several acres for the children to play in and a garden and lots of privacy. *I should be happy.*" In actuality, the move had severed her relationship with her neighbors who had been close personally as well as geographically and had required considerable amounts of exhausting work. Thus, for the time being at least, she had sustained a substantial loss.

The therapist pointed out that she had intensified her feelings of sadness by her self-denunciations. His approach was as follows:

> We have a wide range of feelings. Feelings of sadness usually occur when the losses seem paramount. You reacted to the move in a normal fashion at first—for example, you had an immediate loss of your friends and neighbors and therefore you felt sad. But you then pushed yourself from sadness to depression by applying your "shoulds" and berating yourself. You told yourself, "I should feel happy. . . . Why can't I be happy in our beautiful new home? What's wrong with me?"

The patient was initially surprised to realize that her injunction to feel happy after the move was not realistic. When she accepted the therapist's assessment, however, she was able to contain further sadness by telling herself: "It's natural to feel sad—temporarily. However, there are a number of people in the neighborhood whom I will get to know better. . . . Actually, it makes more sense to think I should feel sad right now rather than glad."

This case illustrates how a person is tyrannized by the code of "shoulds" he absorbs from society. The societal rules dictate that a person should feel happy under circumstances that in actuality are more likely to produce (in the short run, at least) sadness. The person prone to self-debasement then concludes that her lack of the expected pleasure response indicates a serious flaw in her character and that she will *never* be able to be happy. By recognizing that a particular decision (such as moving) is not fatal and that the short-term loss will be offset eventually by long-term gains, the patient is able to mitigate instead of exacerbate her present feelings of sadness.

"Uncontrollable" Crying Spells

Increased periods of crying are a common symptom in depression. This symptom is frequently found with females. At times patients feel better after crying, but more often they become further depressed. Some patients cry to such an extent that their communication with others and the therapist is severely hampered.

Patients often cry at some point in therapy. If the therapist doesn't overreact, this usually does not present a problem. A few patients cry during the session because they believe this is expected from them. The therapist can easily correct this misconception. The therapist should also be on the alert for any shame the patient may experience after crying. Feeling ashamed after crying is more typical of male patients than female.

Excessive crying is usually not the patient's central concern. However, if this symptom is hindering verbal communication, it has to be resolved so that the therapist can obtain crucial information from the patient. The general strategy is for the patient to learn a self-control procedure that gives him control over his crying. This strategy can include diversion training, active self-instruction *not* to cry, and setting a time limit on amount of crying.

One patient cried to such an extent during therapy sessions that almost no therapy was taking place. Excessive crying also posed problems for her outside of treatment; she was unable to carry on a conversation without crying. After trying unsuccessfully several self-control procedures, the therapist structured the interview (with the patient's agreement) so that she would have time allotted for crying for three-minute periods at the beginning, middle, and end of therapy. This procedure was successful in limiting the patient's crying both in and out of therapy. The patient said after several attempts at "structured crying," she realized she could control her crying. Moreover the ability to control her crying gave her an increased sense of mastery and improved her self-image.

Guilty Feelings

Because the sense of "wrongdoing" is based on highly idiosyncratic and arbitrary standards, the therapist has to resist jumping to conclusions about the source of a patient's guilty feelings. One patient, for example, said she felt guilty about sex. Closer examination revealed she didn't feel guilty about her numerous extramarital affairs, but about masturbating. When patients do not admit to a sense of guilt about "antisocial behavior," the therapist should not assume that the patient is simply repressing guilty feelings.

Some patients may feel guilty about their thoughts or wishes rather than special actions. A female patient experienced no feelings of guilt over having an affair with a married man, but felt extremely guilty about wishing that the man's sick wife would die. The therapist pointed out that thoughts are not actions, and that since the patient wasn't omnipotent, her wishes could not influence reality. The therapist also explained that her wish, although contrary to her value system, was understandable in view of the patient's desire to marry her lover.

A patient's sense of guilt is frequently related to his assuming an unrealistic share of responsibilty for the behavior of other people. Simply by asking the patient *why* he is responsible, the therapist often forces the patient to examine the nature of his excessive sense of responsibility. The therapist may wish to provide some additional information that will help to change the patient's guilt-producing interpretation of a situation. This approach was used successfully in the case of a patient who felt guilty about her daughter's suicide.

THERAPIST: Why are you responsible for your daughter's suicide?
PATIENT: I should've known she was going to kill herself.
T: People have been studying suicide for a great number of years, and no one can predict exactly where or when an individual is going to kill himself.
P: But I *should* have been able to know.
T: Believing you should know the unknowable is contrary to the laws of nature. All we know is that your daughter made a

> mistake in deciding to commit suicide and you are making a
> mistake by holding yourself responsible for this.

We have found that mothers (more than fathers) are prone to assume an unrealistic or high degree of responsibility for the presumed deficiencies, disappointments, or "defeats" of their children. In contrast, men are more prone to hold themselves responsible for setbacks in their vocations. The "guilt-ridden mother" frequently comes for treatment during middle age. At this stage, she often feels guilty about her desire to emancipate herself from her children, who are already adults. She generally continues to carry the same sense of obligation and responsibility she had experienced when they were infants.

Some patients believe a sense of guilt prevents one from engaging in self-defeating and antisocial behavior. They fail to realize that there are natural positive consequences for acting in one's best interest (which includes prosocial behavior) and natural negative consequences for acting otherwise. Feelings of guilt often add an unnecessary burden that may increase self-defeating behavior. The alcoholic who drinks, feels guilty, then drinks to cope with the guilty feelings, is a classic example. If the patient is engaging in some self-defeating behavior, such as smoking, drinking, or procrastination, and is feeling guilty over this behavior, his attention should be directed toward controlling the behavior *and* his self-criticisms for lack of success in attaining this goal.

Shame

Many patients experience shame over some "socially undesirable" aspect of their personality or behavior. Unlike guilty feelings which are related to a supposed infraction of the patient's *moral* or *ethical* code, shame stems from the patient's belief that he is judged as childish, weak, foolish, or inferior by others. Thus, acts that he expects to evoke ridicule from others initiate the sequence: "I look like a fool"→"It is awful to appear this way"→shame. Because patients don't readily admit to feeling ashamed, the therapist often has to inquire about this feeling. The therapist can explain that shame, in a sense, is self-created. To illustrate that the patient induces feelings of shame in himself, the therapist can ask the patient: (a) Are there things you were ashamed of in the past and no longer are? (b) Are there things you are ashamed of and others aren't? (c) Are others ashamed of things that you are not?

The patient can be told that if he adopts an "antishame" philosophy, a great deal of pain and discomfort can be avoided. When, for example, the patient makes a mistake that he believes is shameful, he can turn this experience into an antishame exercise by openly acknowledging it instead of hiding it. If he pursues this "open policy" long enough, his proneness to experience counterproductive shame will diminish. Moreover, he will be less inhibited and more flexible and spontaneous in his range of responses.

One way a therapist can help a patient to resolve feelings of shame over being depressed is illustrated in the following excerpt:

PATIENT: If the people at work found out I was depressed they would think badly of me.

THERAPIST: Over 10% of the population is depressed at one time or another. Why is this shameful?

P: Other people think people who become depressed are in-ferior—

T: You are confusing a psychological condition with a social problem. This is a version of blaming the victim. Even if they did think badly of you—either out of their own ignorance or adolescent way of rating people—you do not have to accept their evaluation. You will feel ashamed only if you apply their value system to yourself, that is, if you *really* believe it is shameful.

Other standard procedures, such as having patients list advantages and disadvantages of expressing shame, can be used to deal with this response.

Anger

Excessive feelings of anger are not a typical problem for the depressed patient. Some depressed patients do experience more anger as they start to feel better. This period of excessive anger is usually of short duration and usually indicates the patient is improving. However, there are patients whose anger is an early, persistent, vexing symptom. In these cases, many of the procedures—such as distraction and increasing tolerance—that are used to cope with other negative emotions may be applied to anger. Patients may use relaxation methods as active coping skills when they start to become angry. Goldfried and Davison (1976) give an excellent description of relaxation procedures.

The patient is taught to become task-oriented when his anger starts to develop. As Novaco (1975) points out, the angry person is generally flooded with irrelevant thoughts revolving around intolerance for others and of the necessity for retaliation. The patient is encouraged to use self-talk that "cools him down" rather than self-talk that "heats him up." Patients are frequently taught to increase their ability to empathize with the other person. By empathizing, the patient may shift to a cognitive set of acceptance that is incompatible with anger.

A college student, for example, raged against her father's disapproval of her unconventional life-style. When she role-played her father (in an exercise with the therapist), she realized that he perceived her as making "a terrible mistake" and as likely to ruin her life. She then realized that his behavior reflected his concern and caring for her, and she experienced empathy with him.

Anxiety

Patients frequently report anxiety as a problem that accompanies their depression or as a problem that appears as the depression lifts. Some patients are excessively disturbed by the symptoms of anxiety because they do not label this emotion correctly. The therapist can give these patients relief merely by identifying these symptoms as anxiety and assuring the patients that, while these feelings are uncomfortable, they are not dangerous. This procedure helps to decatastrophize the experience of anxiety and to prevent the patient from having anxiety about anxiety.

The first step in treating anxiety is to encourage the patient to monitor this symptom. In addition to recording situational variables, such as time, place, and precipitating events, the patient is asked to measure the degree of anxiety over a period of time. This procedure is carried out by instructing the patient to graph on a sheet of paper the amount of anxiety in "subjective units of discomfort" from 0 to 100 on one side and the "time" on the other side, usually in half-hour intervals. This graph will provide the therapist with crucial information and will show the patient that anxiety is generally related to external situations and is *time-limited*. Often patients in the midst of an anxiety attack believe that the anxiety will never let up.

Patients may be taught a variety of self-management procedures to control their anxiety. The best antidote to anxiety is generally some type of physical activity. Repetitive physical action such as bouncing a ball, skipping rope, or running are often useful. Some patients find relief through physical activity such as cleaning the house or doing yard work.

Distraction is an effective way to lower anxiety levels. Two members of our team who were caught in a traffic jam were able to reduce their anxiety over the possibility of missing a train by working out a complicated formula to predict how many cars in front of them would go through the traffic light before it changed to red. Patients can be asked to buy pocket puzzles or to focus on advertisements in a subway train to distract them when they become anxious. Those patients who become totally absorbed in their anxiety may have to use more dramatic forms of distraction. Some patients have used bells to ring as a form of distraction from anxiety.

Many of the methods used to modify depressive thoughts are effective in dealing with anxiety. In the standard procedure, the patient rates the degree of anxiety over an anticipated situation, such as making a sales call. Then, after more realistic ways of looking at the situation are discussed, the patient rerates his anticipatory anxiety. Subsequently, he rates the anxiety he experienced in the actual situation. Patients often fail to realize that a person can perform adequately even when he is anxious. Studies have shown that even high levels of anxiety do not necessarily block a person from performing well in anxiety-producing situations.

Patients frequently overlook the "rescue factors" in threatening situations. The patient who is fearful of automobile breakdowns on lonely highways generally does not take into account emergency phones and tow trucks. Similarly, the person with social anxiety disregards the empathy others may have for an anxious person. Moreover, the anxious patient generally fails to recognize that there are a range of neutral or even positive outcomes for most situations; the fact that a salesman does not make a sale does not mean the customer is going to cut his head off.

The therapist generally has to inquire about the anxious patient's visual imagery since patients rarely volunteer information about their fantasies. We generally find that anxious patients exhibit vivid images of a "catastrophe" (Beck, 1976). The patient can use a variety of methods to control these images by changing the visual content. One patient, frightened of her boss, had a visual image of him as a monster. She was able to change this visual image into one of him as a lamb.

As with other negative affect states, the therapist has to discover specifically what is frightening to the patient about a particular situation. Categories such as "airplane phobias" and "school phobias" are too general and diffuse for therapeutic purposes. Often, helping patients to construct specific scenarios of a frightening situation will reveal the major fear. One shop owner, for example, was afraid to go to New York on a buying trip. Closer examination revealed he was afraid of having to say "no" to salesmen. After this problem was pinpointed, the therapist was able to use a role-playing technique to desensitize him to this fear.

Some patients have to learn to increase their tolerance for a certain amount of anxiety. If these patients avoid anxiety-producing situations, they miss a chance to test their unrealistic thoughts. They are told that by plunging into or just "staying with" the experiences they will often become desensitized. Patients often avoid what they perceive as dangerous situations and thus do not reach closure in this area. *

MOTIVATIONAL SYMPTOMS

Loss of Positive Motivation and Increased Avoidance Wishes

The patient's lack of motivation to carry out even the most simple tasks is often a major symptom of severe depression. The patient knows what he has to do but he doesn't have the internal desire or stimulus to carry it out. In most cases, the patient immobilizes himself by believing he is unable to perform the activity or that he will not receive any satisfaction from doing the activity.

---

* An extensive manual for the cognitive treatment of anxiety is available from the Center for Cognitive Therapy (see Appendix).

The loss of positive motivation is generally accompanied by strong desires to *avoid* constructive activity. These active wishes to avoid are highlighted in the patient's negative reactions to homework assignments (see Chapter 13).

The cognitive and behavioral procedures outlined in previous chapters can be used to help the patient overcome his motivational blocks. The general strategy is for the patient to attempt to undertake the avoided activity on an experimental basis. This "experiment" can help to correct the patient's mistaken thinking and provide success experiences. Obvious, immediate success is usually a good motivator. When the patient realizes he has control over some particular aspect of his life, he is more likely to attempt to control other aspects of his life.

Some patients with extreme motivational problems benefit from a self-instructional method developed by Low and his group (1950). In this method, the patient gives himself specific instructions to move his body into action. For example, a patient with trouble getting out of bed in the morning would say, "Legs . . . move . . . hit the floor, . . . Muscles . . . move." Some patients find this active self-instruction exceedingly helpful; others, however, don't. Low's method is discussed further in Chapter 13.

Often the patient wants to escape from or avoid his normal routines and duties. There is usually an attitude of hopelessness underlying this symptom. Because hopelessness, suicide, and the wish to escape are such crucial symptoms of depression, they will be discussed at length in the next chapter.

Increased Dependency

Intensified dependency is a prevalent symptom of depression. The clinically depressed patient often has a strong impulse to seek help from others in carrying out everyday activities. This wish for assistance, which may take the form of a demand or a whining complaint, generally exceeds the patient's realistic needs for help. Although help often gives the patient some temporary emotional relief, it can reinforce the patient's dependency and lack of self-confidence.

It is often useful for the therapist to explain to the patient the difference between "constructive" and "regressive" dependency.

183

Seeking to learn ways to cope with depression represents a form of constructive dependency; the patient has a problem he is unable to solve without assistance and thus seeks expert help. On the other hand, regressive dependency is manifested by seeking help for something that he is capable of handling himself. By engaging in regressive dependency, the patient reinforces his idea of inadequacy.

Patients are sometimes concerned about becoming too dependent on the therapist. The therapist should explain that the purpose of therapy is to give him the tools to become more independent. By learning new ways of thinking and new coping skills, he will be less dependent on other people.

Without safeguards, constructive dependency can deteriorate into destructive dependency. This tendency is illustrated by the patient who learns ways to tolerate his depression, but continues to insist the therapist solve all of his problems. (For ways to handle this specific problem, see Chapter 15 on the termination of therapy.)

Patients with dependency problems are given training in self-reliance (see Emery, in press). This training involves teaching the patient to take increasing responsibility for directing his actions and modifying his emotional reactions. Initially, the patient reinstates his previous self-reliance activities, such as making his own bed. As he improves, he is taught to increase his range of independent activities. The patient who believes he can only experience enjoyment through others is urged to go to movies, museums, and out to dinner alone. In self-reliance training, the patient attempts to do as much as he can of his everyday activities by himself. This may transcend sexual stereotypes. The male may try cooking or doing household chores and the female may attempt mechanical work around the house or on the car.

The patient can use the full range of cognitive techniques to increase his self-reliance. This repertoire includes running experiments to see whether he can do more than he believes he can and actively challenging initiative-killing thoughts such as: "Why bother?" "It's too hard," "Let someone else do it," and "I don't have the time." Often, the patient can radically increase his self-reliance by placing himself in situations in which he is forced to be self-reliant, such as spending a weekend alone in a strange city. Throughout a day a person is confronted with numerous situations in which he can *choose to be either dependent or independent.* A general strategy is for the patient to monitor the number of times he chooses self-reliance and to gradually increase this number.

The role of self-reliance training in the cognitive treatment of depression is similar to the role of assertiveness training in treatment. Prior to becoming depressed, the patient usually had an adequate repertoire of assertive and self-reliant behaviors; however, once depressed he may develop a deficit in these two areas. At this point, his nonassertiveness and dependency become target symptoms, and assertive or self-reliance training is appropriate. When the patient's depression improves, he may no longer require this special form of intervention.

Some patients, however, are still excessively dependent or nonassertive after their depression has lifted. For these patients additional self-reliance or assertiveness training may be needed. In these cases the patient usually still holds maladaptive assumptions revolving around assertiveness or dependency issues. Special training can help to weaken these beliefs. For example, assertiveness training can help the patient who believes it is necessary for his well-being that everyone like him, and self-reliance training can help the patient who believes he is helpless without support from other people.

COGNITIVE SYMPTOMS

The importance of a patient's cognitions in maintaining and exacerbating his depression is described in Chapter 1. Various techniques for dealing with dysfunctional or distorted cognitions are covered in Chapters 2–8. This section will concentrate only on those cognitive problems that are not dealt with elsewhere.

Indecisiveness

Making decisions often presents a problem for depressed patients. The patient often believes his job, family, or other outside situations are *the cause* of his depression and, consequently, that if he leaves the problematic situation, the depression will lift; but he is unsure of the wisdom of this decision. Another common type of problem occurs when the patient has made some move—new job, new area—and is dissatisfied with this move. The patient believes that if he reverses this change, he will no longer be depressed. In general, the therapist tells the patient that it is inadvisable to make major decisions when one is depressed. In nearly every case, the major decision can be postponed without dire consequences. The depressed person is told that when he is functioning below his normal capacity, he is not as able to make long-term decisions as when he is not depressed. Also, he may view his life situation differently when he is over his depression.

For important decisions that cannot or need not be postponed, the therapist and the patient can write out the advantages and disadvantages of each choice and then use this as the guide for making decisions. In this procedure, the patient lists the alternative decisions and the possible consequences of each.

Often the patient will not make *any* decisions because of the negative results he foresees. In cases in which either choice is equally acceptable, the depressed person is encouraged to make decisions. There are several rather simplistic techniques to help people make these types of choices. One is to have the patient list alternatives alphabetically, and then choose whichever one comes first in the alphabet. At other times, the patient can flip a coin. The emphasis is on having the patient make a decision and take action.

Often, depressed people believe they must have absolute certainty of the correctness of a decision. The therapist has to explain that there is no absolute certainty in life. There is no way that one can guarantee that favorable or unfavorable events will happen or will not happen. Some of the alternatives of the decisions, however, can be researched by therapist and patient. The patient should be told that often none of the options is necessarily "wrong," but they are simply different. Each has a different set of consequences. It also is a good policy to see whether the patient has a tendency to structure the decision as a no-win situation. For example, one patient couldn't decide whether to go to a small or a large college. He saw the disadvantages of both choices but not the advantages. In therapy, he was taught to evaluate the advantages of whichever choice he made and ways in which he could modify or cope with the disadvantages. Thus, he changed a no-win situation to a "no-lose" situation.

The following is one way to deal with decisions that have to be made immediately. A patient had been extremely upset for two or three weeks because of a decision she had to make. The decision concerned which of two desirable graduate schools to attend. One school offered a large scholarship, but the other school was more prestigious. In addition, she ruminated over being selfish if she chose the school she wanted, 'and acquiescing to her parents' demands if she chose the other. She' managed to turn a can't lose situation into a can't-win situation.

She decided to accept the school she wanted, which was the one that offered no financial support. On the day she had to make the final irreversible decision, she experienced waves of panicky feelings. At this point, the therapist outlined the following proposal to her:

1. The act of *making* a decision in this instance was more important than either decision.
2. Her behavior was the result of her problem of obsessiveness. She desired absolute certainty. Her anxiety stemmed from the fear that she would not have an absolute guarantee that either choice was "right."
3. The rational response is that no one can expect absolute certainty or "correctness." No one can predict the future. There would be unanticipated consequences (pluses and minuses) no matter which school she chose.
4. There is no need for absolute assurances. She must make a decision and then "cope, not mope."
5. She should anticipate a regret period of about a week no matter what the decision. She should accept her sense of regret and cope with it with the use of cognitive techniques.

After explaining, the therapist took out a coin to flip. He told her heads would be school A and tails school B and he flipped the coin. Before showing her the result, he asked her what she hoped the coin showed. When she answered "school A," the therapist put the coin in his pocket without showing it to her and said that she had made her decision. She then called the school to confirm her acceptance. The therapist structured the situation so that the patient was forced to make a decision. The patient did not have time to ruminate. This strategy necessitated an immediate choice and increased the probability of the patient's choosing from "wants" rather than fears. The technique also provided a dramatic demonstration of how to cut the web of her obsessional indecisiveness.

Guilty feelings often play a role in making decisions. One

patient, for example, couldn't make up his mind about whether or not to buy a new car. He believed he would be depriving his family of money if he bought the car, but he knew he needed a new car for his job.

When working with patients' indecisiveness, the therapist may have to use methods for modifying guilt feelings. The patient has to learn that there are often only partial solutions, but that the cumulative effect of several partial solutions can solve the problem. Then he has to learn to inoculate himself against feelings of guilt arising from his belief that he has made a mistake.

View of Problems as Overwhelming

The "cognitive triad" consists of a negative view of the outside world, the self, and the future. The negative view of the future ("hopelessness") will be dealt with in the next chapter. The first two facets of the triad will be discussed in the next two sections.

The general strategy for dealing with "overwhelming problems" is to have the patient pinpoint a specific problem he wants to work on and to develop constructive procedures for dealing with it. The patient's formulation of his world is reconceptualized from "It is overwhelming" to (1) "What are the specific problems?" (2) "What are the solutions?" The patient may be told that he can do only one thing at a time and therefore cannot pay attention to all the things that he believes he has to do. However, he can list all the problems and set priorities. Activity schedules are often helpful when following priorities poses a problem for the patient. Concrete ways to *begin* activities are given to the patient. The therapist can tell the patient that starting projects is at first difficult for nearly everyone, but that the job becomes easier once the project is underway.

At times creative problem solving is needed. Depressed patients are frequently blocked from thinking of solutions that are obvious to them when they are not depressed. One businessman was overwhelmed by the amount of work he had to do, yet couldn't get out in the field because he had to watch the phone. As a result, he did not leave his office to do the work in the field. The therapist suggested that he buy a telephone-answering machine. This simple intervention helped solve the dilemma. As an alternative strategy, the patient could have been asked what solutions he would offer to another

188

person in this situation. In responding to this question, the patient becomes a consultant to himself.

Many patients take on more work than they need to. Others mistakenly believe that more is expected of them than is the case. This belief can be checked out. A housewife, for example, accepted a full-time volunteer job, became president of a large organization, and made plans to run as candidate for political office. She *believed* that it was impossible for her to reduce or withdraw from any of her commitments. At times such a patient will have to become more assertive to lessen the demands made on her.

Many patients are overwhelmed by their problems because they exaggerate the difficulties and minimize the possibility of corrective action; thus, they take no action at all. The therapist has to show the patient how he can handle some of these situations. The following example illustrates how this can be done.

A depressed patient said she wanted to go swimming but was overwhelmed by the problems this would entail.

PATIENT: There is nowhere I could go swimming.
THERAPIST: How could you find a place?
P: There is a YWCA if I could get there. . . . I'd get my hair wet and get a cold.
T: How could you get there?
P: My husband would take me.
T: How about your wet hair?
P: I couldn't take a hair dryer; someone would steal it.
T: Could you do something about that?
P: They don't have lockers.
T: How do you know?
P: I just don't think they do.
T: For the first step, why don't you call up and see if they do?

The patient did make the necessary inquiries and eventually was able to start swimming again. Her problems had to be spelled out in detail, and then she had to investigate the possibilities.

Patients at times may be accomplishing more than they realize. By recording what they have accomplished, they can correct this cognitive distortion. Patients can be told that simply trying to accomplish something or thinking of ways to accomplish it represents a partial success.

Self-Criticism

As is typical of most people, the depressed patient searches for explanations of his problems. In his notion of causality, the depressed patient is prone to regard some disgraceful deficiency in himself as the source of his psychological disorder. This tendency is often supported by significant others who state that the patient "could get better if he wanted to." Severely depressed patients take the notion of self-causality to seemingly absurd extremes. One patient who was hospitalized for his depression heard a fellow patient across the hall sneeze and had the automatic thought, "I'm to blame. I must be infecting everyone on the floor." This type of unrealistic self-blame serves to make the patient feel worse. Therapists have to treat the self-criticisms of patients with caution as any direct rebuttal may result in the thought, "He doesn't understand my weakness." One patient, after hearing that his self-criticisms were maladaptive, began to blame himself "for blaming himself."

The cognitive approach to self-criticism involves making the patient aware of the pervasiveness of specific self-criticisms, and as a result of this increased awareness, making an objective assessment of the self-blaming thoughts. The recurrent, stereotyped nature of the patient's self-criticisms allows the therapist and patient to make significant gains once the thoughts have been modified. Recognizing his specific self-criticisms is not difficult because the patient usually feels worse immediately after a self-criticism. Thus, when he experiences an increase in dysphoria, he need only "play back" his preceding thoughts to identify the self-criticism.

The next step is to increase the patient's objectivity toward his self-blame. This step is crucial since the patient commonly believes his self-criticism is justified. One method is to ask the patient a question such as, "Suppose I made mistakes the way you do? Would you despise me for it?" Inasmuch as the patient generally recognizes that he would not be so critical of another person, he may realize the exaggerated nature of his self-criticisms. Mildly to moderately depressed patients may recognize the *self-defeating* nature of their self-criticisms if the therapist says, for example,

> How do you think I would feel if somebody were standing over my shoulder evaluating or criticizing everything I did? . . . In a sense,

this is what you are doing to yourself without deliberately wanting to. . . . The net effect, however, is that you not only feel bad, but you can't perform adequately. You will find that you can be free with yourself and more successful if you try to ignore the self-evaluations.

Role-Playing. The process of gaining objectivity toward the destructiveness of the self-criticisms may sometimes be accelerated through role-playing. The therapist, for example, dramatizes the way that the patient sees himself: inadequate, inept, weak. The patient is coached to assume the role of a harsh critic who will verbally attack the "patient" for any demonstration of acknowledgment of a fault. A skillful therapist may play the "weak" role in such a way as to demonstrate the patient's distortions and arbitrary inferences. If the patient is properly "warmed up" to the critic role, he can simultaneously act out the denunciations and observe the extravagance of his negative judgments.

Another method to increase the patient's awareness of his self-criticisms is to reverse the roles: The patient attempts to help the therapist who takes a self-debasing role.

The following case example illustrates the use of role reversal with a 27-year-old depressed inpatient. She had participated in three previous sessions but in the fourth session she continually labeled herself as "too stupid" and "foolish." These self-criticisms seriously interfered with her attempts to begin any new task and, in fact, were disrupting the therapy session itself.

PATIENT: Now that I know I can control my thinking, I feel really stupid for being depressed.

THERAPIST: You have to learn about yourself before you can make changes. Before therapy, you didn't have the knowledge and it doesn't seem reasonable to criticize yourself after the fact.

P: I must be too stupid to pick things up on my own.

T: Do you realize how often you criticize yourself for being "stupid?"

P: If the shoe fits, wear it. I've never been bright enough to pick things up quickly. I can always remember being the dunce of my class when it came to math.

T: I could probably understand if you learned to be critical of yourself when faced with a math problem, even though criticism at that point wouldn't be of much use. But you continuously criticize yourself whenever we attempt something new. Would you be willing to take a look at the "hidden effect" these criticisms have on you?

P: I guess so.

T: Okay, I'd like to do some role-playing. You are quite a good swimmer, so why don't we rehearse what it would be like if you were going to teach me how to swim? I'll listen to your instructions and we can both imagine the scene.

P: Okay, the first thing you need to do is learn how to relax in the water.

T: I'm too stupid to learn that. I haven't been able to learn properly since the fourth grade.

P: Well, you'll have to try and I'll coach you.

T: If I get into the water I'll look stupid.

P: You have to get into the water if you're going to learn how to swim.

T: I'll embarrass you in front of the others because I'll do something foolish. I'm certain. It always happens.

P: You're starting to get me frustrated.

T: Is that because you think I can't learn how to swim? You think I'm too stupid?

P: No, it's *because you think you're too stupid.* I haven't had a chance to even see you in the water. (laughs)

At this point, the patient became aware that objective information was needed for learning and, where indicated, coaching could be useful. However, the entire learning procedure could be thwarted by her continual production of self-criticisms. The therapist's instructions included the self-appeal, "Take one step at a time and make up for *any* inherent lack of ability with extra effort." The therapist and patient had to deal with the patient's fear of embarrassing herself or the therapist by awkward behavior that is expected of any novice, whether a novice swimmer or problem-solver.

Another strategy to attack the patient's self-criticisms is to teach him how to make "automatic" rational responses to any self-deprecatory automatic thoughts. The patient learns to challenge the validity of these negative thoughts and to substitute a more reasonable appraisal of himself. The "triple column" technique, referred to in Chapter 8, enables the patient to pinpoint his negative thought and to specify why it is erroneous or maladaptive. These homework assignments are crucial to implementing the strategies formulated during the therapeutic interview.

The application of the technique of identifying and responding to self-criticism is illustrated in the following case. In this case, the patient was instructed to present positive responses in a role-playing situation.

A depressed woman believed she was incompetent as a wife and mother. This basic belief was manifested in her evaluation of her responsibilities in the home. When she made dinner for the family, she remarked, "I hope this food is good enough. If it's not worth eating, I'll get you something else." The experience of continually devaluing the results of her labor had the effect of reinforcing her negative self-image, particularly as she valued her family responsibilities more than anything else. Her family, however, learned to expect the self-criticisms but always responded with positive supporting comments that the patient did not believe.

The patient identified two aspects of the self-criticisms that had an automatic quality. First, whenever she would undertake a task, she was flooded with images of her husband's being disappointed with her. As a result, she became increasingly anxious and concluded that he should expect "incompetence from an incompetent." Her own self-criticism continued from this point. Second, when she saw her husband (or even her two oldest children), she automatically verbalized her self-criticism "before they can speak." She further criticized herself for not expressing her feelings and always "being defensive."

The first part of the method chosen to deal with this problem was to examine the meaning of her self-criticisms. The meaning was pursued from two perspectives. An attempt was made to examine her self-criticisms objectively using the triple column technique and a lengthy period of discussion about the evidence for her "poor homemaking." For instance, she recalled that guests had often spontaneously complimented her on her baking. The patient recognized that many of her self-criticisms were characterized by exaggeration of minor errors (for instance, she added too much tasteless food coloring to the icing of a cake and concluded, "The cake isn't worth eating").

The second perspective was to examine *alternative responses* to her self-criticisms. The therapist asked the patient to recall the specific message that she *wanted* to communicate to her family. She thought she may have been trying to say, "Tell me how you feel about my efforts" and/or "Pay some attention to the things I do around here." The therapist decided to role-play the situation with the instruction that the patient was to convey any message except a self-critical one. She imagined herself at dinner and said to the therapist ("husband"), "I wanted to bake you a cake that you liked but I made a mistake and added too much coloring, but it should taste okay." At that point she became distressed and said, "He doesn't care about the cake. He probably wonders what's wrong with me that I can't snap out of this depression." She was able to counter this notion with, "You will like the cake even if it isn't perfect."

Absolutistic (All-or-Nothing) Thinking

As pointed out in Chapter 1, the thinking disorder in depression may be analyzed in terms of primitive vs. mature modes of organizing reality. Depressed persons tend to make broad categorical judgments and the meanings they attach to experiences tend to be extreme, unidimensional, and absolute. More mature thinking conceptualizes life situations into *many dimensions* or qualities, uses quantitative rather than qualitative terms, and applies relative rather than absolute standards. Moreover, depressed persons tend to view negative consequences as irreversible.

The categorical, absolutistic thinking may be modified in a number of ways.

Looking for Partial Gains ("Pluses") in Reversals. Depressives often show the typical all-or-nothing response to an adverse event. Thus, their pain tends to be proportional to the symbolic loss. Actually, even an event that appears to be an unmitigated loss may have some benefits. For example, a patient who had been recovering from her depression was dejected after she had asked her employer for a raise and had been turned down. The therapist asked her if there was anything positive about the experience. She initially responded that it was a "totally bad" experience. The therapist then asked her to list some possible benefits. As she reflected, she was able to list the following benefits:

1. It was the first time I got up the nerve to ask, so it will be

easier next time. I need to learn to assert myself sooner or later.

2. Actually, he was very nice and I think it will be easier to talk to him from now on.

3. Come to think of it, he didn't turn me down flatly. He said he'd consider giving me a raise in a few months. So I guess this was a step toward that.

Another example is the expectation of a single (bad) consequence of a particular event. A manufacturer found that he was caught in a tight squeeze between rising costs and diminished income. He could think only of bankruptcy until the therapist asked, "Is it possible that something good might come out of this?" As he thought about it, he realized that the present situation would provide an excellent opportunity for him to sell out an inventory he had accumulated over many years and which he had felt was an obstacle to making a shift in his business. He concluded that he might actually come out ahead—and be able to make a shift in the nature of his business. As it turned out, eventually, he was able to capitalize on this opportunity and shift to a different kind of business.

Use of Self-Questioning. As the patient becomes more amenable to viewing his "primitive" type of judgments more objectively, he can be trained to use a number of techniques, especially self-questioning, in order to shift his mode of thinking to a more nature level.

This technique is illustrated below:

PATIENT'S ABSOLUTE CONCLUSION: I have always been a total failure.

THERAPIST'S QUESTIONS:

1. How do you define failure? What are your standards?

2. Have there been *degrees* of failure: that is, some failures were more total than others?

3. If some experiences were only partial failures, did they also represent partial successes?

4. Were there some areas in your life (friends, family, school work, recreation) in which you did not fail and may, in fact, have reached your goals?

5. Even if you did fail in specific areas, does it follow that you cannot improve and become more successful?

6. Do failures in reaching a goal make you a failure as a person?
7. Should people who have experienced failures be subjected to rejection by other people?
8. Should a person who has suffered defeat subject himself to further pain by rejecting himself?

We have found that by simply asking himself such questions, the patient can open up the tight compartments enclosing his preformed judgments. Once exposed to the fresh air of further scrutiny, these judgments become less arbitrary and less maladaptive.

Difficulties in Concentration and Memory

The patient's problems in concentration and memory are often interrelated. The patient is unable to recall information because he isn't concentrating on the material to be learned. As with other symptoms, the therapist should assure the patient that problems in concentrating and remembering are symptoms of depression. These are problems that the depressed patient is "supposed to have" and they are not signs the patient is losing his mind.

The major problem with the patient's concentration is one of proper focusing. The patient is usually preoccupied with material other than what he desires to concentrate on, for example, a student who wants to concentrate on his teacher's lecture but ruminates about his problems instead. The therapist can help the patient to improve his focusing through a series of structured exercises, for example, by asking him to read short passages aloud from a book in the office or work out a simple math problem. This can also help to correct the patient's belief that he isn't able to concentrate at all. After going through this exercise, the patient is asked to buy a kitchen timer and to practice concentrating on specific assignments between sessions for increasing lengths of time.

A patient who had been unable to concentrate on any household task for more than a few minutes at a time was given a list of steps to execute in washing her car. To her surprise, she found she was able to spend 3 hours on this assignment and did an excellent job.

If the patient has to remember specific material on the job or at school, he can be taught the SQ3R method (Survey, Question, Read, Recite, and Review). First the patient surveys the material he wants to learn. This gives him a blueprint to work from. Next, he writes out specific questions about the material to be remembered; this helps him to focus and give meaning to the material. Then he reads the material or attends to it some other way. This is followed by reciting the material either by making notes or talking out loud. In the last step, the patient reviews the material (Robinson, 1950).

An important byproduct of sharpening, focusing, and task-orientation is the fact that these activities divert the patient from his perseverating negative thinking.

BEHAVIORAL SYMPTOMS

Passivity, Avoidance, and Inertia

Patient inactivity and passivity are central target symptoms. Some approaches to this problem are discussed in the behavioral methods chapter (Chapter 7) and the homework chapter (Chapter 13). A more detailed account is presented in *Cognitive Therapy and the Emotional Disorders* (Beck, 1976, pp. 274–287).

The passivity and inactivity seen in depression have historically been regarded as a form of neurophysiological inhibition: psychomotor retardation. An activity schedule often serves to counteract the apparent passivity and retardation.

Activity Schedules and Projects. A rationally designed activity program has several advantages. Some of these are: (a) The patient's self-concept is changed. He is able to evaluate his experiences more realistically. Concomitantly, with the improvement in his self-concept, he becomes more hopeful about the future. (b) He is distracted from his painful, depressing thoughts and his unpleasant affect by transferring his attention to the activity. (c) The responses of "significant others" become more positive, as they generally reinforce the patient's constructive activity in a beneficial way. (d) He may begin to enjoy the activities and thus receives an immediate reward for engaging in the activities.

Of course, anyone who has treated depressed patients knows that they frequently make efforts to become more active. Typically, their family and friends cajole, prod, or exhort them to be more active—without lasting success. These efforts generally fail because these individuals do not understand the psychology of depression. It is essential, first, to create the *motivation* for activity by explaining a clear rationale that is understandable to the patient. Initially, the therapist must elicit the patient's reasons for inactivity.

There are a number of methods to ascertain the reasons for the patient's inactivity. For example, the therapist may recommend a particular activity or project that is obviously within the patient's capacity. When the patient expresses his reluctance or inability to follow the suggestion, the therapist asks the patient to detail the reasons for his reluctance. These "reasons" are treated as hypotheses to be tested by devising a specified project.

The usual reasons given by depressed patients for their passivity and resistance to engaging in a project are: (a) "It is pointless to try." (b) "I cannot do it." (c) "If I try anything, it won't work out and I'll only feel worse." (d) "I am too tired to do anything." (e) "It is much easier to just sit still."

The patient generally accepts his reasons for inactivity as valid, and it does not occur to him that they may be fallacious or, at least, dysfunctional. Later, when the therapist designs an activity project with the patient, they will test the validity of these "reasons." If the patient achieves the specified goal, it is important that the therapist review whether the success experience contradicts the erroneous attitude (for example, that he is "too weak to do anything").

Before the project is initiated, the meanings and connotations of the symptoms should be explored and discussed. For instance, a connotation of being immobile is that the patient is "lazy." He tends to hold this view of himself, as do the people around him. As a result, he criticizes himself—as do the significant others. By mobilizing the patient into activity, the therapist can help the patient to combat his demeaning self-evaluations.

Since the depressed patient's desire to escape from everyday activities is strong and his negative beliefs are entrenched, it is important for the therapist to state explicitly to the patient how he is unwittingly defeating himself and making himself more miserable by blandly accepting his self-defeating attitudes and yielding to his regressive wishes. The therapist should indicate to the patient, directly or indirectly, that by questioning his ideas, he is likely to feel better.

It is crucial that the therapist present his questions and assertions regarding the patient's self-defeating ideas and wishes in a nonjudgmental, reflective way. He should avoid the appearance of scolding the patient. Because depressed patients generally respond to "criticism" with further self-reproaches and self-immobilization, the therapist should inquire about the patient's reactions in order to determine whether the patient is using the therapist's comments "against himself." The therapist, furthermore, should be aware that his statements may be construed simply as an exhortation to invoke "the power of positive thinking." He should indicate clearly that he and the patient are attempting to *pinpoint a problem* and *provide a specific remedy for it.*

The next stage in the treatment of passivity consists of engaging the patient's interest or curiosity so that he will at least cooperate to the extent of attempting to carry out a simple project. This preliminary goal can be reached through a novel presentation of a specific project, by explaining the rationale for the particular procedure, and by conveying to the patient the idea that there is a less painful alternative to feeling as bad as he does—through collaborating with the therapist by involving himself in a specific activity. When the patient responds to the incentive to cooperate, then a variety of verbal cognitive or behavioral methods can be used to enable the patient to complete this project.

An ultimate goal of this program is to train the patient to identify his negative thoughts prior to or while engaging in the specific project. As the patient realizes how these automatic thoughts are defeating him, he may begin to challenge them spontaneously. At a later stage, he will learn how to correct them and to view his situation in a more reasonable manner.

The therapeutic program may be formulated in terms of the following steps: (1) proposing a specific project to the patient; (2) eliciting his reasons for opposing the proposal; (3) asking the patient to weigh the validity of his "reasons" (or negative attitudes); (4) indicating to the patient why these reasons (or attitudes) may be self-defeating and invalid; (5) stimulating the patient's interest in attempting to perform the proposed assignment; (6) setting up the project in such a way that the patient's performance will test the validity of his ideas. Thus, successful completion of the task will contradict the patient's hypothesis that he is incapable of doing it.

It is important for the therapist to bear in mind that the patient may "fail" at a certain project. Therefore, the experience should be couched in such a way that the information will be useful irrespective of the outcome. Thus, the therapist can elicit the exaggerated generalizations following a "defeat" and point out the cognitive distortion. Then, he and the patient can set a new goal that is more likely to be obtained.

The following case illustrates the therapist's use of an activity schedule in the treatment of a 48-year-old depressed man.

The patient was hospitalized in a general hospital psychiatric ward and his depression was particularly difficult to treat. The man had attempted suicide by carbon monoxide poisoning prior to his admission. He had been treated for depression with tricyclic antidepressants and supportive psychotherapy for eight months prior to hospital admission. He had shown little improvement (with the exception of improved mood in the evening hours) as a result of five electroconvulsive treatments and this treatment was discontinued. The therapist was aware from nurses' observations that the patient had been able at times to complete relatively complex tasks (for example, washing clothes) but remained immobile the rest of the time in the patient's lounge. Thus, the therapist decided to prepare an activity schedule with the patient.

THERAPIST: I understand that you spend most of your day in the lounge. Is that true?

PATIENT: Yes, being quiet gives me the peace of mind I need.

T: When you sit here, how's your mood?

P: I feel awful all the time. I just wish I could fall in a hole somewhere and die.

T: Do you feel better after sitting for two or three hours?

P: No, the same.

T: So you're sitting in the hope that you'll find peace of mind, but it doesn't sound like your depression improves.

P: I get so bored.

T: Would you consider being more active? There are a number of reasons why I think increasing your activity level might help.

P: There's nothing to do around here.

T: Would you consider trying some activities if I could come up with a list?

P: If you think it will help, but I think you're wasting your time. I don't have any interests.

T: Let's find out whether I'm wasting my time. I would like to know whether you feel better or worse after some activities . . . to see how they affect your boredom. As for your interests, we should consider some of the things that please you *in the past* and see what reactions you have now—even though you aren't interested.

The patient and therapist then reviewed a list of potential activities available on the ward. The patient maintained that he wasn't interested in any of the activities (his reason for inactivity). Again, the therapist differentiated between (a) the goal of doing something interesting, and (b) being willing to do something that would break the pattern of inactivity.

THERAPIST: When do you *decide* to go and sit in the lounge?
PATIENT: Right after breakfast.
T: Okay, that's the first time we can concentrate on. Pick an activity that you would be willing to do right after breakfast.
P: Well, not exercise . . . I'd be sick if I exercised right after breakfast.
T: Well, how about an activity that will keep your mind active. We can put exercise down later in the morning if you agree.
P: I guess I could listen to the radio. (The therapist takes note of the slight change in the patient's attitude but recognizes this activity could be completed while sitting in the lounge.)
T: That would be okay if you would be distracted from your worries by the program. Is there some activity that you could do that would get you away from the lounge area?
P: I guess I could go to occupational therapy but I get bored too easily.
T: Going to O.T. sounds like a good idea. You could work on a specific project. What can you think of?
P: Maybe I could make a belt for my son.
T: That's good. Then we can find out more about what makes you feel bored. Do you know what thoughts you have when you get bored?
P: I don't know.
T: Well, why don't we set a goal of finding out? First, let's put occupational therapy on the activity schedule. Then, our second goal will be to "catch" the thoughts you have when you get bored. If you get bored then try to catch these thoughts and write them down. Later you can go on to the other activities,

> say to the exercise group, and then listen to the radio.
> (Therapist records activities on a list.) If you are bored, you
> can try to catch these thoughts . . . What are your reactions to
> this plan?
>
> P: I'm willing to try but I think you're wasting your time with me.

To the surprise of the staff members, the patient went to the occupational therapy program (which was headed by a behaviorally oriented therapist), where he remained for 40 minutes. He was able to notice some "boring" thoughts: "I've got to get out of here. I've got too much work to do at home" and, "If my boss saw me making a belt in here, he'd fire me for sure." These thoughts were discussed in the next therapy session. The patient reported feeling better for the first 30 minutes of the activity schedule but then felt "worse" after a period of ruminating about the consequences of his hospitalization.

It is worth noting that the patient recognized very informative cognitions in association with a sense of boredom. The therapist would not have found out about these depressing thoughts unless the activity schedule had been implemented and the patient assigned the task of recognizing his depressogenic thoughts. The drop in the patient's mood after 30 minutes was not truly a negative experience because it afforded the opportunity for collecting his specific negative cognitions. In the next two sessions, therapy focused on the patient's concern that his employer would criticize him for his depression. The patient continued with his activity-scheduling as homework. Within three days, his "boredom" decreased and later he even found some of the activities to be interesting.

A broader program involving an activity schedule can be used to help the patient who is relatively inactive but not immobile. The hour-to-hour schedule offers a specific, defined alternative to inactivity, and when the additional project of "catching" negative thoughts is included, the patient can use the structure provided by the activity schedule to obtain further useful information.

One of the potential problems with the assignment of an activity schedule is that the patient may react negatively if the schedule is rigid and demanding.

1. He will interpret his failure to maintain time schedules or complete every activity as a "serious sign."

2. He may interpret the need for an activity schedule as evidence of his degree of regression.

We have developed a specific technique (the graded task assignment) on the basis of these clinical experiences and research data. The technique is like the activity schedule in that it is used to increase activity, improve optimism, and elevate mood by demonstrating to the patient that his predictions about his abilities are unrealistically negative.

Graded Task Assignment. The choice of the graded task assignment instead of the standard activity schedule is based on the status of the patient. In general, with the more severely depressed patient, the graded task assignment is used so that the *therapy can monitor each step the patient makes.* The graded task assignment allows the therapist to break down a task into its components and tailor it to the behavioral level of the patient. The standard activity schedule, on the other hand, is more frequently employed with the patient whom the therapist judges to be capable of regular activities. Of course, the present distinction remains somewhat artificial without the knowledge of a particular patient. The two techniques can be employed concurrently when a patient is functioning at an acceptable level of activity but is attempting to master a more difficult task (and therefore could benefit from a graded task approach).

Impaired Coping with "Practical Problems"

The patient frequently presents practical problems he is encountering in his life. These might be difficulty in finding a job, problems with parenting, or general organizational problems. These practical problems, while not symptoms of depression, are discussed under the behavior section because they require that the patient do something to change his environment.

The therapist has to be able to discriminate between the patient's real problems and the patient's distortion of events. These practical problems shouldn't be avoided simply because of their nonpsychological nature. Solving practical problems often can ameliorate or lessen psychological problems. In a number of cases, psychological problems develop out of unresolved practical problems. This is a version of what Beck (1976) calls the "speck in the eye" syndrome: ". . . a person may writhe with pain and be unable to walk, eat, talk at length, or perform minimal constructive activities because of a speck in the eye. The 'speck in the eye' syndrome probably occurs more frequently among psychiatric patients than is generally realized." (p. 227)

One patient, for example, was able to avoid lengthy therapy by use of a simple intervention. The woman came to therapy complaining of fatigue and inability to cope with her everyday duties. An analysis of the problem revealed she was spending nearly all of her time chauffering five children to various activities. This left her little time for her other duties and virtually no free time. After she took the therapist's suggestion to hire a driver for the children, her psychological symptoms quickly disappeared.

If the patient has a problem that is beyond the therapist's competence, he should not hesitate in referring the patient to an expert. This referral might be for medical, legal, financial, or vocational consultation.

Social Skills Deficits

The depressed patient generally does not function at his normal level in nearly all areas of his life, including his social life. The patient may actively avoid others or too readily acquiesce to others' wishes. Usually the patient has adequate social skills but is not using them. The goal, therefore, becomes one of reactivating old skills rather than teaching new ones.

Many of the cognitive/behavioral procedures previously outlined, such as graded task assignments, behavioral rehearsal, and running experiments can be used to accomplish this goal. Standard assertive training methods are also employed. Because there are a number of excellent books on assertive training, these methods will not be described here.

PHYSIOLOGICAL SYMPTOMS

Sleep Disturbance

Sleeping difficulty is one of the most striking symptoms of

depression. The majority of clinically depressed patients have some form of sleep disturbance. These problems include problems in falling asleep, restless sleep, and early morning waking. Generally the patient regains his normal sleeping pattern after his depression lifts.

The therapist usually has to provide the patient with basic information about sleep. Although depressed patients do sleep less than normals, many patients exaggerate the extent of the insomnia. The patient who says he was awake all night was probably in a light sleep for a good part of the time. The patient's minimization of actual time slept is often coupled with the belief that he needs more sleep than he actually does. One patient, for example, believed he was seriously endangering his health by not getting enough sleep. This type of thinking naturally increases the insomnia. The therapist should correct these misconceptions and stress that lost sleep is not a catastrophe since lost sleep can easily be recouped.

The patient can be told that as he improves in other areas of his life he will begin to sleep better. For example, if a patient is spending a large part of his day sitting in a chair, lying on a sofa or taking naps, he probably won't feel like sleeping at night. However, once the patient becomes more active, particularly if this includes some form of physical activity, he will naturally sleep better at night. Although exercise allows the patient to sleep better, this exercise should not be done prior to going to bed as the exercise can activate the patient.

The usual treatment for sleep disturbance is to teach the patient how to relax; this can be done with cassette tape recorders. Some standard relaxation methods are used with the addition of having the patient visualize some pleasant scene while trying to sleep. The patient can also relax by taking deep breaths or using yoga exercises.

The patient is encouraged to discover what his natural sleeping cycle is and to go to bed only when he is tired. A fixed routine right before going to bed, such as having a glass of milk, can be helpful. Stimulants such as coffee or tea should be avoided prior to going to bed. And, finally, if the patient cannot sleep, it is better for him to get out of bed and to do something than to lie awake and experience unpleasant thoughts.

Appetite and Sexual Disturbances

Loss of appetite and loss of interest in sex are often first signs of depression. Both symptoms appear to be manifestations of the patient's generalized loss of pleasure in activities. As the person's depression lifts, his appetite for food and sex usually returns. Simply telling the patient this can be helpful.

Decreased appetite or loss of sexual interest usually doesn't bother the depressed patient to a great extent. For this reason, these symptoms are rarely targeted for change. When they are targeted, sensory awareness exercises and having the patient strongly challenge "kill-joy" thoughts are helpful procedures. The therapist also should be on the alert for any sensual activities in which the patient may be overindulging. Overindulgence in one sensual modality often results in loss of pleasure in other modalities.

Some patients overeat and gain weight when they become depressed, while others gain weight when mildly depressed and lose weight when severely depressed. Patients often are concerned about weight gain. Because undertaking a regimen for losing weight is a difficult process for a depressed patient, the initial goal is to have the patient just maintain his present weight and stop gaining. When the patient begins to feel better, he can attempt to lose weight. Cognitive and behavioral methods are used for weight reduction. For a more detailed discussion of these methods, see Mahoney and Mahoney (1976) and Emery (1977).

SOCIAL CONTEXT OF SYMPTOMS

As pointed out previously, a skillful interviewer is able to weave questions regarding symptoms in and out of those relevant to the patient's actual life situation and his idiosyncratic way of construing his current experiences. Thus, most of the symptoms tend to be related to a specific social setting. The patient's feelings of guilt, reduction of satisfaction, withdrawal, and apparent retardation are generally wrapped up in how he interprets specific external events, how he evaluates himself, and how he believes others evaluate him.

Take, for example, a middle-aged lawyer who says he wants professional help because he wants to separate from his wife. We learn, however, that he has a broad range of symptoms: hopelessness, suicidal wishes, social withdrawal, loss of gratification, guilty feelings, loss of motivation, indecisiveness, self-criticisms, and self-blame.

As his story unfolds we realize that practically all of his symptoms are related to each other and have a definite meaning in terms of the social context. He has *withdrawn* from his associates at his office and from his friends because he believes that he is a bore and a failure and that he imposes a burden on them. He *criticizes* himself for not being more friendly and for "ducking" his responsibilities at his job and at home. He *avoids* carrying out responsibilities and he has no motivation to undertake any activity because he believes he will do a bad job. His *lack of gratification* is related to his constant criticism of himself whenever he engages in professional, social, or solitary activities. He feels *sad* because of his disappointment over his perceived failures. He feels *guilty* because he believes he has let down everyone important to him: his wife, his friends, his law partners, and his clients. He is *hopeless* in that he believes that his present inadequacies are irreversible and he, thus, will continue to fail (if he undertakes anything) and will continue to suffer for his failures. Since his present life is devoid of any satisfactions and is heavily laden with painful feelings of guilt and sadness and he can see no likelihood for any improvement, he seeks a way to escape. The only way out that he can think of is to end his life; thus, he is *suicidal.* All of this patient's symptoms are interrelated because they share a common link to the core psychological problem: the patient's negative view of himself, his future, and his experiences. This negative construction is superimposed on every relationship, activity, or experience that is meaningful to him.

Now, how do we explain the patient's "reason" for seeking help? We find that he wants a separation or divorce because he believes he is a burden on his wife as a result of his many presumed failings. However, as long as he shares a home with her, he cannot avoid her the way he avoids his business associates and friends. By becoming separated from her, he believes he can remove a blight on her life.

In "attacking" the target symptoms, the therapist has to be aware of how they are interrelated and how they are related to interpersonal relationships, role expectations, and activities. Above all, he has to unravel the relationship between the symptoms and the patient's systematic negative bias in evaluating himself and his experiences. In sum, the symptoms have to be viewed concomitantly in a social context (the significant interpersonal relationships) and from a cognitive perspective (the meaning of his experiences). As the therapist helps the patient to design a therapeutic program, he needs to apply each project to a specific situation which is related to the specific symptoms and to the overall negative conceptualizations.

Chapter 10

SPECIFIC TECHNIQUES
FOR THE SUICIDAL PATIENT

Assessing Suicidal Risk

Since suicidal wishes are a prevalent and potentially lethal problem in depressed patients, it is important for the therapist to understand why the patient is considering such a drastic action. The therapist will then be in a better position to select appropriate and effective techniques to deal with this particular problem. However, no anti-suicidal strategy is of any use unless the therapist is able to detect and assess the degree of suicidal intentionality.

Many professionals still believe the myth that questioning a depressed person about the presence of suicidal ideas may "put the idea in his head" or make the idea of suicide more acceptable if he is already thinking about it. Actually, we have found that encouraging a patient to talk about his suicidal ideas generally helps him to view them more objectively, provides necessary information for therapeutic intervention, and offers some degree of relief.

Therapists as well as friends and family members are often surprised by a patient's suicidal attempt because they are aware only of the factors that would (according to their perspective) favor his desire to continue living. Following this suicide attempt, they may say, "He seemed to be in good spirits," "He had everything to live for," or "He was making real progress in therapy." Such statements indicate that the therapist and the persons in the immediate social environment were either oblivious to the clues to suicidal wishes or that the individual was adept at concealing his suicidal thoughts. Further, these statements illustrate the incongruity between the patient's own perception of his life situation and the "more realistic" perception of the significant persons in his social environment.

In assessing the suicidal risk of an individual, the professional must consider such factors as the method contemplated by an individual, his familiarity with lethal dosages of drugs or other forms of self-destruction, and access to the suicide method, such as firearms or an adequate number of sleeping pills. Another factor to be considered is the presence of environmental resources for intervention, which include the likelihood of detection of suicidal intent by another individual, of intervention in time to prevent the suicide attempt, and of assistance in obtaining immediate and adequate medical help following a suicide attempt. Of course, the presence of a viable social support system is a therapeutic resource.

Clues to suicide plans may be detected in overt behaviors such as secretiveness, a sudden decision to make a will, or verbal statements. A suicidal individual may say, for example, "I don't want to go on living" or "I want to end it all." Other statements suggestive of suicidal intent include: "I'm not going to put up with it anymore," "I'm a burden on everyone," "Things will never get better," and "My whole life has been a waste." Sometimes the expression of suicidal intent is indirect and may be pieced together only in retrospect. For example, a depressed patient leaving on a weekend pass from a hospital may say, "I guess I won't be seeing you again" or "I want to thank you for *trying* so hard to help me." Or on retiring for the night, the patient may say "goodbye" instead of "goodnight." It is important to note that 40% of attempted and completed suicides had visited medical and psychiatric services in the week prior to the suicidal action (Yessler, Gibbs, and Becker, 1961).

Some systematic studies have shown that a period of calm may follow a decision to commit suicide (Keith-Spiegel and Spiegel, 1967). A sudden appearance of tranquility in a previously agitated patient is a danger signal that is often misinterpretated by others as a sign of improvement. This misinterpretation leads to a decrease of vigilance, which facilitates a successful suicide attempt.

SUICIDAL INTENT AS A CONTINUUM

A person's degree of suicidal intent may be regarded as a point on a continuum. At one extreme is an absolute intention to kill oneself and at the other extreme is an intention to go on living. Many different forms of intent may be found along the continuum. A gamble with death is exemplified by an individual who plays Russian roulette with a sense of resignation to the probabilities of his dying. Another point on the continuum is illustrated by a rejected woman who took a potentially lethal overdose of a sedative and then called her lover. She thought of leaving it to Fate as to whether her lover would come in time to save her life. Presumably, if he did not love her enough to rush to rescue her, then she would die. Also on the continuum of suicidal intent is the individual who simply wants to stop living. Although statements such as "I cannot stand things anymore" do not necessarily represent a wish to kill oneself, they are frequently a manifestation of a desire to block out all experience or sadness, at least for a period of time. The desire of a depressed patient to escape life may be so great that the idea of suicide represents a relief from his present situation.

Chance factors may operate in tipping the balance in favor of commiting suicide. For example, a man who was chronically suicidal managed to contain his suicidal impulse until his wife informed him that she was pregnant. The prospect of fatherhood tilted him toward a fatal suicide attempt. Similarly, a patient with periodic depressions accompanied by suicidal wishes always turned for support to his physician when he felt his suicidal wishes getting stronger. When his physician cancelled an appointment because of illness, the patient proceeded to commit suicide. His suicide note indicated that he regarded the cancelled appointment as the "last straw" in a series of disappointments.

In contrast, a highly suicidal patient was interrupted in the act of hanging himself by the unexpected arrival of a friend. This accidental demonstration of friendship shifted his thinking away from suicide.

EXPLORING MOTIVES FOR SUICIDE

As we will discuss later, the therapist should start to deal therapeutically with suicidal wishes in the initial interview. The reasons elicited from a patient for his suicide attempt or his current suicide wishes provide a promising point of entry for early intervention.

We have found that the reasons most commonly reported by patients for their recent suicide attempts or suicidal wishes are easily categorized. Some patients state that their goal is to give up and escape from life and to seek surcease: Life is "simply too much" or "not worth living." Their inner mental or emotional distress is intolerable; they see no way out of their problematic situations and are "tired of fighting."

Other suicide attempters report that they have gambled with death in order to produce some interpersonal change. They hoped that the suicide attempt would bring back some emotionally important person, make others realize that "help is needed," resolve some environmental problem, or help them get into the hospital as a temporary respite from their surroundings. We have often observed a combination of the above motives, namely both escape from life and manipulation of others. When the motive is primarily manipulative, the suicide attempt is less serious than when the primary goal is escape from life.

Of the 200 patients in a sample of patients hospitalized for attempted suicide, 111 (56%) reported reasons for their suicide attempt that belonged in the escape/surcease category. In brief, the majority of the patients regarded living as undesirable, wanted to escape from life, and were attracted to suicide as the only viable solution to their problems. In contrast, 13% of the patients indicated that they attempted suicide for the sole purpose of taking a chance on producing some change in others or in the environment.

The remaining 31% of the sample reported varying combinations of escape and manipulative motives for their suicide attempts. Those patients who scored high on hopelessness and high on depression were more likely to report "escape from life" and "surcease" as the reasons for their suicide attempts. In contrast, the less hopeless and less depressed patients tended to designate manipulative reasons for their suicidal acts (Kovacs, Beck, and Weissman, 1975).

As the crucial first stage in helping the suicidal patient, *the therapist must step into his world and view it through the patient's lens.* The type of self-destructive motive that is reported can guide the clinician's decisions regarding therapeutic focus and technique. For example, if the patient's goal is to find surcease, to escape into death through suicide, his hopelessness and lack of positive expectations would be the focal point. If his hopeless outlook is largely based on reality, as for instance in extreme poverty, medical disorder, or social isolation, appropriate social intervention would be indicated.

However, when the pervasive negative expectations, the hallmarks of hopelessness, are based on distorted or pathological ways of viewing oneself and the world, the therapist should focus on the misconceptions and irrational belief systems.

If a patient has attempted suicide in order to affect or influence other people, the therapist could help him to sort out his various manipulative motives. Was the suicide attempt prompted by the desire for love and affection, by the need to take revenge, or by the need to express hostile feelings? Was it related to a breakdown of conventional modes of interpersonal communication? If the goal of influencing another person through the suicide attempt is, for example, related to an inability to communicate his problems, the therapist might focus on identifying maladaptive or deficient interpersonal techniques and teach the patient more adaptive methods of relating to other people.

The therapist must be able to sense why the patient feels driven to kill himself and to experience, to some degree, the patient's despair and frenzy. Such understanding and empathy not only enable the therapist to adapt his helping strategies to the specific needs of the patient but communicate to the patient that he is "understood." The therapist should be able to play with the notion that, given the patient's premises, the suicidal wishes are not "crazy"—but indeed may seem a logical deduction from these premises. Then he can work with the patient to uncover the erroneous assumptions or faulty logic that provides the groundwork for the suicidal impulse.

TIPPING THE BALANCE AGAINST SUICIDE

At the outset, it is important for the therapist to "play for time" until the danger period for suicide has passed. One strategy for influencing the patient to postpone suicide is to get him so involved in the process of therapy that he decides to "stick it out" until he sees where the therapy is going. Thus, the therapist needs to arouse and maintain the patient's curiosity and to stimulate his interest in his therapeutic approach. Further, the therapist should maintain the patient's curiosity and to stimulate his interest in his therapeutic approach. Further, the therapist should maintain a continuity between sessions. He can, for example, build the bridge to the next

213

session by eliciting questions from the patient and then responding with statements such as, "That's an intriguing question. I have some ideas about it now but we will go into it more fully next time. Would you be willing to jot down some of your own thoughts about that question between now and the next appointment?"

It is not necessary, nor even possible in most cases, to obtain a valid commitment from the patient that he will *never* commit suicide. A promise or "contract" to postpone suicide for a week or two may not be honored under the pressure of a strong wish to die. By regarding his wishes objectively and acknowledging the possibility that they may be based on invalid reasoning, the patient may feel motivated to defer acting on his suicidal wishes until he has explored them further with the therapist.

As he formulates his treatment plan, it is useful for the therapist to treat the decision to commit suicide as the outcome of the struggle between the patient's wishes to live versus his wishes to die. As in a declaration of war, an irrevocable decision may be made on the basis of a margin of a single vote, as it were. Initially, therefore, the therapist's efforts should be directed toward shifting the votes in favor of living.

Once the patient has agreed to weigh the pros and cons of suicide, then the therapist can proceed to elicit "Reasons for Living" and "Reasons for Dying." Although the patient may initially have difficulty in offering any reasons for living right now, he is generally able to recall his reasons for living during a previous, happier period. A technical aid is to draw two columns on a blackboard or a sheet of paper. The therapist and patient can then list reasons in favor of living that were valid in the past. The therapist proceeds to ascertain which of the "past" reasons for living are valid in the present or at least might be valid in the future. It is interesting to note that the suicidal patient has often nullified these positive factors in his life: (a) He has forgotten them, (b) ignored them, or (c) discounted their value. By injecting the reasons for living into the patient's appraisal of his life situation, the therapist is able to provide a counterbalance to the reasons for dying.

The therapist should exercise caution in suggesting the positive factors in the patient's life. If the patient senses that the therapist is trying to "talk him out of" suicide, he may become negativistic. Thus, the approach should have an empirical flavor, as if to say,

"Even though you may be convinced that your decision is right, it is worthwhile to list the positive factors in your life and see what you think of them." Then the therapist may suggest that the patient rate how valuable each of these factors is.

After listing the advantages of living, the therapist and patient can then list the advantages and disadvantages of dying. After this procedure, the suicidal patient generally increases his objectivity, and his reasons for dying do not seem as absolute and compelling as previously.

It is essential that the therapist take the patient's reasons for dying seriously and not cavalierly dismiss what might seem to him to be a trivial or irrational reason for suicide. Above all, he should avoid the use of ploys such as stating flippantly, "If you want to kill yourself, go ahead and do it."

The therapist should also recognize that it may be quite painful for the patient to reconsider his decision to kill himself. The patient may have undergone enormous turmoil before arriving at his decision to terminate his suffering via suicide, and reopening the question may mean to him that he will have to go through another period of turmoil and prolong his pain.

Dealing with Hopelessness

When asked why he wants to commit suicide, the seriously suicidal patient generally gives responses such as the following:

1. There is no point to living. I have nothing to look forward to.
2. I just can't stand life. I can never be happy.
3. I am feeling so miserable this is the only way I can escape.
4. I am a burden to my family and they will be better off without me.

Note that all of these statements are related in some sense to hopelessness. The patient typically regards suicide as the most attractive way of dealing with his problems. He sees himself as trapped in a bad situation from which there is no escape and he views continuation in this situation as unbearable. He regards suicide as the only way of dealing with his "insoluble" problems.

If hopelessness is at the core of the suicidal wishes, a variety of methods can be used to convey to the patient that (a) there are alternative interpretations of his life situation and of his future that are less dire than those he entertains, and (b) he has other choices than his current behavior, which may, indeed, be leading to a blind alley. A seemingly prosaic example of nonadaptive behavior is illustrated by a young woman who had become increasingly desperate and suicidal because her boyfriend had not called her for several days. When asked whether there was anything she could do besides sitting by the telephone and waiting for him to call, she brightened and responded, "Well, I could call him."

We attempt to discuss the patient's sense of hopelessness *in the first interview*. Later, we try to induce him to recognize the degree of illogical thinking and erroneous assumptions that go into the hopeless thinking. We have developed a Hopelessness Scale that serves as a useful adjunct for indirectly assessing the degree of suicidal risk (Beck et al., 1974). A high score on this scale is almost always a sign of high suicidal intent and, in fact, is a better predictor of suicidal intent than is depression (Beck et al., 1975). This scale, which takes only a few minutes to complete, may be given to the suicidal patient prior to each interview—in order to provide the therapist with a quick reading of the present suicidal risk.

If the clinical and psychometric assessment indicates a high level of hopelessness and associated suicidal wishes, the therapist must gear his therapeutic approach to *deal with these problems immediately*. He cannot afford the luxury of waiting several sessions for the picture to develop. If the patient's urge to kill himself is not explored promptly, the patient may not be alive at the time of the next scheduled interview. Furthermore, it is often desirable to keep in telephone contact with the patient until the suicidal crisis has passed. Sometimes, it is useful to apprise members of the family, or a friend, of the problem and obtain their cooperation in carrying out a therapeutic regime.

The particular therapeutic strategy used in dealing with the patient's hopelessness is based on the premise that he is locked in by his arbitrary conclusions. It does not occur to him to question these beliefs. Even when they are questioned by the therapist, they appear reasonable to him. However, by engaging his interests in exploring the validity of his fixed notions, we can unlock this closed system. As he reflects on evidence bearing on his fixed belief, he himself may then recall information that contradicts this belief. By introducing "cognitive dissonance," that is, demonstrating the inner contradictions in the belief system, we can open up this closed system to reason and to corrective information. One technique illustrated in some of the cases in this chapter is to introduce evidence that is contradictory to the fixed beliefs. Since the patient's beliefs cannot readily accommodate the anomaly, they become more accessible to modification.

A woman experienced intense suicidal wishes after having broken up with her second husband. When the therapist questioned her regarding why she felt that suicide was the only answer to her problems, she said, "I can't live without Peter." When questioned further, she said, "I just can't get along without a man."

When asked whether she always had needed a man in order to exist, the patient experienced a "cognitive click." With an expression of enlightenment she stated, "Actually the best time in my life was when I was completely alone. My ex-husband was in the army and I was working and living alone." The anomaly in this instance was the fact that she had done well by herself. This bit of evidence undermined her idea, "If I am alone, I am helpless." With her recognition of the fallacy of this idea, her attitude about her own competence began to change. She regained a sense of independence and control over her life and her suicidal wishes gradually disappeared.

Another example of how a patient may become aware of the logical inconsistencies in her belief system is presented in the following interchange with a 25-year-old woman who had made a recent suicide attempt and still wanted to commit suicide. She regarded her life as "finished" since her husband was unfaithful. An interesting aspect of the therapeutic technique is the therapist's consistent use of questions to obtain information contradictory to her conclusions and also to draw her into thinking logically.*

> THERAPIST: Why do you want to end your life?
> PATIENT: Without Raymond, I am nothing . . . I can't be happy without Raymond. . . . But I can't save our marriage.
> T: What has your marriage been like?
> P: It has been miserable from the very beginning . . . Raymond has always been unfaithful . . . I have hardly seen him in the past five years.
> T: You say that you can't be happy without Raymond . . . Have

---

* This transcript is an expanded record of an interview previously printed in *Cognitive Therapy and the Emotional Disorders* (Beck, 1976, pp. 289–291).

you found yourself happy when you are with Raymond?

P: No, we fight all the time and I feel worse.

T: Then why do you feel that Raymond is essential for your living?

P: I guess it's because without Raymond I am nothing.

T: Would you please repeat that?

P: *Without Raymond I am nothing.*

T: What do you think of that idea?

P: . . . Well, now that I think about it, I guess it's not completely true.

T: You said you are "nothing" without Raymond. Before you met Raymond, did you feel you were "nothing"?

P: No, I felt I was somebody.

T: Are you saying then that it's possible to be something without Raymond?

P: I guess that's true. I *can* be something without Raymond.

T: If you were somebody before you knew Raymond, why do you need him to be somebody now?

P: (puzzled) Hmmm . . .

T: You seemed to imply that you couldn't go on living without Raymond.

P: Well, I just don't think that I can find anybody else like him.

T: Did you have male friends before you knew Raymond?

P: I was pretty popular then.

T: If I understand you correctly then, you were able to fall in love before with other men and other men have fallen in love with you.

P: Uh huh.

T: Why do you think you will be unpopular without Raymond now?

P: Because I will not be able to attract any other man.

T: Have any men shown an interest in you since you have been married?

P: A lot of men have made passes at me but I ignore them.

T: If you were free of the marriage, do you think that men might be interested in you—knowing that you were available?

P: I guess that maybe they would be.

T: Is it possible that you might find a man who would be more constant than Raymond?

P: I don't know, . . . I guess it's possible.

T: Do you think there are other men as good as Raymond around?

P: I guess there are men who are better than Raymond because Raymond doesn't love me.

T: You said that you can't stand the idea of losing the marriage. Is it correct that you have hardly seen your husband in the past five years?

P: That's right. I only see him a couple of times a year.

T: Is there any chance of your getting back together with him?

P: No, . . . he has another woman. He doesn't want me.

T: Then what have you actually lost if you break up the marriage?

P: I don't know.

T: Is it possible that you'll get along better if you end the marriage?

P: There is no guarantee of that.

T: Do you have a *real marriage*?

P: I guess not.

T: If you don't have a real marriage, what do you actually lose if you decide to end the marriage?

P: (crying) Nothing, I guess.

T: Well, what do you think your chances are that you can find somebody else?

P: I know what you are getting at and I know you are right. I've actually thought of that myself. . . . There is no reason why I should go on hanging on to Raymond when he doesn't want me. I guess the thing to do is just make a clean break.

T: Do you think that if you make a clean break, you will be able to get attached to another man?

P: I've been able to fall in love with other men before.

T: Well, what do you think—you can again?

P: I guess I'll be able to do it again.

At this point it was apparent from the discussion that the patient was no longer as depressed and, upon inquiry, it was clear that she was no longer suicidal. The thrust of the therapy was to get her to see that she was not losing anything by breaking with Raymond (since the relationship was already dead) and that there were *other options* open to her. The therapist also started to make a dent in her formula: "Unless I am loved, I am nothing."

Following this interview, the patient was more cheerful and it appeared that she was over the suicidal crisis. In a subsequent interview, she stated that the question that really struck home was: How could she be "nothing" without Raymond—when she had lived happily and was an adequate person before she even knew him? On the basis of reviewing the questions posed during the interview, she decided to seek a legal separation. She eventually was divorced and settled down to a more stable life.

In this case, the questioning was directed toward the patient's beliefs that (a) she needed her husband in order to be happy, to function, and to have an identity, (b) that she had a viable—or at least a salvageable—marriage, (c) that the end of the marriage would be a devastating, irreversible loss, and (d) she could have no future life without her husband. The patient was able to recognize the fallacy of her beliefs and her either-or thinking; consequently, she realized she had options other than the two she had considered: *either* trying to preserve a dead marriage *or* committing suicide. In other cases, the therapist needs to work with the patient to generate realistic alternatives to self-destructive courses of action.

Problem-Solving with Suicidal Patients

Many suicidal patients have realistic problems that contribute to their hopelessness and desire to die. These environmental factors cover the entire gamut of human stresses, but there are a few general categories that seem to account for the majority of such factors.

Our analysis of the case histories given by *males* who have attempted suicide suggests that the most common single stressor precipitating the suicidal attempt was related to their performance at work or at school. When there was a large discrepancy between the individual's expectations of himself and his actual performance, he was prone to experience a sharp decline in his self-esteem and outlook for the future. In a typical case of a suicide-prone individual, the loss of self-esteem generalized into a notion such as, "I'm worthless, . . . I've let everybody down." The natural sequence then was: "There's nowhere for me to turn. I just can't make it in this world. There's no way out except to kill myself."

Typical precipitating factors are illustrated by the following males who attempted suicide. A 12-year-old boy whose grade average at preparatory school fell to the point that his scholarship was in jeopardy became increasingly agitated. He thought, "My mother will be disappointed in me . . . I will have to go to public school . . . I'll never be successful . . . I'm a failure." He attempted to hang himself but was rescued in the nick of time.

His mother, indeed, had unreasonably rigid expectations of him and was disappointed and rejecting of him for his "failure" at school. Part of the treatment, thus, was directed toward moderating his mother's demands and disapproval of him. The boy himself had to define his problem: (a) Decide what he wanted to do; that is, whether to transfer to public school where he would be under less competitive pressure or remain in preparatory school where he could get a better education. Thus, he needed to recognize that there were advantages to each course of action and that neither choice would be "disastrous." (b) Learn to cope with his mother by standing up to her and conveying the attitude, "This is my life, not yours."

A contrasting example is provided by a head of a family who had lost his job. His thoughts ran the usual sequence from "I am worthless" to "My family would be better off if I were dead." The type of intervention involved (a) defining the problem in getting another job, and (b) obtaining sufficient funds to support his family until he was re-employed. The psychological intervention consisted of asking him to list the ways in which his family would benefit from his death and then list their feelings at losing him. By playing the role of a member in his family he was able to experience the grief they would feel if he died.

We found that suicide attempts among females were often preceded by friction in or disruption of their relationships with another person. One woman felt disturbed because her husband spent increasingly less time at home. Her sequence of ideas spread from "I'm losing Tom" to "I'd be better off dead." In this case, the realistic problem centered around her realistically difficult relationship with her husband. The patient required some coaching in dealing more effectively with her husband. If this procedure had proved to be insufficient, then marital counseling would have been indicated.

In each of these cases cited above, "real life" problems were involved: (a) making a decision about school, (b) making arrangements for finding a new job and arranging for unemployment compensation, or (c) trying to improve an unsatisfactory relationship with a spouse.

In proposing solutions to these problems, the therapist must bear in mind that the patient's thick layer of pessimism is likely to engulf any constructive alternatives that may be suggested. Since the patient regards his options in a negatively distorted way, the therapist must be wary not to accept at its face value the patient's blanket rejection of a plan. The patient's choice of suicide as a reasonable course of action is often based on his unrealistically negative appraisal of the prognosis for solutions to his problems. This type of "solution" also reflects the patient's dichotomous (either-or) thinking: *"Either* my husband returns to me *or* I will have to commit suicide." *"Either* I obtain a scholarship *or* I will have to drop out of school."

Stress-Inoculation Technique

The types of life situations that seem related to many suicidal attempts do not appear to be very unusual. In fact, most people in our culture have experienced such stresses at some time or another.

Why then do some people think of suicide when confronted with a serious problem, while others either make adaptive attempts to solve the problem or else decide to "live with it," albeit unhappily? Unfortunately, we don't know the complete answer to this question, but we have some hints from our clinical studies.

Suicide-prone individuals have a particular disposition to over-estimate the magnitude and insolubility of problems. Thus, small problems are perceived as large and large problems are overwhelming. Furthermore, these individuals show as incredible lack of confidence in their own resources for solving problems. Finally, they tend to project a resulting picture of doom into the future. Thus, they show the cardinal features of the Cognitive Triad: an exaggerated negative view of the outside world, themselves, and their future.

Another characteristic demarcates suicidal from nonsuicidal patients. The suicide-prone individual has somehow incorporated the notion of the acceptability or desirability of solving problems through death: "All of my problems would be over if I were dead." Whereas the average person may become frustrated at not having any ready solution for a major problem, he has some tolerance for uncertainty: "Maybe I'll be able to solve it and maybe I won't." Furthermore, in the course of time, he attempts a variety of solutions. The suicide-prone person, on the other hand, has a very low tolerance for uncertainty. If he cannot think of an immediate solution, the idea of future doom is triggered, which, in turn, triggers the idea, "Death is the only solution."

The resultant desire to die may reach fantastic proportions. In a sense, suicide serves as a kind of "opiate" for this kind of person and, analogous to the drug-dependent person, the suicide-prone individual regards his own idiosyncratic form of "relief" as highly desirable.

The patient's suicide-proneness should be a major target in therapy. One approach that appears promising consists of training the patient in (a) thinking of solutions to problems and (b) focusing attention away (distraction) from suicidal wishes much as is done with obsessions or pain (Meichenbaum, 1977). Preparation for meeting problems consists of outlining typical stresses that are likely to occur and asking the patient to engage in generating solutions. A "forced fantasy" technique (cognitive rehearsal) can be used with many patients. They are asked to:

1. Imagine themselves in a desperate situation
2. Try to experience the typical despair and suicidal impulses
3. Attempt—despite the distraction of the stimulated "suicidal impulses"—to generate possible solutions to the problems.

The patient is then encouraged to practice this technique in real life situations; that is, actively plunging into an unpleasant situation (for example, confrontations with a spouse) and then attempting to think of realistic solutions to the problems that arise. Along the same lines, the stress-inoculation technique is used to train the patient to distract himself away from his preoccupations with suicide. A somewhat similar approach has been used by Dr. Keith Hawton at Oxford. He attempts to prepare the patient for future crises by the following strategy: He presents the patient with hypothetical but realistic crisis-provoking situations similar to those which the patient has experienced in the past; then, they examine in detail alternative courses of action which could be followed should that situation occur. Similarly, the patient can be induced to re-live previous crises that precipitated suicidal impulses and to imagine applying adaptive coping techniques to those impulses.

INCREASES IN SUICIDAL WISHES DURING THERAPY

The therapist should recognize that wishes to die may fluctuate considerably during the course of treatment. He should convey this fact to the patient and warn him that a sudden recrudescence of suicidal impulses should not be interpreted as a sign that he has not made progress in therapy. Relatively early in the course of treatment, the therapist should review with the suicide-prone patient various strategies that he can use to cope with the sudden arousal or intensification of suicidal impulses. The therapist can prepare the patient with a statement such as the following:

> One of the important goals of therapy is to learn how to cope effectively with suicidal impulses. So you ought to be on the lookout for these wishes. As soon as you become aware of them, you should rehearse the steps to take to cope with them. In this way, your suicidal wishes can provide you with a valuable learning experience. In fact—if you'd like—we can practice right now what you would do in the event that you experience a wish to die.

The therapist should be continuously alert to the effects of traumatic experiences outside of therapy that may arouse or exacerbate suicidal wishes. We have treated several patients who were not notably suicidal at the beginning of therapy but who became suicidal subsequently as the result of adverse events. One patient, for instance, became acutely suicidal after a rejection by her boyfriend. The therapist had to dissect out in meticulous detail why the rejection led inexorably to the decision to die. A nest of unreasonable attitudes was uncovered; for example, the notion, "I can't live without love." "If nobody loves me, I am nothing." "Dying is the only relief for my pain."

Patients who have made suicide attempts prior to therapy are particularly prone to experience an exacerbation of suicidal wishes in the course of therapy; that is, the usual stresses of living are likely to stimulate suicidal wishes or actual suicide attempts—even though the therapy appears to be progressing. Some patients become discouraged if they experience increased suicidal wishes and conclude that they have made no progress in therapy or that therapy is ineffective. Such patients should be informed that suicidal impulses can be used as a valuable focus for therapy. The therapist's stance should be that such an event represents an opportunity rather than a setback: therapy can actually be helped by the recurrences of suicidal wishes, which can then be "worked through" in the therapeutic situations.

Note: The therapist should be sensitive in discriminating whether a recrudescence of suicidal wishes is related to some covert problem in the therapist–patient relationship (for example, the patient's belief that the therapist is rejecting him or that the therapist is incapable of helping) or to problems not directly related to the psychotherapy.

Chapter 11

INTERVIEW WITH A
DEPRESSED SUICIDAL PATIENT

A test of the value of cognitive therapy is the range of its applicability across a broad range of clinical problems and a diversity of patients. In order to pass this test, the system of psychotherapy must provide a sufficiently flexible conceptual framework and an adequate number of techniques to meet the varying requirements of a given patient at various times as well as those of different patients.

Perhaps the most critical challenge to the adequacy of cognitive therapy is its efficacy in dealing with the acutely suicidal patient. In such cases the therapist often has to shift gears and assume a very active role in attempting to penetrate the barrier of hopelessness and resignation. Since his intervention may be decisive in saving the patient's life, he has to draw on his ingenuity and attempt to accomplish a number of immediate goals either concurrently or in rapid sequence: establish a working relationship with the patient, assess the severity of the depression and suicidal wishes, obtain an overview of the patient's life situation, pinpoint his "reasons" for wanting to commit suicide, determine the patient's capacity for self-objectivity, and ferret out some entry point for stepping into the patient's phenomenological world and thus introduce elements of reality.

Such a venture, as illustrated in the following interview, is taxing and demands all the qualities of a "good therapist"—genuine warmth, acceptance, and empathetic understanding—as well as the application of the appropriate strategies drawn from the system of cognitive therapy.

The patient was a 40-year-old clinical psychologist who had recently been left by her boyfriend. She had a history of intermittent depressions since the age of 12 years, had received many courses of psychotherapy, antidepressant drugs, electroconvulsive therapy, and hospitalizations. The patient had been seen by the present therapist (A.T.B.) five times over a period of 7 or 8 months. At the time of this interview, it was obvious that she was depressed and, as indicated by her previous episodes, probably suicidal.

In the first part of the interview, the main thrust was to *ask appropriate questions* in order to make a clinical assessment and also to try to elucidate the major psychological problems. The therapist, first of all, had to make an assessment as to how depressed and how suicidal the patient was. He also had to assess her expectations regarding being helped by the interview (T1;T8) in order to determine how much leverage he had. During this period of time, in order to keep the dialogue going, he also had to repeat the patient's statements.

It was apparent from the emergence of suicidal wishes that this was the salient clinical problem and that her hopelessness (T7) would be the most appropriate point for intervention.

Several points could be made regarding the first part of the interview. The therapist accepted the seriousness of the patient's desire to die but treated it as a topic for further examination, a problem to be discussed. "We can discuss the advantages and disadvantages" (T11). She responded to this statement with some amusement (a favorable sign). The therapist also tried to test the patient's ability to look at herself and her problems with objectivity. He also attempted to test the fixity of her irrational ideas and the degree of her acceptance of his wish to help her (T13–T20).

In the first part of the interview the therapist was not able to make much headway because of the patient's strongly held belief that things could not possibly work out well for her. She had decided that suicide was the only solution, and she resented attempts to "get her to change her mind."

In the next part of the interview, the therapist attempted to isolate the participating factor in her present depression and suicidal ideation, namely, the breakup with her boyfriend. It becomes clear as the therapist tries to explore the significance of the breakup that the meaning to the patient is, "I have nothing" (P23). The therapist then selects, *"I have nothing"* as a target and attempts to elicit from the patient information contradictory to this conclusion. He probes for a previous period of time when she did not believe "I have nothing" and also was not having a relationship with a man. He then proceeds (T26) to probe for other goals and objects that are important to her; he seeks concrete sources of satisfaction (T24–T33). The therapist's attempt to establish that the patient does, indeed, "have something" is parried by the patient's tendency to discount any positive features in her life (P32).

Finally, the patient does join forces with the therapist, and it is apparent in the latter part of the interview that she is willing to separate herself from her problems and consider ways of solving them. The therapist then moves to a consideration of the basic assumptions underlying her hopelessness, namely, "I cannot be happy without a man." By pointing out disconfirming past experiences, he tries to demonstrate the error of this assumption. He also attempts to explain the value of shifting to the assumption, "I can make myself happy." He points out that it is more realistic for her to regard herself as the active agent in seeking out sources of satisfaction than as an inert receptacle dependent for nourishment on the whims of others.

The taped interview, which was edited down from 60 minutes to 35 minutes for practical reasons, is presented verbatim. (The only changes made were to protect the identity of the patient.) The interview is divided into five parts.

PART 1: QUESTIONING TO ELICIT VITAL INFORMATION

1. How depressed is patient? How suicidal?
2. Attitude about coming to appointment (expectancy about therapy).
3. Emergence of suicidal wishes: immediate critical problem.
4. Attempt to find point for therapeutic intervention: hopelessness—negative attitude toward future (P7).
5. Accept seriousness of patient's desire to die but treat is as a topic for further examination—"Discuss advantages and disadvantages" (T11).
6. Test ability to look at herself—objectivity; test fixity of her irrational ideas; test responsiveness to therapist (T13–T20).

Part 2: Broadening Patient's Perspective

1. Isolate the precipitating factor—breakup with boyfriend; reduce use of questioning.
2. Determine meaning to patient of the breakup.
3. Immediate psychological problem: "I have nothing."
4. Question the conclusion, "I have nothing."
5. Probe for other objects that are important to her: concrete sources of satisfaction (T24–T33).
6. Shore up reality-testing and positive self-concept (T35–T37).

Part 3: "Alternative Therapy"

1. Therapist very active in order to engage patient's interest in understanding and dealing with her problem. Induce patient to examine options (T38). "Eliminate" suicide as option.
2. Undermine patient's all-or-nothing thinking by getting her to regard herself, her future, and her experiences in quantitative probabilities (T45).
3. Feedback: important information as to success of interview. Look for (a) affect shift, (b) positive statements about herself, (c) consensus with patient re solution of problem (P47).

Part 4: Obtaining More Accurate Data

1. More therapeutic collaboration: discussion about therapeutic techniques and rationale.
2. Testing her conclusions about "no satisfaction," indirectly disproving her conclusion.
3. Patient's spontaneous statement, "Can I tell you something positive?"
4. Periodic attempts to evoke a mirth response.

PART 5: CLOSURE

1. Reinforce independence (T106), self-help, optimism.

THERAPIST (T1): Well, how have you been feeling since I talked to you last? . . .

PATIENT (P1):   Bad.

T2: You've been feeling bad . . . well, tell me about it?

P2: It started this weekend . . . I just feel like everything is an effort. There's just completely no point to do anything.

T3: So, there's two problems; everything is an effort, and you believe there's no point to doing anything.

P3: It's because there's no point to doing anything that makes everything too hard to do.

T4:   (Repeating her words to maintain interchange. Also to acknowledge her feelings.) Because there's no point and everything feels like an effort . . . And when you were coming down here today, were you feeling the same way?

P4: Well, it doesn't seem as bad when I am working. It's bad on weekends and especially on holidays. I sort of expected that it would happen.

T5: (Eliciting expectancy re session) You expected to have a hard time on holidays . . . And when you left your office to come over here, how were you feeling then?

P5: Kind of the same way. I feel that I *can* do everything that I have to do, but I don't *want* to.

T6: You don't want to do the things you have to.

P6: I don't want to do anything.

T7: Right . . . and what kind of feeling did you have? Feel low?

P7: (hopelessness to be target) I feel that there's no hope for me. I feel my future . . . that everything is futile, that there's no hope.

T8: And what idea did you have about today's interview?

P8: I thought that it would probably help as it has always happened in the past . . . that I would feel better—temporarily. But that makes it worse because then I know that I am going to feel bad again.

T9: That makes it worse in terms of how you feel?

P9: Yes.

T10: And the reason is that it builds you up and then you get let down again?

P10: (Immediate problem—suicide risk) I feel like it's interminable, it will just go this way forever, and I am not getting any better . . . I don't feel any less inclined to kill myself than I ever did in my life ٜ . . . In fact, if anything, *I feel like I'm coming closer to it.*

T11: Perhaps we should talk about that a little bit because we haven't talked about the advantages and disadvantages of killing yourself.

P11: (smiles) You make everything so logical.

T12: (Testing therapeutic alliance) Is that bad? Remember you once wrote something . . . that reason is your greatest ally. Have you become allergic to reason?

P12: But I can't try anymore.

T13: Does it take an effort to be reasonable?

P13: (Typical "automatic thoughts") I know I am being unreasonable; the thoughts seem so real to me . . . that it does take an effort to try to change them.

T14: Now, if it came easy to you—to change the thoughts, do you think that they would last as long?

P14: No . . . see, I don't say that this wouldn't work with other people. I don't try to say that, but I don't feel that it can work with me.

T15: So, do you have any evidence that it did work with you?

P15: It works for specific periods of time, and that's like the Real Me comes through.

T16: Now, is there anything unusual that happened that might have upset the apple cart?

P16: You mean this weekend?

T17: Not necessarily this weekend. As you know, you felt you were making good progress in therapy and you decided that you were going to be like the Cowardly Lion that Found His Heart. What happened after that?

P17: (agitated, bows head) It's too hard . . . it would be easier to die.

T18: (Attempts to restore objectivity. Injects perspective by recalling previous mastery experience.) At the moment, it would be easier to die—as you say. But, let's go back to the history. You're losing sight and losing perspective. Remember when we talked and made a tape of that interview and you liked it. You wrote a letter the next day and you said that you felt you had your Heart and it wasn't any great effort to reach that particular point. Now, you went along reasonably well until you got involved. Correct? Then you got involved with Jim. Is that correct? And then very predictably when your relationship ended, you felt terribly let down. Now, what do you conclude from that?

P18: (Anguish, rejects therapist's venture) My conclusion is that I am always going to have to be alone because I can't stay in a relationship with a man.

T19: All right, that's one possible explanation. What other possible explanations are there?

P19: That's the only explanation.

T20: Is it possible you just weren't *ready* to get deeply involved and then let down?

P20A: But, I feel like I'll never be ready. (weeps)

P20B: I have never given up on him, even when I couldn't see him for a year at a time. He was always in my mind, all the time. So how can I think now that I can just dismiss him.

T21: This was never final until now. There was always the hope that . . .

P21: There wasn't, and he told me very clearly that he could not get involved with me.

T22: Right, but before January, it was very quiescent. You weren't terribly involved with him. It started up in January again. He did show serious interest in you.

P22: For the first time in four years.

T23: (Attempts to restore perspective) All right, so that's when you got involved again. Prior to January, you weren't involved, weren't thinking of him every minute and you weren't in the situation you are in now, and you were happy at times. You wrote that letter to me that you were happy, right? Okay. So that was back in January, you were happy and you did not have Jim. Now comes May, and you're unhappy because you have just broken up with him. Now, why do you still have to be unhappy say in July, August, or September?

P23: (Presents specific target belief) I have nothing.

T24: You weren't unhappy in January, were you?

P24: At first I was, that's why I called.

T25: All right, how about December? December you weren't unhappy. What did you have in December? You had something that made you happy.

P25: I was seeing other men. That made me happy.

T26: There are other things in your life besides men that you said you liked very much.

P26: Yes and I . . .

T27: (Aims at target beliefs. Shows she had and has something.) Well, there were other things you say were important that are not important right now. Is that correct? What were the things that were important to you back in December, November, and October?

P27: Everything was important.

T28: Everything was important. And what were those things?

P28: It's hard to even think of anything that I cared about.

T29: Okay, now how about your job?

P29: My job.

T30: Your job was important. Did you feel that you were accomplishing something on the job?

P30: Most of the time I did.

T31: (Still aiming) Most of the time, you felt you were accomplishing something on the job. And what about now? Do you feel you are accomplishing on the job *now?*

P31: (Discounts positive) Not as much as I could.

T32: (Reintroduces positive) You're not accomplishing as much as you could but even when you are "off," I understand that you do as well or better than many of the other workers. Is that not correct?

P32: (Disqualifies positive statement) I can't understand why you say that. How do you know that? Because *I* told you that. How do you know that's true?

T33: I'm willing to take your word for it.

P33: From somebody who is irrational.

T34: (Presents positive evidence of satisfactions and achievements.) Well, I think that somebody who is as irrationally down on herself as you, is very unlikely to say something positive *about herself* unless the positive thing is so strong that it is unmistakable to anybody . . . In any event, you do get some satisfaction out of the job right now and you do feel you are doing a reasonably good job, although you are not doing as well as you would like to, but as well as you are capable. You're still doing a reasonably good job. You can see for yourself. Your clients' plans are improving? Are they being helped? Does anyone say they are appreciative of your efforts?

P34: Yes.

T35: They do tell you? Yet you are saying you are so irrational that I can't believe anything you say. Do you say, "You're just a dumb client . . . no judgment at all," to your clients?

P35: I wouldn't say that about somebody.

T36: Well, do you think it about yourself?

P36: Yes.

T37: (Points out inconsistency. Underscores her capacity for rationality. Fortifies her professional role.) So, you trust the word of your clients, but you won't trust your own word. You won't think of your clients as being irrational, and yet, you think of you—when you are the client— as being irrational. How can you be rational when you are the therapist and irrational when you are the patient?

P37: I set different standards for myself than what I set for anybody else in the world.

P37B: Suppose I'll never get over it?

T38: (Changes the options—consider nonsuicidal solutions. Sweat it out or fight to solve problem.) Suppose you'll never get over it? Well, we don't know whether you'll never get over it or not . . . so there're two things you can do. One is, you can take it passively and see, and you might find that you will get over it, since almost everybody gets over grief reactions. Or, you can attack the problem aggressively and actively build up a solid basis for yourself. In other words, you can capitalize on the chance . . .

P38: (Thinks of finding another man.) I feel desperate. I feel that I have to find somebody right now—right away.

T39: All right, now if you found somebody right away, what would happen?

P39: The same thing would happen again.

T40: (Omits suicide as one of the options.) Now, remember when we talked about Jim and you said back in January you decided that you would take that chance and you'd chance being involved, with the possibility that something would come of it positively. Now, you have two choices at this time. You can either stick it out now and try to weather the storm with the idea that you are going to keep fighting it, or you can get involved with somebody else and not have the opportunity for this elegant solution. Now, which way do you want to go?

P40: (Compulsion to get involved with somebody.) I don't want to, but I feel driven. I don't know why I keep fighting that, but I do. I'm not involved with anybody now and I don't want to be, but I feel a compulsion.

T41: That's right, because you're hurting very badly. Isn't that correct? If you weren't hurting, you wouldn't feel the compulsion.

P41: But I haven't done anything yet.

T42: (Emphasizes ideal option. Also turning disadvantage into advantage.) Well, you know it's your decision. If you do seek somebody else, nobody is going to fault you on it. But I'm trying to show that there's an opportunity here. There's an unusual opportunity that you may never have again—that is to go it alone . . . to work your way out of the depression.

P42: That's what I'll be doing the rest of my life . . . that's what worries me.

T43: You really just put yourself in a "no-win" situation. You just acknowledged that if you get involved with another man, probably you would feel better.

P43: Temporarily, but then, I'd go through the same thing.

T44: I understand that. So now, you have an opportunity to not have to be dependent on another guy, but you have to pay a price. There's pain now for gain later. Now are you willing to pay the price?

P44: I'm afraid that if I don't involve myself with somebody right away . . . I know that's dichotomous thinking . . . I think if I don't get immediately involved, that I will never have anybody.

T45: That's all-or-nothing thinking.

P45: I know.

T46: (Seeking a consensus on nonsuicidal option.) That's all-or-nothing thinking. Now, if you are going to do it on the basis of all-or-nothing thinking, that's not very sensible. If you are going to do it on the basis of, "The pain is so great that I just don't want to stick it out anymore," all right. Then you take your aspirin temporarily and you'll just have to work it out at a later date. The thing is—do you want to stick it out right now? Now, what's the point of sticking it out now?

P46: I don't know.

T47: You don't really believe this.

P47: (Reaching a consensus.) Theoretically, I know I could prove to myself that I could, in fact, be happy without a man, so that if I were to have a relationship with a man in the future, I would go into it not feeling desperate, and I would probably eliminate a lot of anxiety and depression that have in the past been connected to this relationship.

T48: So, at least you agree, theoretically, on a logical basis this could happen. If you try to stick it out . . . Now, what do you think is the probability that this could happen?

P48: For me?

T49: For you.

P49: For another person I'd say the probability is excellent.

T50: For one of your clients?

P50: Yeah.

T51: For the average depressed person that comes to the Mood Clinic . . . most of whom have been depressed seven years or more. You would still give them a high probability.

P51: Listen, I've been depressed all of my life. I thought of killing myself when I was 14 years old.

T52: (Undermining absolutistic thinking by suggesting probabilities.) Well, many of the other people that have come here too have felt this way. Some of the people that have come here are quite young and so have not had time to be depressed very long . . . Okay, back to this. Hypothetically, this could happen. This could happen with almost anybody else, this could happen with anybody else. But you don't think it can happen to you. Right . . . It can't happen to you. But what is the possibility . . . (you know, when we talked about the possibility with Jim, we thought it was probably five in a hundred that a good thing could come from it) . . . that you could weather the storm and come out a stronger person and be less dependent on men than you had been before?

P52: I'd say that the possibility was minimal.

T53: All right, now is it minimal like 1 in a hundred, one in a million . . . ?

P53: Well, maybe a 10% chance.

T54: 10% chance. So, you have one chance in ten of emerging from this stronger.

P54: (More perspective; disqualifies evidence.) Do you know why I say that . . . I say that on the basis of having gone through that whole summer without a man and being happy . . . and then getting to the point where I am now. That's not progress.

T55: (Using data base.) I'd say that that is evidence. That summer is very powerful evidence.

P55: (Discredits data.) Well, look where I am right now.

T56: The thing is, you did very well that summer and proved as far as any scientist is concerned that you could function on your own. But you didn't prove it to your own self. You wiped out that experience as soon as you got involved with a man. That experience of independence became a nullity in your mind after that summer.

P56: (Mood shift. A good sign.) Is that what happened?

T57: Of course. When I talked to you the first time I saw you, you said, "I cannot be happy without a man." We went over that for about 35 or 40 minutes until I finally said, "Has there ever been a time when you didn't have a man?" And you said, "My God, that time when I went to graduate school." You know, suddenly a beam of light comes in. You almost sold me on the idea that you couldn't function without a man. But that's *evidence*. I mean, if I told you I couldn't walk across the room, and you were able to demonstrate to me that I could walk across the room, would you buy my notion that I could not walk across the room? You know, there is an objective reality here. I'm not giving you information that isn't valid. There are people. . .

P57: I would say, how could you negate that if it didn't happen?

T58: What?

P58: (Asks for explanation. A good sign.) I'd say what's wrong with my mind, having once happened, how can I negate it?

T59: (Alliance with patient's rationality.) Because it's human nature, unfortunately, to negate experiences that are not consistent with the prevailing attitude. And that is what attitude therapy is all about. You have a very strong attitude, and anything that is inconsistent with that attitude stirs up cognitive dissonance. I'm sure you have heard of that, and people don't like to have cognitive dissonance. So, they throw out anything that's not consistent with their prevailing belief.

P59: (Consensus gels.) I understand that.

T60: (Optimistic sally.) You have a prevailing belief. It just happens, fortunately, that that prevailing belief is wrong. Isn't that marvelous? To have a prevailing belief that makes you unhappy, and it happens to be wrong! But it's going to take a lot of effort and demonstration to indicate to you, to convince you that it is wrong. And why is that?

P60: I don't know.

T61: (Since patient is now collaborating, he shifts to didactic strategy. Purpose is to strengthen patient's rationality.) Do you want to know why? Because you've always had it. Why? First of all, this belief came on at a very early age. We're not going into your childhood, but obviously, you made a suicide attempt or thought about it when you were young. It's a belief that was in there at a very young age. It was very deeply implanted at a very young age, because you were so vulnerable then. And it's been repeated how many times since then in your own head?

P61: A million times

T62: A million times. So do you expect that five hours of talking with me is going to reverse in itself something that has been going a million times in the past?

P62: Like I said, and you agreed, my reason was my ally. Doesn't my intelligence enter into it? Why can't I make my intelligence help?

T63: Yeah, that's the reason intelligence comes into it, but that's exactly what I'm trying to get you to do. To use your intelligence.

P63: There's nothing wrong with my intelligence. I know that.

T64: I understand that. Intelligence is fine, but intelligence has to have tools, just as you may have the physical strength to lift up a chair, but if you don't believe at the time that you have the strength to do it, you're not going to try. You're going to say, "It's pointless." On the other hand, to give you a stronger example, you may have the physical strength to lift a heavy boulder, but in order to really lift it, you might have to use a crowbar. So, it's a matter of having the correct tool. It isn't simply a matter of having naked, raw intelligence, it's a matter of using the right tools. A person who has intelligence cannot solve a problem in calculus, can he?

P64: If she knows how to. (smiles)

T65: (Reinforces confidence in maturity.) All right. Okay. You need to have the formulas, that's what you're coming in here for. If you weren't intelligent, you wouldn't be able to understand the formulas, and you know very well you understand the formulas. Not only that, but you use them on your own clients with much more confidence than you use them on yourself.

P65: (Self-praise, confirms therapist's statement.) You wouldn't believe me if you heard me tell things to people. You'd think I was a different person. Because I can be so optimistic about other people. I was encouraging a therapist yesterday who was about to give up on a client. I said, "You can't do that." I said, "You haven't tried everything yet," and I wouldn't let her give up.

T66: All right, so you didn't even have a chance to use the tools this weekend because you had the structure set in your mind, and then due to some accidental factor you were unable to do it. But you concluded on the weekend that the tools don't work for, "I am so incapable that I can't use the tools." It wasn't even a test was it? Now for the next weekend. . .

P66: (Agrees.) . . . It wasn't a true test. . .

T67: No, it wasn't even a fair test of what you could do or what the tools could do. Now for weekends, what you want to do is prepare yourself for the Fourth of July. You prepare for the weekends by having the structure written down, and you have to have some backup plans in case it gets loused up. You know you really do have a number of things in your network that can bring you satisfaction. *What are some of the things you have gotten satisfaction from last week?*

P67: I took Margaret to the movies.

T68: What did you see?

P68: It was a comedy.

T69: What?

P69: A comedy.

T70: That's a good idea. What did you see?

P70: (smiles) It was called *Mother, Jugs and Speed.*

T71: Yeah, I saw that.

P71: Did you see that?

T72: Yeah, I saw that on Friday.

P72: (smiles): I liked it.

T73: It was pretty good. A lot of action in that. So you enjoyed that. Do you think you could still enjoy a good movie?

P73: I can. If I get distracted, I'm all right.

T74: So what's wrong with that?

P74: Because then what happens . . . while I'm distracted the pain is building up and then the impact is greater when it hits me. Like last night I had two friends over for dinner. That was fine. While they're there . . . I'm deliberately planning all these activities to keep myself busy . . . and while they were there I was fine. But when they left. . .

T75: That's beautiful.

P75: The result was that the impact was greater because all this pain had accumulated. . .

T76: We don't know because you didn't run a control, but there is no doubt there is a letdown after you've had satisfactory experience . . . so that what you have to do is set up a mechanism for handling the letdown. See what you did is you downed yourself, you knocked yourself and said, "Well . . . it's worse now than if I hadn't had them at all." Rather than just taking it phenomenologically: "They were here and I felt good when they were here, then I felt let down afterward." So then obviously the thing to pinpoint is what? The letdown afterward. So what time did they leave?

P76: About 9.

T77: And what time do you ordinarily go to bed?

P77: About 10.

T78: So you just had one hour to plan on.

P78: To feel bad. . .

T79: All right, one hour to feel bad. That's one way to look at it. That's not so bad, is it? It's only one hour.

P79: But then I feel so bad during the hour. That's when I think that I want to die.

T80: All right, what's so bad about feeling bad? You know what we've done with some of the people? And it's really worked. We've assigned them. We've said, "Now we want to give you one hour a day in which to feel bad." Have I told you about that? "I want you to feel just as bad as you can," and in fact sometimes we even rehearse it in the session. I don't have time today but maybe another time.

P80: It's time-limited.

T81: (Alliance with patient as a fellow therapist.) Yeah, and we have the people—I'd say, "Why don't you feel as bad as you can—just think of a situation, the most horribly devastating, emotionally depleting situation you can. Why don't you feel as bad as you possibly can?" And they really can do it during a session. They go out and after that they can't feel bad again even though they may even want to. It's as though they've depleted themselves of the thing and they also get a certain degree of objectivity toward it.

P81: (Helping out.) It has to be done in a controlled. . .

T82: It has to be done in a structured situation.

P82: It has to be controlled.

T83: That's true. It has to—that's why I say, "Do it in here, first."

P83: —

T84: Then, I can pull them out of it . . . You need to have a safety valve.

P84: If you do it at home . . . you might. . .

T85: Right, the therapist has to structure it in a particular way. I'm just saying that one hour of badness a day is not necessarily anti-therapeutic. And so it doesn't mean you have to kill yourself because you have one bad hour. What you want to do is to think of this as "my one bad hour for today." That's one way of looking at it. And then you go to sleep at 10 o'clock and it's over. You've had one bad hour out of 12. That's not so terrible. Well, you told yourself during that time something like this. "See, I've had a pretty good day and now I've had this bad hour and it means I'm sick, I'm full of holes, my ego is. . ."

P85: See I'm thinking, "It never ends."

T86: For one hour, but yeah, but that's not even true because you thought that you couldn't have any good times in the past, and yet as recently as yesterday you had a good day.

P86P: But what gives it momentum is that thought that it's not going to end.

T87: Maybe the thought's incorrect. How do you know the thought is incorrect?

P87: I don't know.

T88: (Retrospective hypothesis-testing.) Well, let's operationalize it. What does it mean, "It's not going to end?" Does that mean that you're never going to feel good again in your whole life? Or does that mean that you're going to have an unremitting, unrelenting, inexorable sadness day in, day out, hour after hour, minute after minute. I understand that is your belief. That's a hypothesis for the moment. Well, let's test the hypothesis retrospectively. Now you have that thought: "This is never going to end." You had that thought when? Yesterday at 9 a.m.

P88: Yes.

T89: Now that means that if that hypothesis is correct, every minute since you awoke this morning, you should have had unending, unrelenting, unremitting, inevitable, inexorable sadness and unhappiness.

P89: (Refutes hypothesis.) That's not true.

T90: It's incorrect.

P90: Well, you see, when I wake up in the morning, even before I'm fully awake the first thing that comes to my mind inevitably is that I don't want to get up. That I have nothing that I want to live for. And that's no way to start the day.

T91: That's the way a person who has a depression starts the day. That's the perfectly appropriate way to start the day if you're feeling depressed.

P91: Even before you're awake?

T92: Of course. When people are asleep they even have had dreams. You've read the article on dreams. Even their dreams are bad. So how do you expect them to wake up feeling good after they have had a whole night of bad dreams? And what happens in depression as the day goes on? They tend to get better. You know why? Because they get a better feel of reality—reality starts getting into their beliefs.

P92: Is that what it is?

T93: Of course.

P93: I always thought it was because the day was getting over and I could go to sleep again.

T94: Go to sleep to have more bad dreams? The reality encroaches and it disproves this negative belief.

P94: That's why it's diurnal.

T95: Of course, and we have already disproven the negative belief, haven't we? You had that very strong belief last night—strong enough to make you want to commit suicide—that this would be unremitting, unrelenting, inevitable, and inexorable.

P95: (cheerful) Can I tell you something very positive I did this morning?

T96: (Kidding) No, I hate to hear positive things. I'm allergic. Okay. I'll tolerate it. (Laughs)

P96: (Recalls rational self instruction.) I got that thought before I was even awake, and I said, "Will you stop it, just give yourself a chance and stop telling yourself things like that."

T97: So what's wrong with saying that?

P97: I know. I thought that was a very positive thing to do. (Laughs)

T98: (Underscores statement.) That's terrific. Well, say it again so I can remember.

P98: I said, "Stop it and give yourself a chance."

T99: (More hopeful prediction. Self-sufficiency.) When you had your friends over, you found intrinsic meaning there. This was in the context of *no man* . . . Now when the pain of the breakup has washed off completely, do you think you're going to be capable of finding all these goodies, yourself, under your own power, and attaching the true meaning to them?

P99: I suppose if the pain is less . . .

T100: Well, the pain's less right now.

P100: Does it matter?

T101: Yeah.

P101: But that doesn't mean it won't continue.

T102: Well, in the course of time, you know, it's human nature that people get over painful episodes. You've been over painful episodes in the past.

P102: Suppose I keep on missing him forever.

T103: What?

P103: Suppose I keep on missing him forever?

T104: There's no reason to expect you to miss him forever. That isn't the way people are constructed. People are constructed to forget after a while and then get involved in other things. You had them before.

P104: You spoke of a man who missed a mother for 25 years.

T105: (Emphasizes self-sufficiency.) Well, I don't know . . . this may have been one little hangup he had, but, I don't know that case . . . In general, that isn't the way people function. They get over lost love. All right? And one of the ways we can speed the process is by you, yourself, attaching meaning to things that are in your environment that you are capable of responding to . . . You demonstrated that. . .

P105: Not by trying to replace a lost love right away?

T106: (Reinforcing independence.) Replace it? What you're trying to do is find another instrument to happiness. He's become your mechanism for reaching happiness. That's what's bad about the whole man hangup. It is that you are interposing some other unreliable entity between you and happiness. And all you have to do is to move this entity out of the way, and there's nothing to prevent you from getting happiness. But you want to keep pulling it back in. I say, leave it out there for a while, and then you'll see. Just in the past week you found that when you didn't have a man, you were able to find happiness without a man. And if you leave the man out of the picture for a long enough period of time, you'll see that you don't need him. Then if you want to bring him in as one of the *many* things that can bring satisfaction, that's fine, you can do that. But if you see him as the *only* conduit between you and happiness, then you are right back to where you were before.

P106: Is it an erroneous thing to think that if I get to the point where I really believe that I don't need him, that I won't want him?

T107: Oh, you're talking about him. I think it will just. . .

P107: Any man . . . any man?

T108: (Undermines regressive dependency.) . . . Well, you might still want him, like you might like to go to a movie, or read a good book, or have your friends over for dinner. You know, you still have to have relationships with your friends. But if they didn't come over for dinner last night it wouldn't plunge you into a deep despond. I'm not underestimating the satisfaction that one gets from other people . . . but it's not a necessity . . . It's something that you, yourself, can relate to on a one-to-one basis . . . but one does, as one individual to another. You're relating to a man the way a child does to a parent, or the way a drug addict does to his drugs. He sees the drug as the mechanism for achieving happiness. And you know you can't achieve happiness artificially. And you have been using men in an artificial way. As though *they* are going to bring you happiness . . . rather than they are simply one of the things external to yourself by which you, yourself, can bring yourself happiness. *You* must bring *you* happiness.

P108: I can . . . I've been focusing on dependency.

241

T109: (Emphasizing available pleasures.) Well, you've done it. You've brought yourself happiness by going to the movies, by working with your clients, by having friends over for dinner, by getting up in the morning and doing things with your daughter. You have brought you happiness . . . but you can't depend on somebody else to bring you happiness the way a little girl depends on a parent. It doesn't work. I'm not opposed to it . . . I have no religious objection to it . . . It just doesn't work. Pragmatically, it is a very unwise way to conduct one's life. And in some utopian society after this, children will be *trained* not to depend on others as the mechanism for happiness. In fact, you can even demonstrate that to your daughter . . . through your own behavior, she can find that out.

P109: She's a very independent child.

T110: (Probing for adverse reaction to interview.) Well, she's already found that out. Okay, now do you have any questions? Anything that we discussed today? Is there anything that I said today that rubbed you the wrong way?

P110: You said it would be damaging . . . not damaging . . . but you think it would deprive me of more opportunity to test this out if I did not go to another man.

T111: Well, it's an unusual opportunity. . .

P11: It's not so unusual, because I might get involved with somebody else.

T112: (Turning disadvantage into advantage.) Well, yes, but this is like the worst—you said this is the worst—depression you felt for a long time. It's a very *unusual* opportunity to be able to demonstrate how you were able to pull yourself from the very deepest depths of depression onto a very solid independent position. You may not have that opportunity again, really, and it would be such a very sharp contrast. Now, you don't have to do it, but I'm saying it's really a very rich chance, and it does mean possibly a lot of gain. I don't want to make any self-fulfilling hypotheses, but you've got to expect the pain and not get discouraged by it. What are you going to say to yourself . . . if you feel the pain tonight? Suppose you feel pain after you leave the interview today, what are you going to say to yourself?

P112: "Present pain for future gain."

T113: Now where are you now on the hopelessness scale?

P113: Down to 15%.

T114: It's down to 15% from 95%, but you have to remember that the pain is handled in a structured way, the way I told you about the people who make themselves feel sad during that one period. It has to be structured. If you can structure your pain, this pain is something that's going to build you up in the future, and, indeed it will. But if you see yourself as just being victimized by these forces you have no control over, . . . you're just helpless in terms of the internal things and external things, . . . then you are going to feel terrible . . . And what you have to do is, convert yourself from somebody who feels helpless, right? . . . And you are the only person who can do it . . . I can't make you strong and independent . . . I can show you the way, but if you do it, you haven't done it by taking anything from me; you've done it by drawing on resources within yourself.

P114: How does it follow then that I feel stronger when I have a man? If things are going. . .

T115: (Counteracts assumption about getting strength from another person. Empirical test.) You mean you make yourself feel strong because you yourself think, "Well, I've got this man that's a pillar of strength, and since I have him to lean on, therefore, I feel strong." But, actually, nobody else can give you strength. That's a fallacy that you feel stronger having a man, but you can't trust your feelings. What you're doing is just probably drawing on your own strength. You have the definition in your mind. "I'm stronger if I have a man." But the converse of that is very dangerous . . . which is, "I am weak if I don't have the man . . ." What you have to do, if you want to get over this is to disprove the converse, "I am weak if I don't have a man." Now, are you willing to subject that to the acid test? Then you will know. Okay, well suppose you give me a call tomorrow and let me know how you're going and then we can go over some of the other assignments.

It was apparent by the end of the interview that the acute suicidal crisis had passed. The patient felt substantially better, was more optimistic, and had decided to confront and solve her problems. She subsequently became involved in cognitive therapy on a more regular basis and worked with one of the junior staff in identifying and coping with her intrapersonal and interpersonal problems.

This interview is typical of our crisis intervention strategies but is a departure from the more systematic approach used during the less dramatic phases of the patient's depression. We generally attempt to adhere to the principle of collaborative empiricism (Chapter 1) in our routine interviews and deviate from standard procedures for a limited period of time only. Once the crisis is over, the therapist returns to a less intrusive and less active role and structures the interview in such a way that the patient assumes a greater responsibility for clarifying and devising possible solutions to his problems.

Chapter 12

DEPRESSOGENIC ASSUMPTIONS

As therapy progresses and the patient's symptoms lessen, the focus of therapy shifts to changing his faulty assumptions—those basic beliefs that predispose the person to depression. Changing his erroneous or dysfunctional assumptions has a direct effect upon the patient's ability to avoid future depressions.

Although common themes can be found in the belief systems of depressed patients, each patient has a unique set of personal rules. Time and effort are required to discover and modify the specific dysfunctional assumptions of a particular patient. For both practical and therapeutic reasons, the patient has to be actively involved in this therapeutic process. To emphasize the importance of changing these rules, the therapist may tell the patient that even when the symptoms of depression have abated, he will remain vulnerable to future depressions until these beliefs are identified and changed.

The unarticulated rules by which the individual attempts to integrate and assign value to the raw data of experience are based on fundamental assumptions that shape his automatic thought patterns. During his developmental period, each individual learns rules or formulas by which he attempts to "make sense" of the world. These formulas determine how the individual organizes perceptions into cognitions, how he sets goals, how he evaluates and modifies his behavior, and how he understands or comes to terms with the events in his life. In essence, these basic assumptions form a personal matrix of meaning and value, the backdrop against which everyday events acquire relevance, importance, and significance. Maladaptive assumptions differ from adaptive ones in that they are inappropriate, rigid, and excessive. Beck (1976) has written on the nature of these maladaptive rules:

> Such characteristic thinking aberrations as exaggeration, over-generalization, and absoluteness are built into the framework of the

rule and, consequently, press the person to make an exaggerated, overgeneralized, absolute conclusion. (Of course, in normal states, there are also more flexible rules, which tend to mitigate the more extreme rules that are prepotent in states of disturbance.) When the theme of the patient's preoccupation is related to his specific sensitivities, the more primitive rules tend to displace the more mature concepts. Once the patient accepts the validity of an extreme conclusion, he is more susceptible to an ever-increasing expansion of the primitive rules. . . . Since the rules tend to be couched in extreme words, they lead to an extreme conclusion. They are applied as though in a syllogism.

Major Premise: "If I don't have love, I am worthless."
Special Case: "Raymond doesn't love me."
Conclusion: "I am worthless."

Of course, the patient does not experience a sequence of thoughts in the form of a syllogism. The major premise is already part of his cognitive organization and is applied to the presenting circumstances. The patient may ruminate over the minor premise (the specific situation) and is certainly aware of the conclusion. (p. 100)

These rules are active in situations that impinge on areas relevant to the person's specific vulnerabilities, such as acceptance–rejection, success–failure, health–sickness, or gain–loss. For example, a patient who harbored the belief that he had to be perfect placed high value on performance. He measured his own worth by how well he could accomplish something or by the number of different goals he could achieve. Value to him was dictated by his assumptions, which determined what events to attend to and how to evaluate them.

These assumptions are learned and at one time may have been articulated. They may be derived from childhood experiences, or from attitudes and opinions of peers or parents. Many of these assumptions are based on family rules. For example, a parent might say to a child, "Be nice, or Nancy won't like you." The child may repeat this out loud at first, later to himself. After a while, the child develops the underlying rule: "My worth depends on what others think of me." Furthermore, many of these maladaptive assumptions are culturally reinforced.

Beck (1976) specified some of the assumptions which predispose to excessive depression or sadness (pp. 255–256). Examples are:

1. In order to be happy, I have to be successful in whatever I undertake.
2. To be happy, I must be accepted by all people at all times.
3. If I make a mistake, it means that I am inept.
4. I can't live without you.
5. If somebody disagrees with me, it means he doesn't like me.
6. My value as a person depends on what others think of me.

If a patient has been depressed for a long time, he holds to these assumptions and their negative conclusions with great tenacity. The patient rarely examines or doubts these views. They are as much a part of his identity as being a male or a female. If the therapist challenges these views, his questioning may be construed by the patient as an attack on him or as showing a lack of empathy. The certainty with which these negative beliefs are held is likely to covary with the intensity of the depression.

Identifying Dysfunctional Assumptions

The patient and therapist work together to uncover these assumptions. The collaborative nature of this endeavor is important for a variety of reasons. First, there is the practical consideration of the therapist's time and energy. Because cognitive therapy is active and directive, there is more work involved than in other forms of therapy.

Patients, in turn, benefit by taking an active role in recognizing and correcting their self-defeating assumptions. Some patients can be told that they have problems mainly because in the past they have relied on others to do their thinking for them. Their assumptions don't add up because they have "let others do their arithmetic." By recognizing and testing and changing their mistaken beliefs, patients *learn to think for themselves.*

The patient has to identify his own assumptions to make the learning process plausible. The therapist can guide the patient in this exploration by helping the patient to infer the assumptions from his dysfunctional cognitions, and then by checking out these inferred rules with the patient.

If the therapist leaps prematurely to the identification of a basic belief, he runs the risk of confusing the patient. The patient may agree with the therapist's formulation out of compliance, rather than conviction, or he may dismiss it out of hand and thereby close the door to discovery of the same belief. The therapist has to remember that assumptions, for the most part, are not articulated by the patient without considerable introspection. He will probably run into problems if he tells the patient, "You're telling yourself 'I have to be perfect',"or "You're telling yourself, 'Everyone has to love me'." The patient can readily observe his automatic thoughts but not his assumptions.

Finally, because the assumptions are abstract and impalpable, the patient needs to be actively involved in identifying them. Once therapy moves beyond the concrete data of automatic thoughts and observable behaviors, there is a danger that therapeutic intervention will miss the mark. At this point, therapists are particularly vulnerable to the risk of presenting their own biases—what *they* speculate the patient's beliefs are. If the therapist, however, will listen to and work with the patient, therapy is more likely to stay on target.

The therapist initially draws inferences or develops hypotheses about the patient's assumptions. Information about these assumptions is gathered by observing how the patient justifies a specific cognition or how he is disturbed by a specific thought. The therapist must continually refrain from jumping to conclusions about the patient's assumptions. He remains naïve, unknowing, and curious about the content of the formula that shapes a particular disturbing thought.

One way to help the patient to become aware of his basic assumptions is to work from the specific and explicit to the general and inferred. There are three stages in this process. In the first stage, the patient recognizes and reports his automatic thoughts. The second stage involves identifying the general themes abstracted from automatic thoughts. The final stage focuses on delineating or formulating the patient's central rules or equations about his life.

When the patient has reported a sufficient number of automatic thoughts, themes will emerge, such as the belief that he is unlovable, inadequate, ugly, or helpless. The patient's automatic thoughts frequently stem from an *implicit assumption* upon which the cognition itself logically rests. Although this assumption is rarely articulated,

247

the rule governing the patient's outlook can be inferred from a list of cognitions and events that lead to dysphoria.

For example, these upsetting cognitions were reported by a 38-year-old engineer:

1. My work is of poor quality.
2. I can't fix the bicycle.
3. I can't cut the grass.
4. I can't make a sale.
5. The wallpaper wasn't lined up well enough.

Themes inferred from these cognitions involved (a) performance and (b) perfectionistic standards. The perfectionistic standards become evident when the bases for some of the cognitions are elicited. For instance, the cognition, "I can't cut the grass" was based on the objective data that although he did cut the grass, the edger was broken so some of the trimming wasn't done. The imperfection in the wallpaper wasn't noticeable to anyone else. The therapist verbalized assumptions such as, "If I am not accomplishing or succeeding, I am a loser," and "If I make a mistake, I am inept. Doing an incomplete or imperfect job is as bad as not doing it at all." He checked with the patient to see whether they fit. Precisely pinpointing the assumptions requires considerable "fine tuning."

The types of thinking errors the patient habitually makes (overgeneralization, arbitrary conclusions, dichotomous reasoning) can be a clue to underlying assumptions. For example, the patient who chronically overgeneralizes regarding a particular type of event is likely to have corresponding assumptions that are similarly characterized by overgeneralizations.

Another clue to the patient's belief system is his frequent use of particular kinds of words. Global and vague words that the patient customarily uses are particularly helpful in discovering assumptions. Because the basic assumptions are often learned in early life, childish, global words such as "stupid" and "dumb" can be useful clues to these assumptions. Once these high-frequency words have been identified, they have to be explored further. The patient needs to spell out the meanings concretely.

Although cognitive therapy is quite structured in general, allowing the patient to ramble occasionally may point the direction to underlying assumptions. On these occasions, the therapist attempts to understand the patient's world view rather than to correct his distortions. In the same vein, cognitive therapy is concerned primarily with present problems, but having the patient discuss important incidents in his past may lead to the discovery of basic assumptions. Vivid childhood recollections, bedtime stories the patient remembers from childhood, and family sayings can be useful in revealing these assumptions.

When the patient seems to be usually happy about some event, questions about his thinkng may lead to his base rules. Many of the dysfunctional formulas "pay off" for the patient when they appear to be working. For example, the person who identifies himself with his job may be exuberant when his work is praised. (He gets into trouble with himself when he perceives his performance as below his standards.)

A final clue to the patient's underlying belief system is the way the patient views the behavior of others. Attributions such as "Mary is happy because she has a husband," can be particularly useful. In this case, it suggests the patient's belief, "I cannot be happy unless I have a husband."

In the following case, the therapist used various methods to discover the primary and secondary assumptions of a severely depressed patient. The patient was a recently divorced 33-year-old woman with two children. Her present depression began following her divorce, at which time she moved from a rural to an urban setting. Her children had trouble adjusting to the new area.

During the first phase of treatment, the patient was asked to record the automatic thoughts which preceded her negative affect. She was able to do this: some examples of her automatic thoughts are presented in Figure 3. Next she was taught to answer these thoughts with more realistic and positive thoughts.

During the next stage of treatment, general themes of the negative automatic thoughts were abstracted. One general theme was how she appeared to others. She believed she must appear "nice" to other people. "Nice" was one of her frequently used words, and the therapist asked her to explain what she meant by this word. To her, being "nice" was appearing bright and attractive to others.

One general theme involved her tendency to blame herself when things went wrong. Examples of "bad things" ranged from getting a divorce to having a flat tire. In a number of these incidents, she

249

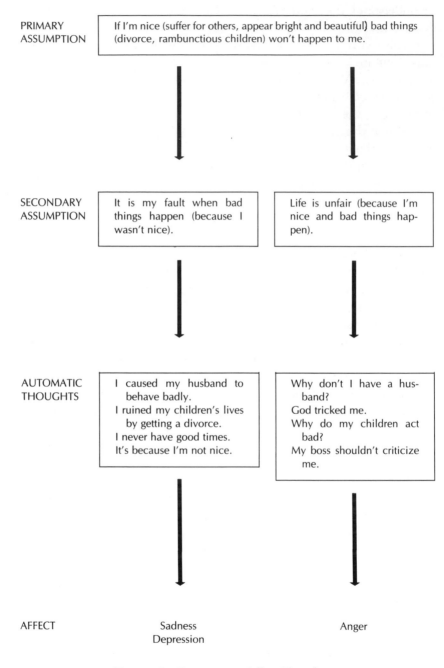

FIGURE 3. Cognition—Affect Flowchart

thought she had a reason for blaming herself. For example, one of her children was having trouble in school. She believed this problem was the result of bad mothering. This general theme of self-blame led to feelings of sadness and depression.

A second theme involved the "unfairness" of life. This theme centered on things other people had which she did not have, such as a husband, good times, money. These thoughts led to feelings of anger.

The following interchange uncovered a basic belief:

THERAPIST: Your automatic thought was, "Your children shouldn't fight and act up." And because they do, "I must be a rotten mother." Why shouldn't your children act up?

PATIENT: They shouldn't act up because . . . I'm so nice to them.

T: What do you mean?

P: Well, if you're nice, bad things shouldn't happen to you. (At this point the patient's eyes lit up.)

Patients' formulas can be used to explore in a variety of directions. In this case, the woman believed, "Bad things have happened to me; therefore, this means I am not nice." This followed logically from her false premise that one can avoid misfortune by "acting nice."

The therapist asked, "Who told you, if you're nice, bad things won't happen?" She said that her mother had always told her this. She also said this rule was reinforced in school where teachers told her that if she was nice she would be rewarded. The teachers also told her she was bright and "should go places."

Early in treatment, the therapist discusses with the patient the role these formulas play in depression and asks the patient to be on the lookout for these assumptions. When the therapist has an accurate idea of the patient's assumptions and the time is appropriate, he can say, "I've been thinking about you and what one of your assumptions or rules might be. Write this down, and think about it between now and the next session. Also write out your thoughts about it and the ways it should be modified."

Therapists can use diagrams or flowcharts, similar to the one shown in Figure 3, to aid in identifying and presenting assumptions. The therapist can give the patient a partially completed chart or a sample chart to help in the process. These charts are constructed by listing the negative emotions and the preceding automatic thoughts. When constructing these charts, the therapist can keep in mind that most negative emotions can be ultimately traced back to self-defeating assumptions.

MODIFYING ASSUMPTIONS

Identifying the patient's assumptions is the first step in changing them. Once these assumptions are verbalized, and thus no longer hidden, many patients immediately see their absurdity or maladaptiveness. This is not surprising considering that many people hold these unspoken assumptions as certainties beyond question.

The therapist can use a variety of arguments and exercises to help patients examine the validity of self-defeating beliefs. Patients do not change their beliefs because of the *number* of counterarguments, but rather because particular arguments make sense to them. One or two new ways of looking at a situation can be instrumental in changing long-held beliefs. What causes patients to change these beliefs is often surprisingly simple. When patients indicate a change in a belief, the therapist should, as a matter of course, ask what led to this change.

The best evidence against these assumptions is that which the patient develops on his own or in collaboration with the therapist. For this reason, challenges to the patient's assumptions should be presented in the form of questions, and suggestions of *alternative assumptions*, rather than in the form of a lecture. Arguments against a patient's belief system are more effective when they are tied in with the patient's adaptive beliefs. For example, a patient believed that others' disagreeing with him meant that they disliked him. He also believed that he couldn't be all things to all people. By applying the second belief to the first, he was able to accept the "new belief" that whether others agreed with him was not a crucial concern. Thus, an adaptive belief was used to counter the other beliefs.

ASSUMPTIONS AS "TARGETS"

Many of the cognitive and behavioral interventions outlined

earlier to modify automatic thoughts are used to change hidden assumptions. However, the difference between these two targets, as the following case illustrates, necessitates contrasting methods of intervention.

The patient was an attractive woman in her early twenties. Her depression of 18 months' duration was precipitated by her boyfriend's leaving her. She had numerous automatic thoughts that she was ugly and undesirable. These automatic thoughts were handled in the following manner:

THERAPIST: Other than your subjective opinion, what evidence do you have that you are ugly?

PATIENT: Well, my sister always said I was ugly.

T: Was she always right in these matters?

P: No. Actually, she had her own reasons for telling me this. But the *real reason* I know I'm ugly is that men don't ask me out. If I weren't ugly, I'd be dating now.

T: That is a possible reason why you're not dating. But there's an alternative explanation. You told me that you work in an office by yourself all day and spend your nights alone at home. It doesn't seem like you're giving yourself opportunities to meet men.

P: I can see what you're saying but still, if I weren't ugly, men would ask me out.

T: I suggest we run an experiment: that is, for you to become more socially active, stop turning down invitations to parties and social events and see what happens.

After the patient became more active and had more opportunities to meet men, she started to date. At this point, she no longer believed she was ugly.

Therapy then focused on her basic assumption that one's worth is determined by one's appearance. She readily agreed this didn't make sense. She also saw the falseness of the assumption that one must be beautiful in order to attract men or be loved. This discussion led to her basic assumption that she could not be happy without love (or attention from men). The latter part of treatment focused on helping her to change this belief.

T: On what do you base this belief that you can't be happy without a man?

P: I was really depressed for a year and a half when I didn't have a man.

T: Is there another reason why you were depressed?

P: As we discussed, I was looking at everything in a distorted way. But I still don't know if I could be happy if no one was interested in me.

T: I don't know either. Is there a way we could find out?

P: Well, as an experiment, I could not go out on dates for a while and see how I feel.

T: I think that's a good idea. Although it has its flaws, the experimental method is still the best way currently available to discover the facts. You're fortunate in being able to run this type of experiment. Now, for the first time in your adult life you aren't attached to a man. If you find you can be happy without a man, this will greatly strengthen you and also make your future relationships all the better.

In this case, the patient was able to stick to a "cold turkey" regimen. After a brief period of dysphoria, she was delighted to find that her well-being was not dependent on another person.

There were similarities between both of these interventions. In both, the distorted conclusion or assumption was delineated and the patient was asked for evidence to support it. An experiment to gather data was also suggested in both instances. However, in order to achieve the results, contrasting versions of the same experimental situation were required.

MODIFICATION OF THE "SHOULDS"

A recurrent theme in the assumptions of depressives is the heavy reliance on the "shoulds," or rules of living. The patient is certain that these rules apply to all situations. They are part of the cognitive structure by which daily experience is organized. Frequently, patients mentally compare what they "should" do with what they "are" doing. In this comparison, they usually judge their behavior and themselves to be inadequate in relation to this set of ideal standards. The standards are usually phrased in absolute terms. Furthermore, the depressed patient overapplies the rules of what he should do or be. This overapplication is reflected both in the *intensity* with which he maintains that he "should" do something and in the large number of situations to which he applies his rules of what he "should" do or be.

Often patients find some support for these rules from personal experience. From the patient's point of view, these rules function to prevent something undesirable from happening; for example, "I *should* listen to those in authority or they won't like me." The patient dominated by "shoulds" is readily recognizable. The cognitions collected as homework, as well as verbalizations in the therapy session, contain a high frequency of "should," "have to," or must." These arbitrary rules (a) prevent the patient from identifying or enjoying his own successes, (b) prevent him from setting priorities as to what he "must" do next, and (c) prevent him from deciding what he *wants* to do for himself. By continually giving himself absolute orders in the form of "shoulds," he becomes chronically anxious, frustrated, and disappointed in himself since he can't carry out all of these commands.

Several techniques are available to modify these "shoulds." One behavioral strategy, "response prevention," has been successfully used in the treatment of compulsions. This strategy trains the patient to find out what will happen if he doesn't follow a command: for example, "I *must* wash my hands every ten minutes or I'll get a fatal infection." This sort of assumption can be invalidated when it is empirically tested.

A variation of response-prevention may be used with the depressed patient. The therapist guides the patient to (a) verbalize the "should," (b) predict what would happen if the "should" was *not* followed, (c) carry out an experiment to test the prediction, and (d) according to the results of the experiment, revise the rule.

The following case illustrates how this procedure can be carried out. The patient was depressed, anxious, chronically irritable, and had difficulty asserting himself with his wife. He was asked what would happen if he told his wife about his unhappiness with the way she treated him. He said his wife would become angry and would threaten to leave him. He believed, "If you want people to like you, you should always be nice to them." "If you find fault, they will punish you." And further, he believed this rule applied at all times and in all situations.

In order to suspend the operation of the rule, the patient was given a series of graded tasks, which ran counter to the "should."

First, he was to confront his wife on a minor difference and gradually move on to more crucial confrontations. In order to prepare the patient, the therapist engaged him in rehearsing the confrontations. The therapist suggested that he imagine what it might be like to state his complaints and how his wife might act toward him. How long would she be angry or sad? Would that permanently or transiently affect the relationship? In this technique, his fantasies about the presumed dire consequences of foregoing the "shoulds" are explored and made more explicit. The patient in this instance fantasized that his wife would leave him. After he engaged in his first confrontation with his wife, she became angry at him and he thought, "I was wrong to criticize. I should have followed my rule of being nice all the time." Later, however, when her anger had subsided, she conceded that he had made a good point.

This positive feedback encouraged him to take a greater risk. He managed to overcome the internal resistance presented by his "shoulds" and raised issues of greater gravity. Again, the confrontation resulted in his wife's becoming angry. However, she soon realized that their happiness depended on working out some of these problems and thus they reached a compromise on several issues. The upshot of these experiences was that the patient realized (a) the rule of being indiscriminately "nice" was a handicap, (b) that no disastrous consequences occurred when he broke the rule, and (c) by adopting a more flexible rule, he could have better relationships with other people.

Assumptions as "Personal Contracts"

Therapy can focus on changing the conditionality of assumptions. Most assumptions have an implied "contractual" basis: If I do X (win others' approval, never make a mistake, prove to be the best), then Y will occur (I'll be happy, have no problems, be worthy.)

When discussing this concept, therapists can cite work done by Canadian social psychologist Lerner (1969), who asserts, with supporting experimental data, that "deserving" and its counterpart, "justice," are the central organizing themes in the lives of most people. On the development of "deserving," he writes:

One reasonable possibility is that the issue of deserving begins to gain meaning when the child encounters his physical and social environment. . . . As the child begins to orient himself to the world on the basis of the "reality" rather than the "pleasure" principle, he seems to be making a kind of contract with himself. By the terms of this "personal contract" he agrees to give up the immediate and direct use of the power he has at hand to meet his wants and desires. The greater the deprivation and effort, that is, his investments, the more valuable should be the outcome. (pp. 5–6)

Many depressed patients run into problems because their "personal contracts" are too severe, too absolute, and too rigid. The job of the therapist is to help the patient to "renegotiate" his contracts or to abandon them altogether if they are unworkable.

The following excerpt illustrates how this concept was presented to one patient.

THERAPIST: Do you see how this concept of personal contract applies to your belief system?

PATIENT: My contract is: "If I work hard, people will respect me," and "Without their respect, I can't be happy."

T: When did you draw up these contracts?

P: As we discussed, probably when I was pretty young.

T: If you had a business, would you let a child draw up the contracts on how it would operate?

P: That is what I seem to have done in my life, and they're contracts that give controlling interests of the business to others.

The therapist can stress that these contracts are not permanent and can be changed.

These contracts are unworkable and maladaptive largely because the terms of the contract are vague and open-ended. In this case, "working hard" is a relative concept, as is "others' respect." There is no end to how hard one would have to work and no measure of how much respect one would need to be happy.

Patients often discuss the issue of justice in terms of "fairness." Often, basic underlying assumptions revolve around the concept of fairness—what one or others deserve when certain acts are performed. Because this expectation is an illusion, many believe the world, God, and society are grossly unfair.

A common concern of patients revolves around the sufferings of others and those treated unjustly. At first, this reaction appears to be empathy, but if questioned, the patient will often discover he is projecting himself into the situation. He is applying his own idiosyncratic assumptions to others. For example, one patient became extremely concerned when a friend's husband died. On closer questioning, she revealed her thoughts were: "What if my husband died? That would be the worst thing that could happen!" Her assumption was that one has to have complete control over all life's events. Conversely, loss of control over a particular event equaled a disaster. Through projection she applied this rule to the other woman.

There are a number of ways to handle in therapy the issue of fairness. One way is to agree with the person that life is unfair. Many situations in the world are unfair because there is no symmetry in the way the good things in life are distributed. People are born with different abilities. Fortunate and unfortunate circumstances and experiences appear to be randomly distributed. Nobody can make a special claim to favored treatment or expect to be magically protected against adversity.

An alternative approach is to ask the patient to list situations that are unfair and then ask him what he could do to change them. The therapist can also ask how worrying about these situations will change them. Most patients concede they can change their attitude even if they can't change the external situation. Often, however, they *can* change the situation.

The therapist can say,

> "I know you think things should be different, but this is just an added burden you're giving yourself—worrying about what others should or shouldn't do. It might be better for you to use that energy more constructively rather than burden yourself with other people's problems. This is not to say that you should not try to make the world a better place if you can."

Another strategy is to discuss how fairness is often a matter of personal opinion or bias. The employee believes, "I do the work around here. I produce the product. I should receive more money. It's not fair"—while the owner believes, "I produce the capital. I invested it. I took the risk. I should get more money instead of having to give it to workers." In nearly every case, fairness can be looked at from two or more points of view.

The final way of dealing with concern about "unfairness" is to discuss fairness as an abstraction. There is actually no concrete entity such as fairness. It is a hypothetical construct, an abstraction. *Fairness* and *unfairness* are general terms that no one can define, yet they can cause great irritation and unhappiness. The therapist can tell patients that viewing the world in these vague and abstract terms limits their perceptions and thus is often counterproductive. It is better for the person to make a pragmatic judgment as to what he wants and what steps would be necessary to get it. When the goal seems attainable and worth the effort, he has a better chance of reaching it if he is not bogged down with concerns about being treated fairly.

The operation of the "shoulds" was readily apparent in the behavior of another patient who believed that if she sacrificed for others (coworkers, husband, and children), they would love her. The therapist sensed that the patient was deceiving herself with this rule. He gave the following homework assignment. She was to observe and record for a week the reactions of others to her self-sacrificing behavior; that is, she was to follow the dictates of the "shoulds" and observe the results.

The patient found that the actual consequences of her self-sacrificing behavior differed greatly from what she expected. Instead of appreciating her, people often discounted her. She decided that she should change her philosophy from "The meek shall inherit the earth" to "The meek shall inherit dirt." The therapist pointed out that this turnabout also represented an extreme way of looking at the world. He stressed that behavior has a range of consequences—some desirable, some not—and that many consequences are unanticipated. He suggested that they work on a series of flexible guidelines that would allow her to have rewarding relationships without automatically subordinating her own interests.

ASSUMPTIONS AS SELF-FULFILLING PROPHESIES

Many, or perhaps most, depressogenic assumptions are self-fulfilling. If a patient believes he will be unhappy without recognition, he probably *will* be unhappy when denied it. By predicting the consequences, he brings them about. Therapy can help a patient change this type of belief by demonstrating how it becomes a self-fulfilling prophecy, trapping the believer in the very circumstances which the belief was designed to help him avoid. The following excerpt illustrates how the therapist clarifies the self-actualizing assumptions:

> PATIENT: Not being loved leads automatically to unhappiness.
> THERAPIST: Not being loved is a "nonevent." How can a nonevent lead automatically to something?
> P: I just don't believe anyone could be happy without being loved.
> T: This is your belief. If you believe something, this belief will dictate your emotional reactions.
> P: I don't understand that.
> T: If you believe something, you're going to act and feel as if it were true, whether it is or not.
> P: You mean if I believe I'll be unhappy without love, it's only my belief causing my unhappiness?
> T: And when you feel unhappy, you probably say to yourself, "See, I was right. If I don't have love, I am bound to be unhappy."
> P: How can I get out of this trap?
> T: You could experiment with your belief about having to be loved. Force yourself to suspend this belief and see what happens. Pay attention to the natural consequences of not being loved, not the consequences created by your belief. For example, can you picture yourself on a tropical island with all the delicious fruits and other food available?
> P: Yes, it looks pretty good.
> T: Now, imagine that there are primitive people on the island. They are friendly and helpful, but they do not love you. None of them loves you.
> P: I can picture that.
> T: How do you feel in your fantasy?
> P: Relaxed and comfortable.
> T: So you can see that it does not necessarily follow that if you aren't loved, you will be unhappy.

TABLE 1
COGNITIVE ERRORS DERIVED FROM ASSUMPTIONS

Cognitive Error	Assumption	Intervention
1. Overgeneralizing	If it's true in one case, it applies to any case which is even slightly similar.	Exposure of faulty logic. Establish criteria of which cases are "similar" and to what degree.
2. Selective abstraction	The only events that matter are failures, deprivation, etc. Should measure self by errors, weaknesses, etc.	Use "log" to identify successes patient forgot.
3. Excessive responsibility (Assuming personal causality)	I am responsible for all bad things, failures, etc.	Disattribution technique.
4. Assuming Temporal Causality (Predicting without sufficient evidence)	If it has been true in the past, then it's always going to be true.	Expose faulty logic. Specify factors which could influence outcome other than past events.
5. Self-references	I am the center of everyone's attention—especially my bad performances. I am the cause of misfortunes.	Establish criteria to determine when patient is *the* focus of attention and also the probable facts that cause bad experiences.
6. "Catastrophizing"	Always think of the worst. It's most likely to happen to you.	Calculate *real* probabilities. Focus on evidence that the worst did not happen.
7. Dichotomous thinking	Everything either is one extreme or another (black or white; good or bad).	Demonstrate that events may be evaluated on a continuum.

ASSUMPTIONS UNDERLYING COGNITIVE ERRORS

Patients' cognitive errors are derived from some type of assumption. For example, the cognitive distortion labeled "overgeneralization" (Beck, 1963) is based on the assumption that if something is

261

true in one case, it is true in all similar cases. These overgeneralizing assumptions can be modified in the same way as other assumptions. Table 1 outlines the applied assumptions in the cognitive errors and suggestions for therapeutic interventions.

LIST ADVANTAGES VS. DISADVANTAGES OF DYSFUNCTIONAL ASSUMPTIONS

At times the patient will be hesitant to discard self-defeating assumptions because of the belief that something important will be lost. Although the patient can see the advantages of changing the belief, the disadvantages seem greater to him. Many depressed people structure their world as a no-win trap with the disadvantages on both sides of an issue outweighing any possible advantages.

The standard procedure, as in other no-win situations, is to have the patient list the advantages and disadvantages of a particular assumption and then to correct the distortions (if there are any) in those listings.

The following is an example of how this procedure was used to modify a patient's basic assumption that in order to be happy she had to be perfect: "Never make a mistake or show a flaw."

She listed the following *advantages* to giving up this belief.

a. Without this belief I could do a lot of things I've been avoiding—like learning to drive a car.
b. If I were more open I would have more friends.
c. I wouldn't be so anxious about making mistakes or depressed because I did make one.
d. I would be able to accept the reality that I'm not a perfect person.

She listed the following *disadvantages* to changing this belief:

a. I've been able to do exceptionally well in school and on my job.
b. What I do, I do well.
c. Because I avoid a lot of things, I've avoided a lot of trouble and problems.

The therapist then discussed these disadvantages with her.

THERAPIST: This belief may have helped you on your present job, but how about in your long-range career?

PATIENT: Actually, it's held me back. I feel I am overqualified for this job. If I had more courage, I'd work for a bigger company in a more challenging position.

T: Dread of making mistakes often blocks people from taking chances. What about this belief—"What you do, you must do well?"

P: That's true. I have the highest ratings at work.

T: Is there a point of diminishing return?

P: Yes. I told you, I bring work home every night and go in on the weekends. I do a lot more than is demanded or expected of me.

T: Sometimes it is a good idea to stand one's beliefs on their heads and see if they make more sense. For example, is it more reasonable to think, "I have to be *imperfect*" than "I have to be perfect?"

P: You mean anything worth doing is worth doing poorly?

T: Let me ask you—if learning to ski or learning to make friends is worth doing, is it worth doing poorly?

P: I guess it would be better than not doing it at all.

T: Further, your work habits are now consistent and reasonable. Just because you soften the demands on yourself, that doesn't mean your work will become shoddy. Your habits will stay.

P: What about the idea that I avoid trouble?

T: When you avoid a problem you often *create others*. Mental health includes a large portion of taking risks. Is there any way you can avoid all problems?

P: No.

The technique of listing the advantages and disadvantages of adhering to a given assumption may appear to be overly simple. However, it has proven to be one of the most effective procedures in long-term modification of the way an individual handles his problems. Since the depressed patient thinks in a closed and limited way, this procedure usually expands the boundaries of his thinking and allows him to experiment with new approaches.

THE ROLE OF ACTION IN CHANGING ASSUMPTIONS

The patient is encouraged to challenge his basic assumptions actively in his ordinary daily experiences. He does this (a) by tracing his automatic thoughts to the assumptive level and then challenging the assumption, and (b) by acting against his assumption.

Acting against an assumption is the most powerful way to change it. The action is tied to the patient's assumption. The therapist suggests that the patient who is afraid to make mistakes seek out situations in which there is a high probability of his making mistakes. He proposes that the patient who feels compelled to be with others force himself to be alone. The patient who places the highest value on acceptance is urged to go places where the probability of being accepted is slight. The patient afraid of making a fool of himself ,is asked to do something outlandish. The patient usually discovers that this behavior is not outlandish to others. One patient, for example, had to force himself to go to his first costume party. He was concerned that would look foolish in his "weird" costume. To his surprise, only a few people at the party made passing comments about his costume.

In reference to changing beliefs, Ellis and Harper (1975) write:

> It takes more than self-talk. In the final analysis, you often would better literally force yourself, propel yourself, push yourself, into action. Often, you can make yourself—yes, *make yourself*—undertake specific acts of courage: beard an employer in his office, ask a very attractive person to dance, take your idea for a book to a publisher. And keep forcing yourself into action long enough and often enough until the action itself proves easier and easier, even enjoyable. (p. 95)

Patients are extremely reluctant to act against these beliefs. The therapist has to motivate the patient to do this. These patients can act against these beliefs at a gradual rate, or jump right in. In either event, they are likely to experience discomfort when they attempt to break long-established "rules."

The following interchange illustrates one way in which this idea was presented to a patient.

THERAPIST: Can you set yourself a goal of doing one thing a day that goes against seeking the approval of others?

PATIENT: I *tell* myself to act this way, but it doesn't work.

T: You have to force yourself. Tell yourself, "If I die, I'll die, but I'll do it."

P: I get really anxious.

T: That's because you've acted on this belief for so long it has become a part of your total system—your mind, emotions, and body. Anxiety won't kill you. Anxiety is like weak muscles. If you stay with the anxiety and practice building up your tolerance, it will harden into courage.

P: I have a difficult time seeing these situations at the time. Afterward I realize I could have acted differently.

T: In these situations you have to be on the lookout for a voice that whispers, "This isn't the right time," or "There is this or that reason for not doing it." These excuses will cripple your efforts. You have to ignore this voice and force yourself to jump in. You also have to keep in mind that because this isn't your normal way of acting, you'll feel strange. If you stay with this long enough, however, the sense of strangeness and acting will go away.

The patient put this suggestion into practice—first at her work and later with her family. And she found (as the therapist predicted) that it became increasingly easier to do.

USING THE PATIENT TO SUPPLY COUNTERARGUMENTS

Patients are a rich source of information which can be used to dispute their assumptions. Pointed questioning by the therapist is one way this information can be obtained. Following are two examples in which the therapist's questioning brought out information that helped modify the patient's belief.

PATIENT: I think anyone who isn't concerned with what others think would be socially retarded and functioning at a pretty low level.

THERAPIST: Who are the two people you admire most? (The therapist knew the answer from previous discussion.)

P: My best friend and my boss.

T: Are these two overconcerned with others' opinions?

P: No, I don't think either one cares at all what others think.

T: Are they socially retarded and ineffective?

P: I see your point. Both have good social skills and function at high levels.

In the following instance, the impact of the insight was greater because the patient generated the information.

P: The only way I could ever be happy is if I could be a great writer.
T: What level of writing would you have to reach?
P: I would have to be as good as (the patient named a poet).
T: Did this poet achieve great happiness?
P: No, I guess not. She killed herself.

ATTACKING ASSUMPTIONS REGARDING SELF-WORTH

Many depression-prone patients believe that the determinants of their worth lie outside of them. The patient's happiness and unhappiness are contingent on external factors—for example, whether others approve of him or how they evaluate him.

The therapist can discuss with the patient the consequences of such formulas in terms of self-acceptance. By viewing his image of himself through the eyes of others, the patient is placing himself in a one-down position. One of the most vulnerable positions involves the patient who believes he has to be loved to be happy. He believes a sense of self-acceptance and self-worth can only be obtained indirectly—from the love of others. In these cases, the therapist can ask if the patient has ever been happy when he wasn't in a love relationship. In most cases, there has been some period of time when the patient was happy on his own.

The therapist can also ask what, on a day-to-day basis, makes the patient happy. The patient's activity schedule can be useful for finding activities he enjoys alone. The therapist can also point out that happiness varies from hour to hour and is not a stable condition.

The therapist can discuss with the patient those persons he knows are married, appear to be in love, yet are not happy. Most patients will agree that love can bring sadness as well as enjoyment. The romantic myth that love solves all problems can be discussed.

The notion of self-acceptance based on extrinsic (as opposed to intrinsic) factors is readily apparent in the patient who believes he has been rejected. The following is one way the therapist can handle this problem.

266

PATIENT: Anyone would be depressed if they were put down by someone they love.

THERAPIST: No one can be put down unless *he is asking someone to hold him up*. Dependence on another person for approval is a form of trying to accept yourself through someone else. "If that person loves me, I'm great, and if he doesn't, I'm worthless." As long as one is self-sufficient and accepts himself, he will not be depressed if someone chooses not to be with him.

P: But she rejected me.

T: No one can totally reject you. That person can only choose to see you or not to see you.

P: If there wasn't something wrong with me, she'd be with me.

T: It's a value choice. One person might like Cadillacs, another Volkswagens. It is a matter of taste. Some people like classical music, others don't. It doesn't necessarily have anything to do with your personality.

P: I still think it's something I did.

T: That is a possibility. . . . There are a number of other ways of looking at the experience. For example, (a) "I feel sorry for her, she is missing out on me," (b) "Well, someone else will come along," (c) "This is all for the better," or (d) not to think about it at all.

The concept of self-worth can be discussed with the patient. Ellis and Harper (1975) have written at great length on this concept. Ellis's writing on self-worth can be given as a homework assignment and his ideas used to discuss this concept.

There are at least three direct approaches to evaluating self-worth. One is to balance positive points about oneself against negative points. The second is to rate oneself as "good" just because one is alive. And the third is not to bother to make these generalizations because the concept of worth is an unmeasurable hypothetical construct: one can grade behaviors but not human beings.

When depressed, many persons begin taking inventory. Because of the distortions intrinsic to depression, this is not a good time to take inventory. Rather, this is the time to concentrate on action and doing. Although self-monitoring often helps depressed patients, self-evaluation generally makes them feel worse. The therapist can use an example to clarify this concept.

When someone says, "Dr. So-and-So is good," what does that

mean? Does it mean he is good in all realms of a medical doctor, or in special areas? Does it mean that he is a good clinician? Is he good with patients? Is he good at research? Is he good at emergencies? Or does it mean he is a good husband, father, neighbor, church member, and bridge player?

One can measure traits or behaviors if one cares to, but measuring *worth* is impossible and will often lead to trouble. There is no way to measure, let alone prove, worth or worthlessness.

Basing one's worth on outside criteria often leads to self-defeating comparisons. There is nearly always someone who has more of the particular factor that is being evaluated (money, status, love, beauty). The high school graduate who drops out of college compares himself unfavorably with the college graduate. The chairman of a physics department compares himself unfavorably with the Nobel Prize winner. Therapists can point out the counterproductiveness of making these comparisons.

Because the criteria of self-worth are vague and ill-defined, the patient never feels satisfied. The pleasures of the moment are bypassed in favor of the chase. The following is the way a therapist pointed out how the patient's assumption regarding self-worth led to insatiability.

The patient believed he had to be on top (make a great deal of money) to be happy.

THERAPIST: How much money would you need to make you happy?

PATIENT: I don't know, more than I have now.

T: Earlier in your life did you think that if you had as much as you now have that you'd be happy?

P: Yes, I probably did.

T: Successes, achievements, money are all open-ended. It's not like painting a wall or building a table. There is no end point.

P: But I believe if I could get the amount of money I need, I would be content.

T: Is this a real need? If you believed you need something that you really don't need, you will never be able to get enough of it. You can't get enough of something you don't need but believe you do.

EXPOSING THE ARBITRARINESS OF ASSUMPTIONS

The patient is often unaware that the internal rules that dominate him are arbitrary. The therapist can help the patient to modify these rules by pointing out and discussing their arbitrariness. Patients will often agree that the belief is arbitrary but will then go on behaving as if the belief were absolute truth. For this reason, the therapist has to illustrate in a number of ways that these personal rules are not universal laws.

The therapist can discuss the difference between beliefs and facts. Many patients confuse the two. The therapist can tell the patient that dogmatism limits one's vision. A person excludes from perceptions and considerations facts that go against this belief. Because belief can only frame a limited amount of truth, more is excluded than included. The therapist can cite Bertrand Russell's observation that the degree of certainty with which one holds a belief is inversely related to the truth of that belief. Fanatics are true believers, scientists are skeptics.

The arbitrariness of these assumptions is readily apparent when they concern happiness. Many patients believe that if they have X (perfection, beauty, fame) they will be happy. This formula contains a number of mistaken notions about happiness that can be discussed. The rules make the "either/or" mistake. Instead of seeing happiness as a continuum, the patient believes one is either happy *or* unhappy. The rules imply that happiness is a static, durable state rather than dynamic and transient. The rules imply that happiness is a pure state rather than a condition varying in degrees, including a certain amount of unpleasantness (for example, one can be happy at the beach, but there are also sand and traffic to put up with).

These rules state that happiness is a consequence of worthiness, rather than a by-product of some pleasurable activity. This last mistake can lead to circular reasoning which can spiral into further depression; for example, "If I'm worthy, I'll be happy. I'm not happy, therefore, I must not be worthy. I'm not worthy, therefore, I cannot be happy."

The therapist can tell the patient that one positive aspect of the arbitrariness of these rules is that they can easily be modified and changed.

269

LONG- VS. SHORT-TERM UTILITY OF ASSUMPTIONS

The therapist can ask the patient to examine the long-term effectiveness of his assumptions. This is particularly important when the dysfunctional assumption currently appears to be working in the person's favor. That is, many who believe that they need the approval of everyone are often extremely happy when they think they have this approval. Others who believe their value depends on their performance are often overjoyed when they are performing well. The job of the therapist is to help the patient see the *long-term effects* of operating under these rules.

The following is an excerpt from a session with a 50-year-old insurance salesman who at one time had been a well-known local entertainer. At this point in therapy, he was asymptomatic and doing well at his job. He still, however, believed he had to perform perfectly and win everyone's approval in order to be a worthwhile person.

> THERAPIST: I'm glad you're doing well and selling a lot of insurance, but this doesn't make you a wonderful person.
>
> PATIENT: What do you mean? Why not?
>
> T: For the same reason that when people were not buying your insurance you were not worthless. Why weren't you?
>
> P: If people don't buy my insurance, they aren't rejecting me but my insurance. And my selling ability is not me, but only one of my traits.
>
> T: Right. There is no agreed-on way to evaluate ourselves. We can only evaluate our traits. And to equate one's traits, such as selling ability, with one's total self is a gross overgeneralization that is likely to lead to trouble.
>
> P: Are you saying I should ignore it when I'm doing well, and not feel happy?
>
> T: No. If you are performing well in one area, it's appropriate to feel good, and to evaluate this performance realistically so you can continue to perform well. And if you're not performing well, it is a good idea to evaluate this realistically, too, so you can improve. But in both cases, the performance has nothing to do with your worth, which can't be measured or evaluated.
>
> P: You mean if I think I'm a great person when I'm doing well, I'm likely to think I'm no good if I'm not doing well?

T: Yes. And because you or no one else is perfect, there will be times when people won't approve of you and when you won't perform perfectly. . . . Another way of looking at this is: "I have (or am developing) a skill in selling. The skill brings me pleasure when I make a sale. Having it doesn't make me a wonderful person. Similarly, if I don't have the skill—or for some reason it isn't bringing me results—that doesn't mean I'm terrible or a failure. The worst it means is that perhaps I don't have this specific skill." To be happy, do those things you enjoy—usually, they are the things you are good at.

We have found that patients who continue to chip away at their dysfunctional assumptions become less prone to depressions. However, the motivation to change is weak when the formulas are working: that is, when rating oneself as wonderful leads to euphoria or when avoiding unpleasant situations relieves anxiety. Hence, it is necessary for the patient to recognize the long-range harm produced by these assumptions.

Chapter 13

INTEGRATION OF HOMEWORK
INTO THERAPY

Several writers have emphasized the importance of homework in effective psychotherapy (Ellis, 1962; Beck, 1976; Shelton and Ackerman, 1974): Since it makes psychotherapy more concrete and specific, it enhances the communications between patient and therapist. The systematic completion of homework appears to be important in assuring that the patient's improvement is maintained after termination of treatment. Longer-lasting changes are more easily accomplished if the patient is actively involved in experiences outside the office. Moreover, he is likely to continue to apply the special techniques and skills that he had previously learned during therapy.

Homework assignments directly relate to several different aspects of cognitive therapy. Therefore, some points covered in this chapter have already been mentioned in earlier chapters.

In cognitive therapy, homework is a significant vehicle from which data which disconfirm many negative thoughts and beliefs can be obtained. Furthermore, data provided by homework shift the focus of therapy from subjective, abstract conceptualizations to more objective, realistic, and detailed accounts. This procedure allows the therapist and patient to review the previous week's activities at a glance; and it helps the therapist to relate the session to specific tasks, thereby avoiding side issues.

PROVIDING A RATIONALE FOR DOING HOMEWORK

The patient is encouraged to view homework as an *integral, vital component* of treatment. Homework is not just an elective, adjunct procedure. The therapist usually spends time presenting the rationale for each assignment. The importance of carrying out each assignment is stressed frequently throughout treatment. We find that patients are more likely to complete a task if they understand the reasons for each assignment and if they are given an opportunity to ventilate their objections to carrying it out.

Homework serves to reinforce and supplement the educational aspects of cognitive therapy. Educators have long noted that homework reinforces the learning process. In cognitive therapy, patients are learning more realistic and effective ways of thinking and acting. Those patients who systematically carry out their homework assignments seem to derive greater benefits from therapy compared to those who neglect their assignments. A recent study (Maultsby, 1971b) reported that diligence in fulfilling homework assignments was a significant factor in success with outpatient psychotherapy. The therapist might tell the patient about this study in order to reinforce his motivation.

The therapist should investigate the patient's attitude toward homework, since it is important that the patient perceive the homework as serving a useful purpose. The therapist clarifies the reasons for doing each homework assignment and gives specific instructions for carrying out each task. The therapist and patient formulate the homework assignments together. This strategy allows the therapist to shape the homework to the individual patient's situation. This team approach converts the homework into an unwritten agreement, and therapy avoids power struggles between the patient and therapist. The patient should see that he has an important role in formulating the homework assignment, or at the very least, that he has been consulted.

Whenever possible, the therapist presents the scientific and therapeutic rationale for the homework. For instance, patients may be told that cognitive therapy, like science, is concerned with converting mysteries into problems, because problems, unlike mysteries, are designed to be solved. The steps to problem-solving are spelled out to the patient: (1) specify the problem; (2) identify a hypothesis about the cause of the problem (therapist might want to call this a "hunch" or an "idea"); (3) design a test of the hypothesis; (4) evaluate the results of the test; and (5) accept, reject, or modify the hypothesis to account for the results of the test.

It is important to state the hypothesis in operational terms (in concrete ways that can be tested empirically). For example, a salesman might avoid making phone calls (specified problem) because he believes he is "inept." The evidence he offers for this belief consists of a series of past incidents which he recalls and conceptualizes in terms of his being "unable to talk to customers so I lost the sales." This belief (hypothesis) may be operationalized concretely in several different ways. Once the belief ("I am inept") is operationalized ("I will fail at making phone calls"), it can be tested. For instance, he might be asked to make three phone calls to potential customers and to record his subjective estimate of his sense of mastery with each call. It is essential that both the patient and therapist agree in advance on the criteria used to evaluate the experiment. In general, behavioral criteria are best. After the completion of the assignment, the patient and therapist would try to identify specific aspects of each phone call which the patient construes as evidence for success or failure (for example, whether the customer sounded interested, promised to come in, etc.). Finally, they decide whether the hypothesis should be accepted, rejected, or modified.

A high degree of compliance with homework can be achieved if the therapist presents the assignment as an experiment. Instead of saying, "This will work for you," the therapist might say, "Why not try it on for size?" or "What do you have to lose and what do you have to gain?" or "Let's see if we can figure out a way to check out these thoughts." An exchange between therapist and patient might run as follows:

THERAPIST: I'd like to have you count on a wrist counter the number of times you say "should" to yourself this week. What do you think of the idea?

PATIENT: It sounds a little stupid to me. Why would I want to do that?

T: We've found that counting automatic negative thoughts makes one more aware of them and thus easier to answer. Also, merely counting tends to decrease their influence. (The therapist might also say, "Recording helps put distance between yourself and your thoughts, and gives you feedback and evaluation in changing thoughts.")

P: I don't think this will work for me.

T: I'm glad you are questioning me. This shows you are using your reasoning powers. There is no reason you should automatically believe something just because I say it. I'm not positive this will work in your case, but I have a hunch—or a *hypothesis,* to give it a scientific sound—that it will work. I'd like to test this hypothesis out.

P: What do you mean "test your hypothesis"?

T: I have a hypothesis that it will help you and you have a hypothesis that it won't. I don't know for sure who is right. Do you?

P: No, I don't.

T: I suggest we run an experiment for a week, gather some data, and see which point of view conforms more closely to the facts. How does that sound to you?

It is often useful for the therapist to employ an analogy which fits the particular patient. For example, if the patient has an interest in sports, the therapist might liken himself or herself to a coach helping the person to develop and sharpen new skills. Homework is presented as the practice that is needed to improve the performance. When possible, an analogy developed by the patient is most effective. A school teacher receiving cognitive therapy compared homework assignments to suggestions she would receive at staff meetings and doing the homework as implementation of the suggestions.

ASSIGNING HOMEWORK

Each homework is tailored to the individual patient. Simpler assignments are preferred with more depressed patients. It is important that the patient experience each assignment as a relative success. Whenever possible, the therapist should try to anticipate problems in carrying out the homework. For example, if the assignment involves outdoor activities for a weekend, alternative activities should be scheduled in case of inclement weather.

The therapist should be as clear and specific as possible when giving the assignment. It is better to say, "Write down 10 to 20 negative automatic thoughts," than "Bring in some thoughts." It is often useful to have the patient repeat the assignment in his own words and to describe any problems he might anticipate. Some patients can be induced to imagine undertaking the assignment in the office so that problems which the patient might anticipate can be identified and dealt with by careful planning.

Following the suggestion of Shelton and Ackerman (1974), we write the homework in duplicate on "No Carbon Required" (NCR) paper so that both the therapist and the client have a copy. We also follow their suggestion that the *therapist give himself a homework assignment,* thereby enhancing the cooperative values of therapy. Homework for the therapist might include reviewing techniques, rereading a passage in a manual, bringing in a handout, reviewing notes, and listening to an audiotape of the session.

The following is an example of the format which has been adapted from Shelton and Ackerman:

DATE: *3-27-77*
Homework for Therapist:
1. Listen to session tape.
2. Bring in handout on "Shame" for the patient.
Homework for Jim:
1. Record number of "should" self-statements on counter. Graph each day's total. (Stipulations: (a) watch for conclusion: "incurable" if thought continues after counting; (b) watch for tendency to blame self for having many "should" thoughts; (c) watch for tendency to interpret increase in number as "I'm getting worse.")
2. Bring in graphs and schedule for next session.
NEXT MEETING, FRIDAY, MARCH 31, 3:30 p.m.

The therapist's interest in the homework assignments tends to influence the completion of future assignments. Each homework assignment should be reviewed at the beginning of each session. New homework should be assigned in the latter part of each session. By reviewing each assignment, the therapist is socially reinforcing the patient for completing the task. In addition, this review provides an opportunity to determine whether the homework instructions were clear.

It is important to examine the thoughts (cognitions) generated by the homework itself. For example, does the patient see the homework as too simple, too difficult, or does he think of it as busy work? Although the therapist might see the homework as familiar or simple, the patient may experience it as alien, complicated, too demanding, or dull.

The therapist should be alert to identify and correct the patient's conclusion that homework which was attempted but not completed represents a failure. Rather, *any* attempt at a new task is a success in its own right. Data which patients report about incomplete assignments often are as useful as a completed assignment. Whenever the patient doesn't attempt the homework, the therapist should find out whether the instructions were clear and whether the patient saw how the assignment was relevant to helping him with his problems.

FACILITATING CARRYING OUT ASSIGNMENTS

There are varous ways to assist patients in doing the homework. Of course, the best aids are those developed by patients on their own. Some patients will develop personal sayings or phrases that remind them to do homework. This particular type of self-help is often of special value. One patient felt better if he wrote an activity schedule in the evening, and followed this schedule the next day. However, he often forgot either to make the schedule or to follow through with it. He developed the verbal cue: "To cope with depression, I have to plan my work and work my plan," which he repeated to himself frequently to remind himself to do the homework.

Other patients have developed verbal cues which prompt them to begin writing and answering automatic thoughts. When one patient started to feel bad, he would say to himself, "I'm talking myself into being sick." This cue was an impetus for him to start writing down and answering his automatic thoughts.

There are a number of self-control procedures that the patient can use to promote completion of homework assignments. If the homework involves writing, the patient may select a specific time of day or a specific place in his house in which to work on the homework or complete the homework. By setting a kitchen timer to mark the 15 to 20 minutes to be spent on writing, and charting and monitoring the time actually spent in doing homework, he can make homework a habit.

Another strategy is to remove everything that might distract the patient from doing the homework. For instance, he might turn off the television or radio while doing the writing assignments. One patient found that her bed was a distracting temptation. She would start to get involved in her activity schedule; but when she walked by her room and saw her bed, she would lie down. She solved the problem by taking the mattress off the bed in the morning.

To promote completion of assignments, patients can employ external "reward-and-punishment" behavioral reinforcements. For example, the patient may "contract" to work on the assignment before engaging in a pleasant activity (for example: watching a favorite TV show, having a cigarette, or calling a friend). Patients can also use aversive techniques: If they don't do the homework, they have to get up an hour earlier, or they have to clean out their closets. Sometimes, a follow-up call by the therapist is helpful in promoting adherence to the "rules" when all else fails. Simply informing the patient that he has to do the homework because it is part of therapy is effective, particularly if the therapist follows up this direction with a telephone call.

An effective coping technique used by some patients to help them carry out homework assignments involves learning to "talk to their muscles." This procedure was adapted from work by Abraham Low, who instructed his patients to give commands to their muscles in certain problematic situations.

For example,

> She commanded her muscles to lie quietly in bed when she was tense and restless, to walk on when she felt exhausted, to eat when the mere sight of food produced nausea, and to speak forcefully when the throat felt choked. And, after the muscles swung into action, disregarding the "symptomatic idiom" of the organs, Harriette's brain was instantly convinced that exhausted muscles can do a fine piece of walking . . . (1950, p. 67)

The following exchange is an example of how this procedure can be used to help patients do their homework:

PATIENT: Sometimes I feel so bad that I can't get up the energy to write down these thoughts and answer them.
THERAPIST: When this happens, do you feel like you are being invaded by a foreign force?
P: That's exactly how I feel.
T: In a certain sense, you *are* being invaded by these internal forces. Are there any benefits to passively giving in to this force?
P: No. But I can't do anything about it. Most people do give in to these internal forces.
T: A few fortunate people are able to fight them and win. Consequently, they are all the stronger for it.
P: How can I do that?

T: You have to see these inner forces as an invading army. The first thing invaders do is try to capture the radio station so they can control communications. To counteract this, you have to give yourself loud, direct, simple orders. The best orders are those telling your muscles what to do.

P: Like, "Muscles, get up, go to the desk and start writing?"

T: Right. You can be even more specific. "Legs, *move;* arms, *pick up the pencil.*" It is important that those orders be loud enough to drown out the "enemy's" communication. It is also extremely important that you act immediately on these orders. If you wait too long the "enemy" will take over the communication.

This method, besides being a self-instruction coping strategy, serves as a distractor for the patients. If they are telling their muscles to do their homework, they aren't thinking of all the reasons why they can't do their homework.

IDENTIFYING DYSFUNCTIONAL REACTIONS TO HOMEWORK

Patients may fail to undertake or complete homework, or they may complete the homework assignments only half-heartedly because of certain negative attitudes toward the homework. These negative attitudes underlie *strong wishes to avoid activity*—one of the cardinal symptoms of depression. These attitudes are evident in the self-defeating thoughts related to completing assignments. The patients can learn to challenge these thoughts much as other distorted cognitions are challenged. We have found it helpful to ask patients with chronic problems regarding homework to fill out a questionnaire listing the common negative attitudes about undertaking assignments. (See the form Possible Reasons for Not Doing Homework Assignments in the Appendix.)

The following examples represent some particularly troublesome attitudes. Some patients believe that, "by nature," they are not record-keepers. The therapist can challenge this notion by asking whether there were times in the past when they kept written lists (for example: when they were getting ready for a trip). Some patients need to be introduced to the idea that keeping written records is a useful skill that can be learned. By developing this skill the patient is helping both himself and the therapist, since these records provide data essential to treatment.

279

Some patients believe their problems are too complex or too deep-seated to be solved by simple assignments. These patients can be told that even the most complex endeavors, such as putting a man in space, begin with and consist of simple concrete steps. Some authors have said that although they can't write a book, they can write a paragraph: If enough paragraphs are written, a book results. Patients can also be induced to consider the advantages and disadvantages of believing that their problems cannot be solved by doing homework. For example, the therapist can ask, "Is it useful to believe, even before trying, that the homework won't work?"

Some patients say they don't do the homework because it hasn't helped in the past. The therapist should keep an open mind about this, inasmuch as the previous assignments may not have been beneficial. Admitting that his "hunch" was proven wrong in this instance, he can point out that there are many different forms of homework. In some cases, the patient may be mistaken about the amount of help he received from previous assignments. If data are available (for example: notes, reports, depression measures), the therapist and patient can review these data together.

Many patients resent having homework assigned to them in an authoritarian manner—another indication of the importance of therapist–patient collaboration. However, a few patients will view even collaboration as authoritarianism. The therapist has several options in these cases.

First, it is a good policy to present therapy in accordance with a "consumer model." The patient wants to reach a certain goal (overcome his depression), and the therapist has certain methods to offer for reaching his goal. The patient is totally free to use or reject the methods, just as he is free to buy or not buy in the marketplace.

Another option is for the therapist and patient to devise several alternative homework strategies. The patient is allowed to choose a particular strategy. Again, the patient may choose not to do any of them. A way to structure the assignment as a fail-proof activity is to plan noncompliance with the other strategies as one of the choices the patient can make. The following example illustrates this last option.

In the previous session the therapist and patient had planned a weekend activity schedule for the patient. Instead of following the schedule, the patient had spent the weekend in bed.

THERAPIST: What do you have planned for this weekend?

PATIENT: Larry is coming over Friday to spend the night.

T: What about Saturday?

P: I'll be depressed Saturday morning and start a fight with Larry. He'll get mad and leave. Then after he is gone, I'll be even more depressed and will go back to bed.

T: What will you say to yourself Saturday morning to depress yourself?

P: "He doesn't love me . . . All he cares about is sex . . . I have no respect for myself."

T: I'd like you to write these thoughts down and also write specifically how you'll react to Larry Saturday morning.

P: Well, I'll be cold to him when he wakes up, and refuse to have sex. Then I'll start on him for not coming around more often. Then he'll get mad and leave.

T: What will you say to yourself after he leaves?

P: "I screwed it up again . . . He won't be back for a long time, if ever. I'm all to blame" . . . Then I'll feel terrible and go back to bed.

T: It sounds like you have a plan, we'll call it Plan A. Can you think of another plan which would lead to your feeling differently?

P: Well, I could be nice to him in the morning.

T: Okay, write this down and call it Plan B.

P: In the morning, I could have sex with him, which I enjoy. I could cook him a nice breakfast.

T: What could you say to yourself?

P: I could say I do enjoy him when he is here and try to make it as pleasant as possible. After all, he is a free person and we're not married.

T: What could you do after he left?

P: I could leave the house and go shopping.

T: Okay, you have a choice of Plan A and Plan B. The choice is totally yours. The only thing I ask is that you stick with whichever plan you decide on.

In this case, the patient chose the adaptive Plan B and was able to follow it 80% of the time. If she had chosen the other plan, the reasons leading to this choice and the *consequences of the choice would be discussed.* Even if the patient makes a maladaptive choice, it is important to use this as an opportunity to demonstrate that a choice exists, to examine the thinking behind a maladaptive choice, and to review the consequences at the next session. The patient can learn that he does have options, and he can hope that next time, by exercising those options more adaptively, he may embark upon a more realistic course of action.

Some patients are hesitant to turn in written homework because of embarrassment or shame over grammar, penmanship, or spelling. The therapist should check to see whether noncompliance with homework assignments is due to one of these factors. Simply telling the patient that the *form* of the homework is irrelevant to its *purpose* may solve this problem. Discussion of the concept of shame is also helpful. Therapists can point out that *shame* is an abstraction—it does not exist in the universe as an independent entity, but rather is an emotion a person experiences, and people have some degree of choice as to whether they feel ashamed or not. If the patient is ashamed to turn in written homework, the therapist might try to show the patient the advantages of risking the embarrassment for the possible advantage of progressing in therapy. The following is one way in which this was done:

> THERAPIST: Generally, if one is going to make an error, it is better to err on the side of inclusion than exclusion. For example, if you are not sure whether or not you're invited to a party, it is better to go and endure whatever embarrassment you might have than to miss the chance of having a good time.
>
> PATIENT: I can see that.
>
> T: How does the principle relate to your fear of handing in written homework?
>
> P: Well, it would be better to have you think poorly of me than miss out on a chance to get help by having you read my homework.

In extreme cases, the patient may not be moved by this argument and may still refuse to turn in written material. If such is the case, the patient can read the material to the therapist. In a similar vein, patients extremely reluctant to talk in therapy can be asked to write out scripts of what they want to say and then read these in therapy.

At times patients will not bring in homework. They may say they forget it. It is fruitless to speculate about their "unconscious" reasons for forgetting. It is best to consider the error innocent until proven otherwise. At other times the patient will say he did not have the time to complete his assignment. This leads into a discussion of priorities.

CONSTRUCTING ACTIVITY SCHEDULES

Activity scheduling is often an important part of the early sessions in cognitive therapy. Several general rules to assigning activity schedules are as follows:

1. After the first interview, patients fill out the activity schedule showing how they are currently spending their time. This schedule gives the therapist baseline information on the level and type of activity. The patient records what he does on an hour-by-hour basis.

2. After this baseline recording, the activity schedule is used to plan activities for some patients.

3. This planning is done with some flexibility. If an unexpected event occurs (for example: arrival of an out-of-town visitor), the patient may change the schedule. Alternative plans should be made if something unexpected occurs (for example: it rains when outdoor activities are planned).

4. If the patient fails to engage in an activity which was planned, it is not necessary to go back and make up the missed activity.

5. If a patient finishes an activity earlier than planned (for example: the laundry takes 45 minutes instead of the anticipated hour), the patient does not necessarily begin activities scheduled for later. Rather, he has the option to engage in some type of pleasurable activity in the extra time.

6. Patients may rely on written or introspective self-instructions to assist in initiating and performing specific activities. This self-instruction might be in the form of "talking to their muscles," for example.

7. In selecting activities, the patient should list short-term pleasurable activities in addition to "mastery" activities. Activities are chosen to decrease depressed mood.

8. In order to prevent regression, we follow a general rule of

thumb: "Beds are for sleeping; sofas are for sitting. Do not stay in bed when awake."

9. Activity schedules should be related to the patient's normal routines. The therapist asks the patient to list typical ways that he acted before he became depressed. The patient tries to perform these activities in ways that he did when he was not depressed. The therapist urges the patient to take on this role as an experiment to see whether his mood and outlook can be changed, if only for a brief while.

10. The patient should record his activities without being too specific (I went downstairs, opened the car door), or too general (I went out for the day). The goal lies somewhere between these two (I went to the store, visited friends for two hours and then came home).

11. The therapist helps the patient recognize that he is always doing something. Instead of the report, "I did nothing," a more accurate account would be, "I sat in the chair and drank coffee and read the paper." Even a passive activity is still an activity. The therapist and the patient can be misled by accepting the conclusion that the patient did "nothing."

SCHEDULING ACTIVITIES TO INCREASE PLEASURE

In the early stages of treatment, the patient may have difficulty in listing activities which he finds pleasurable or enjoys. One way to overcome this difficulty is to ask the patient to select potentially pleasurable activities from a specially designed list. Specific questions have been found useful in constructing this list.

What types of things did you enjoy learning *before* you got depressed? (For example: sports, crafts, languages)

What types of day trips did you enjoy? (For example: to the shore, to the mountains, to the country)

What types of things do you think you could enjoy if you had no inhibitions about them? (For example: painting, acting in a play, playing the piano)

What did you used to enjoy doing alone? (For example: long walks, playing the piano, sewing)

What did you enjoy doing with others? (For example: talking

on the telephone, going to dinner with a friend, playing handball)

What did you enjoy doing that costs no money? (For example: playing with my dog, going to the library, reading)

What did you enjoy doing that costs under $5.00? (For example: going to a movie, riding in a cab, going to the museum)

What did you enjoy doing when money was no object? (For example: buying a new suit, going to New York, going out for a nice dinner)

What activities did you enjoy at different times? (For example: in the morning, on Sunday, in the fall)

These questions are used to generate a list of activities. Then, the patient is asked to rank and select activities that are most likely to bring pleasure now.

SCHEDULING ACTIVITIES TO INCREASE A SENSE OF MASTERY

There are a number of ways to find out what activities increase a patient's sense of mastery. Mastery is the result of engaging in a constructive or creative activity that is difficult for the patient at this time, or one that he resists performing or does not feel motivated to attempt. In order to identify experiences which contribute to a sense of mastery, the therapist is advised to ask specific rather than general questions: for example, "What can you do between 2 and 3 p.m. that will give you a sense of satisfaction?" If the patient is unable to list mastery activities, the question should be rephrased. One patient, unable to list any mastery activities, was asked: "What things are you unable to do now because you are depressed?" The patient was then able to list various activities which would provide a sense of mastery.

Once mastery activities are identified, they are arranged in a hierarchy by degree of difficulty and the patient is assigned the most easily performed activities at first. Restoring the premorbid level of functioning is usually a step-by-step process. As an alternative to forming a hierarchy of mastery experiences, the patient can prepare a list of problematic activities and then attempt one each day.

"Mastery" is a relative concept. What may seem simple to the therapist may be extremely difficult for the depressed patient. For this reason, the patient is asked to rate the degree of mastery involved in carrying out each assignment. Since patients often discount their actual mastery experiences, these ratings of degree of mastery may show the patient how he underrates his actual accomplishments.

The following example shows how this tendency to disqualify achievements is encountered in the session. The patient was actively discounting important steps she had taken up the hierarchy of mastery experiences.

> PATIENT: Anyone can wash the dishes.
> THERAPIST: When you were not depressed, was there any problem with washing the dishes?
> P: None at all.
> T: And now that you are depressed?
> P: It is very difficult.
> T: When you are depressed many things are difficult. This is part of depression. However, you have been using a rating system based on your concept of mastery and difficulty from times when you were not depressed. I want you to review your ratings of these activities and consider rating them based on their current degree of difficulty.

Throughout therapy, the therapist must guard against being misled by the patient's distortion. A therapist without an understanding of the relative difficulty of even simple tasks might believe that boiling an egg could be a simple matter for his patient—when it might involve considerable planning and concentration.

In the construction of a mastery list with the patient, it is most useful to have the patient write down the items himself. This procedure tends to involve the patient more actively in the assignment. In fact, devising and writing the list may in itself constitute a mastery experience. Therefore, it is desirable to begin by scheduling initial structured activities right during the therapy session.

WRITTEN RECORDS AND DUTIES

Written records tend to help the patient examine his thoughts and feelings with increased objectivity and also facilitate recall of important events. Consequently, it is routine to include some writing in most of the homework assignments. The following examples illustrate a few of these assignments. Following the first or second session, the patient is often asked to write a short autobiography. By obtaining these background data, the therapist is free to concentrate on present problems. For the more depressed patients, a brief chronological outline is sufficient.

The Daily Record of Dysfunctional Thoughts is an integral part of cognitive therapy. Initially, patients are asked to complete the first three columns of this record (see Figure 4). Situations that precede unpleasant emotions are recorded along with the emotions and the automatic thoughts. This assignment helps the patient: learn to self-monitor affect changes; learn to correctly label emotions; and learn to recognize automatic thoughts and their relation to emotions. Once the patient has mastered these skills, he is ready to begin answering automatic thoughts. The therapist should make sure the patient knows how to use the form—a completed sample form can be given to the patient (see Figure 4). The therapist should retain copies of record forms which the patient has completed (they will be invaluable in discovering underlying assumptions). And the patient should have copies to refer to.

Patients are at times asked to write essays on particular themes. This technique is most often used in dealing with underlying assumptions. For example, a patient who believed she had to be perfect was asked to write an essay on what she would be like if she were perfect.

PATIENT'S ROLE IN DESIGNING HOMEWORK

The patient's participation in the design of homework assignments increases as treatment progresses. The final goal is for the patient to design and carry out his homework assignment. This goal is pursued to help the patient "shape" his own behavior.

The patient had made steady progress in treatment, but three weeks before the end of treatment her symptoms worsened. Her Beck Depression Inventory (BDI) score was 19. The patient had a recurrent tendency to let others define and solve her problems. However, the therapist was relatively confident that she had the capacity to overcome this particular tendency. She was given the following assignment.

> THERAPIST: For your homework, I'd like you to become less depressed by Friday. Today is Wednesday, so you have two

DAILY RECORD OF DYSFUNCTIONAL THOUGHTS

DATE	SITUATION Describe: 1. Actual event leading to unpleasant emotion, or 2. Stream of thoughts, daydream, or recollection, leading to unpleasant emotion.	EMOTION(S) 1. Specify sad/anxious/angry, etc. 2. Rate degree of emotion, 1-100.	AUTOMATIC THOUGHT(S) 1. Write automatic thought(s) that preceded emotion(s). 2. Rate belief in automatic thought(s), 0-100%.	RATIONAL RESPONSE 1. Write rational response to automatic thought(s). 2. Rate belief in rational response, 0-100%.	OUTCOME 1. Re-rate belief in automatic thought(s), 0-100%. 2. Specify and rate subsequent emotions, 0-100.
9/8	Received a letter from a friend who was recently married	Guilty 60	"I should have gone to her wedding" 90%	It was inconvenient; she wouldn't be writing if she was angry about it 95%	10% Guilty 20
9/9	Was thinking of all the things I wanted to get done over the weekend	Anxious 40	"I'll never get all of this done." "It is too much for me." 100%	I've done more than this before, and there is no law that says I have to get it all done 80%	25% Anxious 20
9/11	Made a mistake ordering supplies	Anxious 60	Pictured my boss yelling at me 100%	There is no evidence my boss will be angry, and even if he is I don't have to be upset 100%	0% Relieved 50
9/12	Pictured myself being depressed forever	Sad/ Anxious 90	"I'll never get better."	I have gotten better in the past. Just because I think something doesn't make it true 80%	40% Sad/ Anxious 60
9/15	My date called and said he couldn't go out with me because he had to work	Sad 95	"He doesn't like me. NO ONE could ever like me." 90%	He asked me out for next weekend so he must like me. He probably did have to work. Even if he didn't like me, it doesn't follow that "no one could ever like me." 90%	30% Sad 50

EXPLANATION: When you experience an unpleasant emotion, note the situation that seemed to stimulate the emotion. (If the emotion occurred while you were thinking, daydreaming, etc., please note this.) Then note the automatic thought associated with the emotion. Record the degree to which you believe this thought: 0%=not at all; 100%=completely. In rating degree of emotion: 1=a trace; 100=the most intense possible.

FIGURE 4. Daily Record of Dysfunctional Thoughts.

days. I'll give you some blank Depression Inventories with which to measure your mood.

PATIENT: How am I supposed to get better? I told you everything is rotten, and things aren't going to get better in two days.

T: Let's look at this homework assignment as an experiment. Because I've seen you overcome these moods in the past, I believe you can do it again. I'd like you to test this idea out.

P: But what am I supposed to do?

T: Do you recall in the beginning when I said this was your journey and that I was the guide and you had to do the walking?

P: Yes.

T: Well, we are at the point where you start becoming your own guide.

At the next session the patient reported she had successfully completed her homework by overcoming her depression in two days. She did this by implementing strategies that she had used in the past—becoming more socially active and refuting her automatic thoughts. By selecting and employing her own strategies, the patient gained more self-confidence and skill than if the therapist had outlined what to do.

The patient's increased participation in designing novel assignments results in effective ways of doing homework. It is often useful to help the patient translate these novel ideas into concrete plans. For example, one patient thought of recording thoughts on a tape recorder. The therapist encouraged him to carry out this idea by providing an audio tape cassette. Also, the therapist can subtly reward novel ideas by asking the patient to write down his procedure for use by other patients.

Alternatively, the therapist may modify the patient's initial idea to improve the therapeutic value of the assignment.

P: You know how I've been postponing analyzing my negative thoughts until seven in the evening instead of thinking about them all day long? I've heard of a technique called a "Wednesday box" which might help. During the week you write your problems on slips of paper and put them in the box. On Wednesday you tear up those that are no longer problems. You put the others that are still problems back in the box for next Wednesday.

T: How could you use this technique?

P: The same, I guess.

T: I have a suggestion to add to your idea. Do you recall when we talked about the difference between pseudo-problems and real problems?

P: Yes. Real problems are circumstances you can change or learn to live with. Pseudo-problems are ones that we create in our minds—like the idea I couldn't live without my girlfriend.

T: Before you put problems in the Wednesday box, I'd like you to write on the paper whether you think it is a real problem or a pseudo-problem. When you take the problem out Wednesday, see if you have changed your mind about what type of problem it is. And I'd like to see the problems.

This patient had trouble discriminating between real problems that require problem-solving skills and self-created problems. The therapist expanded on the patient's idea to help the patient learn to make finer distinctions between these two types of problems.

SPECIALIZED HOMEWORK ASSIGNMENTS

Bibliotherapy

Books and articles have high credibility for some patients. Bibliotherapy is an easy and effective way to reinforce selected material covered in the sessions. Books can be read at the patient's convenience, thereby saving therapeutic time. Before assigning readings, the therapist should find out whether the patient likes to read and should choose material keyed to an appropriate level of understanding.

Asking the patient about the material to see whether he has read and understood it gives him an opportunity to discuss relevant items from the reading.

The choice of reading materials will depend on the therapist's past experience. An experimental approach of trying out a variety of materials is worthwhile. Materials which we often have found useful are: Beck's *Cognitive Therapy and the Emotional Disorders* (1976); Maultsby's *Handbook of Rational Self-Counseling* (1971a); Ellis and Harper's *A New Guide to Rational Living* (1975); and McMullin and Casey's *Talk Sense to Yourself* (1975).

At times the suggested books can be tailored to the patient's individual concern. One patient, for example, did not believe anyone could live through his horrible life and not be depressed. He was given Frankl's *Man's Search for Meaning* (1963) to show how one could live through much worse conditions without totally succumbing to depression.

Assigning patients specific passages is an effective homework assignment. One college student was depressed about his inability to find the meaning of life. He was assigned specific pages from the *Handbook of Rational Self-Counseling,* and this material was discussed in the subsequent therapy hour. He was then asked to underline, make notes, and comment on the passages for the next session.

Another patient who believed everyone in the world was happy but himself was assigned a section in Lazarus and Fay's *I Can If I Want To* (1975) that dealt with this mistaken notion. He credited this handout with being a major element in overcoming this long-held belief.

Chapters of this monograph may also be given to the patients as reading assignments. This approach has proven to be helpful in a number of cases. One patient, for example, was worried about the prospect of ending therapy. She was asked to read the chapter on termination, where she found many of her specific concerns discussed. The assignment not only helped her resolve some of her questions, but it also saved valuable therapy time. By asking the patient to read parts of the treatment manual, the therapist reinforces the collaborative nature of treatment.

Tape Recording

Having a patient listen to an audiotape of the session can be effective when a great deal of material has been covered and the therapist wants to be sure the patient has heard it. Some patients will criticize themselves when they listen to the audiotapes. These self-critical thoughts should be written down and brought in for discussion.

Patients can be told to listen closely and note for discussion at the next session mistakes the therapist made. This reinforces the patient's attention to the material and shows him that making and admitting a mistake is not a catastrophe.

Both Ellis and Maultsby routinely give their patients tape recordings of the session. Although we have not incorporated this procedure for all patients, we believe that it may be of enormous value to some.

Patients may be assigned theme-oriented cassette tapes. These have included tapes by Albert Ellis, relaxation tapes, and tapes on sensory awareness.

Preparing for Anticipated Problems

Once the patient is free from depression, it is important to develop ways for him to use the skills learned in therapy to cope with critical situations in the future. First, the therapist and patient list those events that have recurrently led the patient to become anxious or depressed in the past. These problematic events might include visiting parents, school examinations, interpersonal friction, or rejection. Alternatively, a list can be made of those events antici-pated in the next few months which might cause problems; for example, a new job, becoming engaged, moving to a new city. These potential problems are pencilled into a calendar or log along with a list of coping techniques to be used.

As an illustration, let us consider one patient who was most likely to become depressed on Saturdays and Sundays or holidays (when her time was not structured). She wrote a reminder, in her calendar, to plan activities on these days. She was the editor of a monthly newspaper and was prone to anxiety when the paper had to go to press. She wrote on her calendar for these dates, "Review old homework—analyze thoughts." She was also expecting a visit from her mother, who had dominated her in the past. For days in advance of the time when her mother was expected to visit, she wrote, "Be assertive." The patient carried the calendar with her as a means of self-instruction and updated the calendar as the need arose.

SUGGESTED OUTLINE OF HOMEWORK ASSIGNMENTS

After First Session

1. Record activities on Activity Schedule (to obtain baseline).
2. Read *Coping with Depression* (Beck and Greenberg, 1974)
3. Write autobiographical sketch outline.
4. Listen to audiotape of first interview (optional).

After Second Session

1. Plan and record activities on Activity Schedule.
2. Check off negative automatic thoughts on wrist counter. (See Chapter 8)

After Third Session

1. Continue with Activity Schedule and rate Mastery (M) and Pleasure (P).
2. Continue with wrist counter.
3. Record affect and automatic thoughts in relevant columns on Daily Record of Dysfunctional Thoughts.

After Fourth Session

1. Activity Schedule: continue with M and P.
2. Wrist counter.
3. Fill in rational response column on Daily Record of Dysfunctional Thoughts.

From Fifth Session to Termination (usually Fifteenth Session)

1. Continue with Activity Schedule as long as useful.
2. Continue with wrist counter as long as useful.

3. Fill in all columns of Daily Record of Dysfunctional Thoughts.

Optional throughout Treatment

1. Bibliotherapy.
2. Special handouts on specific problems.
3. Listen to audiotape of interview.
4. Keep diary or log.

Chapter 14

TECHNICAL PROBLEMS

The course of therapy, like true love, is not always smooth. Some patients do not return calls; others call incessantly. Some patients talk too much in therapy; others not at all. Some are chronically late for appointments; others resist terminating an interview. Some spend the time during therapeutic interviews arguing with the therapist about his technique; others pay lip service to therapist's suggestions but do nothing to implement them. Some patients protest that cognitive therapy won't work and demand a "money-back guarantee." In short, patients can behave in a variety of ways or manifest a variety of attitudes that slow down therapy. This chapter will present the "underground" of cognitive therapy: strategies and guidelines for dealing with the technical problems arising from patients' counterproductive ideas and behavior.

Every patient could be placed on a continuum with respect to the number of technical problems he presents. At one end of the continuum are those who present none or few of these problems. Aside from the symptoms and dysfunctional behavior related to their depression, these patients lead reasonably well-adjusted lives. Because of their general cooperativeness and repertoire of adaptive behaviors, therapy usually runs smoothly. The therapist and patient can concentrate on the specific problems relevant to the depression and collaborate on selecting and applying appropriate strategies.

At the other end are the patients who present many of these problems, usually with great intensity and rigidity. These patients often have histories that include previous unsuccessful therapy, hospitalizations, poor work histories, nonexistent or combative social relationships, and a range of maladaptive patterns of interpersonal behavior that encroach on their work with the therapist. These patients have been given labels such as chronic neurotics, "borderlines," character disorders, passive–aggressive, negativistic, "hysterical," and unstable. These terms generally do not improve the therapist's understanding of the patient but indicate the patient has personality problems that make him difficult to work with. For want of a better term, we have used the label "the difficult patient" to designate a member this group. If these patients stay in treatment, cognitive therapy can help them to lead more comfortable and adaptive lives. Treatment with this population, however, takes longer, and the patient's overall improvement is usually less stable than that of other patients. Since they are also more prone to relapse, they require more booster sessions. Furthermore, a larger portion of the interview has to be devoted to the patient's negative reactions to the therapist, his resistance to doing homework assignments, his frequent life crises, and to repetitive setting of guidelines for the therapy. To be successful with difficult patients, the therapist usually has to be prepared to invest considerable extra time, energy, and ingenuity.

THERAPIST GUIDELINES

The following suggestions may be useful to the therapist when working with difficult patients.

1. Avoid stereotyping the patient.

A patient has, creates, and presents problems, but the patient himself is not the problem. Once the therapist begins to think of the patient as *the* problem or as a psychiatric anomaly, he closes off potential solutions to these problems. Even the most difficult patient has strengths that can be used to offset his antitherapeutic reactions.

2. Remain optimistic.

One observer of a cognitive therapy session remarked, "The difference between your therapy and others is that you don't give up." There is some truth to this observation. Hopelessness, whether in the patient or the therapist, is a powerful block to problem solving, and is rarely, if ever, warranted. Unless the therapist has exhausted his repertoire, there is always the chance of achieving a breakthrough.

Many difficult patients who eventually recover report that the therapist's refusal to give up was the most helpful element of therapy. Of course, if there is no progress or an actual worsening of the patient's condition, then consultation or referral to another therapist is indicated. Moreover, a different type of treatment might be more successful with this particular patient.

3. *Identify and deal with your own dysfunctional cognitions.*

When encountering difficult patients, the therapist should be vigilant in detecting his own self-defeating thoughts. Common self-defeating thoughts of therapists are: "The patient isn't getting any better so I must be a lousy therapist." "The patient shouldn't act that way." "After all I've done for him, he is ungrateful and gives me a hard time." The therapist has to remember that he does not need to be upset by the patient's counterproductive behavior. The patient, not the therapist, is ultimately responsible for his own counterproductive actions; the therapist can guide the patient but cannot expect to mold his behavior. However, the therapist should utilize his ingenuity to capitalize on idiosyncratic behaviors or attitudes. For example, the therapist may be able to utilize a patient's mistrust of him to test out with the patient some hypotheses regarding this issue and also to utilize the patient's wariness and build his self-sufficiency.

A therapist often mistakenly believes that the more he does for a patient, the more the patient should appreciate him. The reverse of this is often true. The therapist is confusing how he wants the patient to act with the way the patient is likely to act. Therapy is work, and there are generally rewards intrinsic to the work.

4. *Maintain a high tolerance for frustration.*

The therapist is better able to solve the "special difficulties" if he develops and maintains a high tolerance for frustration and a high threshold for the patient's dysphoria. When working with difficult patients, the therapist should expect to be thwarted frequently. He can also keep in mind that because these problems present a challenge and prevent therapy from becoming routine, they provide the therapist with an opportunity to apply his creativity to these problems. He can also increase his frustration tolerance by not giving up on patients and by remaining focused on the task, instead of blaming the patient for the obstacles to therapy.

5. *Maintain a problem-solving attitude.*

A problem-solving approach will enable the therapist to handle most of these difficulties as they arise. First, the problem should be specified and then verified by the patient. The therapist and patient then generate a variety of solutions. These solutions are then tried on an experimental basis.

The therapist's approach to these problems is structured but not rigid. It should be reasonable, flexible and applied in a "customized" way to the specific patient. A rigid approach, in contrast, mistakenly assumes a uniformity among patients. Pat, rehearsed therapeutic responses are generally ineffective. Therapists' interventions should take into account the patient's unique history, life-style, and way of relating to others.

By following these guidelines, the therapist provides a strong model for the patient. For example, he can demonstrate by his own behavior that frustration does not automatically lead to discouragement or anger.

The following is just a sample of countertherapeutic beliefs and actions of patients. The list, however, does contain many recurring issues found in therapy. A number of suggestions are given for resolving these issues. The suggestions are far from conclusive. When discussing these problems, the therapist may at times be at a loss for ideas. In these cases, he can tell the patient that he will have to think more about the problem and discuss it at the next session.

There may be issues that the patient and therapist cannot agree on. The therapist can suggest, if the issue is crucial, that they discuss it later in therapy. If the issue is not crucial, the therapist and patient may have to agree to disagree.

PATIENTS' COUNTERTHERAPEUTIC BELIEFS

1. *"Cognitive therapy is a rehash of 'the power of positive thinking'."*

The therapist can agree that there are a few superficial similarities between cognitive therapy and schools of "positive thinking." Both hold that thoughts influence feelings and behavior. However, an obvious problem with "positive thinking" is that the positive thoughts are not necessarily valid or accurate. A person may deceive himself for a while with unrealistically positive thoughts, but he will eventually become disillusioned as the law of diminishing returns goes into operation. Positive thoughts lead to positive feelings only when the person is convinced they are true.

Cognitive therapy can be called the power of *realistic* thinking. A half glass of water may be from a pessimist's viewpoint half empty or from an optimist's viewpoint half full, but from an objective point of view, is simply 4 ounces of water in an 8-ounce glass. When a patient says his life is "bad," the therapist doesn't try to convince him his life is "good." Rather, the main thrust is on *gathering accurate information to pinpoint and counteract distortions.*

In cognitive therapy, the therapist tries to induce a shift away from vague moralistic labels such as, "I'm terrible" (power of negative thinking). These self-judgments imply the existence of a host of negative or positive traits. There is little the patient or therapist can do to change these abstract, globally defined "character traits." However, when the problems are broken down into particulars, solutions become apparent. Therapist and patient shift from global judgments to observation of specific problems. "Positive thinking," in contrast, consists of substituting one global abstraction, "I'm a wonderful person," for another, "I'm a bad person."

Schools of "positive thinking" are based on an authoritative approach, as when someone says, "Cheer up, things aren't that bad." Cognitive therapy, on the other hand, stresses that one shouldn't accept a statement on the basis of authority. A person should test statements empirically or figure them out logically—not accept uncritically the beliefs of others.

Many of the principles of "positive thinking" contain distortions or half-truths, e.g., "Every day, in every way, things are getting better and better." From a cognitive therapist's perspective, saying that everything is going to get better is as unrealistic as saying that everything is going to get worse. What one wants and needs is *accurate information in order to make adaptive decisions.* The patient also can be commended for not automatically agreeing with an authority.

2. *"I'm not depressed because I distort reality, but because things really are bad. Anyone would become depressed."*

The therapist can say he does not know whether things are or are not as bad as the patient paints them, but that he wants to check the facts and see. After these preliminaries, the therapist pinpoints concrete instances and discusses the reasonableness of each. The major premise in cognitive therapy is to speak from the data—not attempt to convince the patient through force of argument.

The first part of the patient's belief, that "things are bad," may or may not be true. In any event, therapist and patient have to agree on a working definition of "bad." The second part, that "anyone would be depressed" is generally incorrect. Most people become frustrated and unhappy over negative events but *do not become clinically depressed.* The therapist can ask the patient whether he knows anyone who has gone through similar situations without becoming depressed.

The therapist can help the patient separate real problems from psuedoproblems. A pseudoproblem is one the patient creates entirely himself. An example of a pseudoproblem is a patient's belief that he can't go to a concert because he anticipates that he will not know anybody else in the audience. Actually, the important objective is to enjoy the performance, not to be welcomed by friends.

If the patient has a real problem (for example, he can't go to work because his car is broken), then he can counteract his discouragement and passivity by adopting a problem-solving approach. In this instance, for example, the patient could consider alternative modes of transportation, requesting a ride from a friend, etc. The first step is to "decatastrophize" the problem and avoid task-irrelevant thoughts and actions. The therapist can tell the patient that if he assumes a problem-solving attitude, he can take care of his problems.

The therapist should not be reluctant to refer patients to other professional services. One therapist, for example, referred a battered wife to a women's organization that provided support in this area and to the District Attorney's office for legal help.

3. *"I know I look at things in a negative way, but I can't change my personality."*

First, the therapist wants to know why the patient believes he can't change. The patient might propose any number of reasons to support this belief: (a) He is too stupid to change. (b) Change takes too long. (c) Any change would only be superficial. (d) Something irreversible happened to him in childhood that prevents change. (e) He is too old to change. Once the reason for the belief is discovered, the therapist can apply standard procedures: for example, seek evidence and data to prove or disprove the belief.

In general, the therapist can tell the patient that it is not necessary (or even possible) to change his whole personality but only several of his habitual ways of thinking and acting. The therapist can explain that many depressed people believe they cannot change or get better; this belief is part of depression and is to be expected. The therapist can also tell the patient that once corrective action takes place, dramatic changes may occur.

The therapist can then ask whether the patient has changed any of his beliefs in the past—ideas that teachers, parents, or childhood friends may have told him, for example. He can also suggest that the patient list specific behaviors that he has changed in the past. Often, after the patient has reflected on beliefs and habits he has changed in the past, he gains confidence in his present ability to change. The therapist can ask the patient whether there were difficult situations in the past that he was able to handle. Most patients are able to report some difficult problems that they were able to solve successfully in the past. This exercise lets the patient know that he has strengths available to effect change. The therapist can also emphasize that depression is a psychiatric condition (a "state") not a character "trait," and, therefore, is relatively amenable to change.

The following illustrates how a therapist worked with a patient who was convinced he couldn't change.

PATIENT: I'm weak. I'll never be able to change.

THERAPIST: You have 40 years of coping well—I might add under difficult conditions—versus only two years of being depressed. In fact, you coped well during part of those two years.

P: It's so hard to change.

T: That's true. Change can be difficult, particularly the first few steps, but it is not impossible. Many people have changed extremely difficult habits.

P: I just don't believe I can change.

T: The belief that one can't change is the strongest obstacle to change. It's an escape clause that can prevent one from trying to change.

P: My problems are too ingrained to change.

T: Your problems may be ingrained in the sense they are of long duration. But they are not ingrained in that you can't change them on an everyday basis. A person can change even lifelong habits, such as particular ways of speaking, eating behaviors, or habitual postural patterns.

Throughout therapy, the patient can use himself or people he knows of as models. A coping model is generally better than a mastery model. The coping model, in contrast to the mastery model, has to struggle with the problem before coming to a satisfactory resolution.

4. *"I believe what you are saying intellectually, but not emotionally."*

Patients often confuse the terms "thinking" and "feeling." This semantic problem is most obvious when the patient mistakenly uses the word "feel" for "believe," for example, "I feel you're wrong." The therapist can tell the patient that a person cannot believe anything "emotionally." Emotions include feelings, sensations; thoughts and beliefs lead to emotions. When the patient says he believes or does not believe something emotionally, he is talking about *degree of belief.* He has two minds about some issues. On the one hand, for example, he believes that making a mistake is human; on the other hand, he believes it's unacceptable. When a patient sees the point a therapist is making, he is not necessarily convinced and then may talk about not believing it "emotionally." This degree of belief is often contingent upon the situation, the time, and the patient's condition. When a person says, "I know I'm not worthless but I don't believe it emotionally," he is indicating that his dysfunctional or distorted thoughts of worthlessness are so overpowering that he believes them.

At this point, the therapist can say,

What you're really saying is that you don't truly believe my explanation is correct. You don't have a real gut feeling for it, and it is to be expected. These ideas feel foreign to you. What you can do is act upon my suggestions, test them out, see if they're true, discuss them with yourself, look at the other alternatives, consider the evidence. I certainly do not want you to believe it just because I say it or take it on faith; rather, just to try it on for size. Try to have an open mind.

The therapist can tell the patient that cognitive therapy teaches a person how to change unrealistic beliefs that are making him uncomfortable and unhappy. He changes these beliefs by strengthening the adaptive beliefs. To reach this degree of belief, the patient, with the help of the therapist, has to challenge his old maladaptive beliefs actively and act on new adaptive beliefs. (For further elaboration of this point, see the sections on dealing with underlying assumptions in Chapter 12.)

5. *"I can't think of rational answers to my automatic thoughts when I'm emotionally upset."*

The therapist can explain that this difficulty may occur because the patient is mentally and physically in a state that makes reasoning difficult. The patient should be on the lookout for thoughts that aggravate this problem, such as, "Since this technique doesn't work, nothing will work."

There are several ways to help the patient handle this problem. One is for the patient to wait until he is less upset before attempting to write the rational or reasonable answer to the automatic thought. The patient can engage in some kind of activity or distraction in the interval. He can also be told that with practice he will be able to think of rational responses more quickly. It is unreasonable for the patient to expect rational answers to come easily when he is upset.

The therapist can tell the patient that those times when he is able to calm himself down immediately will give him the most confidence; however, the ability to correct distortions immediately is a skill that has to be developed over a period of time.

6. *"Since I don't like these negative thoughts, the reason they come must be that I want to be depressed."*

The therapist can explain that these negative thoughts are automatic and are not conjured up because the patient wants them; rather, they come involuntarily as though by reflex. Since having automatic negative thoughts is an inherent aspect of being depressed, the occurrence of this type of thinking does not indicate a desire to be depressed.

The patient can be told that these thoughts are not continual (unless he is severely depressed), but generally are triggered by certain events, certain stresses, and by certain associations. The origin of these thoughts is not completely understood at this time. The most plausible explanation is that automatic thoughts are the result of some underlying assumption (schema) that is particularly salient at the present time. As the patient and therapist discover and modify these underlying assumptions, we find that patients have fewer negative thoughts.

Many patients have been told by others that they are depressed *because they want to be depressed* and consequently they believe this notion. The following is one way this can be handled.

PATIENT: My wife says I love to be miserable, that this is my fault. It must be true.

THERAPIST: Do you want to be miserable?

P: No, not really.

T: Is there any payoff from being depressed?

P: I can't think of any.

T: Many people enjoy sympathy and attention and at times people seek attention when they have bad moods. They want consolation to make themselves better. But clinical depression is quantitatively and qualitatively different from this type of condition. Although many depressed people may want others to know they are suffering, other people may misconstrue this communication as a basic desire to be depressed.

7. *"I'm afraid once I'm over being depressed, I'll become anxious like I was before."*

The patient can be told that anxiety, on occasion, does occur or become exacerbated as the depression lifts. Anxiety, therefore, may be a sign that depression is lifting. Simply telling the patient that anxiety sometimes often follows depression, but in most cases is usually a short-term process, may be helpful. The patient can be told that anxiety is not dangerous; the strange experiences associated with anxiety do not mean he is going crazy or that anything "awful" is going to happen to him. Although anxiety may be very unpleasant there are many procedures for handling it. These include modifying anxiety-producing thoughts, distraction, relaxation exercises, and increasing one's anxiety tolerance.

8. *"I want a guarantee this therapy will cure my depression."*

Depressed people often demand a degree of certainty that cannot exist in reality. Patients can be told that we live in a problematic world where there are no *absolute* guarantees in any undertaking. However, the therapist can explain that most depressed patients in our clinic believe (erroneously) they will not be helped. Our research indicates that low expectation of being helped does not forecast an unfavorable outcome from therapy. In fact, patients improve whether they expect to or not. However, to obtain the optimum results, the patient does have to apply himself and work on his therapy assignments. In fact—and this is a good time for the therapist to mention it—the amount of effort put into therapy is directly related to how much the patient gets out of it.

Patients' countertherapeutic actions can be used in a variety of therapeutic ways. The following exchange shows how this was done with a patient who wanted an absolute assurance that therapy would work:

THERAPIST: I think if I gave you a 100% guarantee you wouldn't believe me.
PATIENT: No, I'd believe you. You're the authority.
T: Do you think it makes much sense to believe me just because I'm an authority?
P: Who better to believe?
T: Yourself, for one. By using your own judgment, you learn to be more self-reliant.
P: How would I know anything if I didn't take people's word?
T: True. At times you have to rely on others for information, but for some of the best information you have to help yourself. As far as this type of therapy goes, the best way to find out is to try it and see. You will be able to see for yourself whether or not you make progress.

9. *"Cognitive therapy is concerned with mundane things in life and not with the serious problems that make me depressed."*

The patient's expectations of therapy should be taken into consideration. The therapist shouldn't say, "We cannot talk about these things, they are not important." Any issues that are important to the patient are topics for discussion. But they can be discussed in an adaptive way that leads to self-understanding and problem-solving.

The therapist should be sure that he and the patient are in accord about the goals and methods of therapy. Patients have to believe therapy makes sense; so the therapist should check periodically with the patient that they are together on these questions. For example, the patient has to understand that cognitive therapy concentrates on concrete incidents because it is easy to become lost in rhetoric and metaphysical ideas. The therapist can explain that he wants to understand the patient, and that the best way to do this is to make communication concrete, clear, and unambiguous. Concrete, specific references enhance communication while the use of abstractions fosters a multiplicity of diverse meanings.

Patients are often concerned about the emphasis on everyday experiences early in treatment. The therapist can tell the patient that philosophical issues can be discussed later but that it is important for the patient to become more active and to get back to his normal state. Many of these philosophical issues (Who am I? Where am I going? What is existence all about?) may appear irrelevant, but if they are important to the patient, they should be discussed eventually. Cognitive therapy is flexible, and the therapist should keep in mind the patient's expectations from therapy. Dreams, childhood experiences, and expression of feelings can be discussed. If there is a problem or an issue the patient believes is important, some time in therapy can be spent in this area.

Dreams can be interpreted cognitively (see Beck, 1967, pp. 208–217; and Freeman, in press). Generally, the themes of dreams have some bearing on the way the person construes his experiences. The therapist could talk about the content of the dreams, as well as past experiences.

10. *"If negative cognitive distortions make me unhappy, does that mean positive cognitive distortions make me happy?"*

This question may be asked by the more intelligent patient. The therapist can say that in a manic reaction, cognitive distortions are very much present. However, people can be happy without distorting reality. People seem to be most happy when engaged in activities they do well or having experiences that are meaningful and satisfying. There seem to be no distortions at these times.

There are times when people obtain pleasure through rating themselves: "I'm great because that person gave me a compliment," or

"I'm wonderful because I achieved this." These high self-evaluations are related to the kinds of assumptions that predispose some persons to depression and anxiety. The most lasting enjoyment is probably gained from the intrinsic satisfaction of engaging in an activity for its own sake, not from praise from others or from competing with others.

11. *"I have been coming to therapy for four weeks and I'm not any better."*

The patient can be told it is unrealistic to expect to be over depression in this short a time. Further, many patients improve without realizing it. One of the reasons for giving the Beck Depression Inventory is to show how much the patient has improved over a period of time. This measurement helps patients start to think in relative rather than absolute terms.

The therapist should indicate that therapy often *follows an uneven course*, with ups and downs. There are individual differences: some persons overcome depression quickly, but for most it is a zig-zag recovery. Most depressed persons want immediate results; but therapy is a process involving persistent effort, and to expect immediate recovery is unrealistic.

The following is a way one therapist handled this problem.

PATIENT: It's been five weeks and I'm not any better. I have a friend who went to a psychiatrist and got over his depression in four visits.

THERAPIST: Do you know how long he had been depressed?

P: I think a couple of months.

T: How long have you been depressed?

P: Three years.

T: Do you think it is realistic to expect to overcome a three-year depression in five weeks?

P: No, I guess not.

12. *"You can't treat my depression without seeing my wife, too. She caused the depression."*

First, the therapist should address the fallacy: "My wife caused the depression." The therapist often has to demonstrate, in a variety of ways, that the interpretation of events plays a primary role in precipitating depression. The therapist has to guard against the notion that another person can produce depression.

However, it is generally a good idea for the therapist to see others of significance in the patient's life. This may be a spouse, roommate, friend, or parent (if patient is living at home). These people can be used as "auxiliary therapists." The therapist can teach them to help the patient to follow activity schedules, to monitor his automatic thoughts, and to question and challenge these thoughts. When marriage partners are brought in, the patient should be told, "I am not going to take sides. I want to listen to both of you objectively, and try to get an accurate picture of what is happening. I'll talk to both of you straightforwardly rather than be on one side or the other."

The therapist obviously can't force a spouse to come to therapy. In this case, the patient can be told,

> I can't do marriage counseling with one person. However, we can work on changing those things within your power that are causing you trouble. For the time being, we will just have to take your spouse's behavior as a given and work with you. Later, if it seems indicated, you can do some things that might change your spouse's maladaptive behavior.

The therapist has to be careful not to make adverse judgments about the absent spouse. The patient will probably relay any adverse statements, and as a result the therapist will have an enemy—not an ally—at home.

13. *"I'm smarter than the therapist. How can he help me?"*

This attitude can be a problem in all forms of therapy. The therapist can tell the patient that in some areas the patient may be more successful or brighter than the therapist, but that at present the patient requires specialized help with specific types of problems. And since the therapist is skilled in this area, he is qualified to help the highly intelligent patient. They can form an ideal working partnership in which the combination of their respective skills and abilities can enhance the effectiveness of the therapy. Thus, the therapist should underscore the rationale of the therapeutic collaboration as opposed to the authoritarian approach, in which one person (the therapist) imposes his ideas on another (the patient). This same explanation may be utilized to reassure a patient who believes that the therapist is "too young" to help him.

The therapist can tell the patient that cognitive therapy works best when the therapist is well trained in this therapy, but it does not require a high intelligence on the part of either the therapist or patient.

The patient who believes he is brighter than the therapist often wants to engage the therapist in an intellectual debate. The therapist can point out that this type of activity is not productive. To illustrate this, the therapist can ask whether the patient's intellectualizing in the past solved his emotional problems.

14. *"You are more interested in doing research than in helping me."*

A patient engaged in a treatment-outcome study may secretly harbor the belief that he is simply being "used as a guinea pig" unless the therapist inquires about it. The therapist has to be continually aware of the fact that depressed patients may distort any of the therapist's actions. Many potential problems can be avoided if the therapist explains the reason for his actions. For example, a therapist interviewed a depressed patient in front of a group. Knowing that some members of the group would have to leave in the middle of the session, the therapist told the patient at the beginning, "Some of the people will have to leave before we are done. They'll do this, not because they dislike you, but because they have other appointments."

When conducting research in conjunction with therapy, the therapist has to explain fully the purpose of this research. He should explain the ways in which the research is beneficial to therapy; the questionnaires and outside evaluations, for example, give the therapist a more complete report on the patient than the therapist's own observations.

15. *"Cognitive therapy won't work because my depression is biological."*

Many patients believe that only drugs can help depression. This belief may be partly offset by a patient's previous unsuccessful experience with medication. When discussing this issue, and others, the therapist has to provide the most accurate information currently available. The therapist's credibility is especially crucial in regard to this question.

The following is one way the biological issue can be discussed with the patient.

THERAPIST: No one knows for sure all the causes of depression, especially in an individual case. There is a good chance that certain types of depression do have a biological basis.

PATIENT: If it does, how can cognitive therapy work?

T: Our research has shown that it can help your type of depression.

P: How can a psychological approach treat a biological problem?

T: It is an old-fashioned idea that the mind and body are separate. Many scientists *now* believe the mind and body work so closely together that it is possible to affect physiological processes through psychological methods.

With the more intelligent patient, the therapist can discuss the electrochemical nature of thinking. Because thinking involves electrochemical activity, cognitive therapy can be seen as a type of biological intervention.

16. *"I have to assert my independence by not letting the therapist get the best of me."*

Patients present different versions of this belief. Essentially, the patient believes that if he fights the therapist, he is demonstrating independence. The patient's previous (or current) behavior with other authority figures (parents and teachers) frequently has followed this same pattern.

There is often a brief honeymoon period in therapy: the patient may say, "You're better than other therapists who have tried to help me." The therapist is advised to take such flattering comments with a great deal of caution. Eventually, such a patient may begin taking a contrary point of view toward nearly everything the therapist says and may refuse to cooperate. The patient wants to argue in order to triumph over the therapist, not to gather information. (The therapist should be aware that many patients argue as a form of reality-testing, or to fill in gaps of knowledge. In these instances, arguing with the patient is an effective intervention.)

The therapist can present a strong defense of his position to the argumentative patient but should avoid lengthy arguments. If the therapist engages in a prolonged power struggle with this patient, the therapy usually suffers. It is better to set up projects or experiments to test the patient's and therapist's hypotheses. The therapist can convey the idea that he cannot force the patient to believe or do anything and that consequently there is no point to doing battle with his ideas. The patient is ultimately responsible for his own beliefs, his behavior, and their consequences. The therapist can give suggestions as to how the patient can change these consequences by changing certain maladaptive beliefs and behaviors, but he does not have the power to force him to change his beliefs. The therapist's degree of effectiveness with these patients is often in proportion to his nondefensive handling of the patient's negative behavior. However, the therapist should be flexible and ready to acknowledge that the patient may have a valid point.

The therapist can explain that contentiousness is not the hallmark of independence: saying "no" to everything can undermine independent action as much as saying "yes" to everything.

The therapist's strategy with the dependent patient who is striving for independence by rejecting the therapist is to help the patient to think for himself. The patient is asked for his suggestions, opinions, and methods for making changes. The following is an example of how this can be done.

> THERAPIST: What would you like to discuss today?
> PATIENT: I'm having trouble with my roommate.
> T: First, shall we list what these problems are?
> P: Okay. (The patient and therapist then make a list of specific problems.)
> T: Do you want to discuss some solutions to these problems?
> P: No, my roommate's not my real problem. I don't want to talk about this.
> T: Okay. I'll put this list in my desk, and when you want to discuss it, I'll get it out. Now what would you like to talk about?

An effective technique for this type of situation is to ask the patient to investigate the cost–benefit ratio for acting on this conception of independence. The patient is asked to weigh the ego-satisfying gains from fighting the therapist against losing the chance to work with him to overcome the emotional problems. If the patient believes the balance is tipped in favor of "fighting," the therapist should agree with the proviso that they evaluate the benefits at the end of specified time. The patient often comes to realize his victories over others are hollow and that in the process he has lost a great deal of time which can never be recovered.

Patient's Countertherapeutic Behaviors

1. *The patient will not (or cannot) talk in therapy.*

There are a variety of methods to encourage the patient to communicate in therapy. The therapist can reinforce verbally and nonverbally what the patient does say. He can also tell the patient, "You do not have to talk. I'll be happy to do the talking for a while." Taking off the pressure to talk may counteract the anxiety that is blocking the patient.

The patient can be asked to write down and bring in material to read or for the therapist to read regarding what is bothering him. If the patient is extremely reluctant to talk, he can use hand signals to answer questions or to indicate agreement/disagreement with what the therapist says. The therapist can say, "Raise your right hand if I'm on target, your left if I'm off . . . now let's test out the system. Are you thinking about not being able to talk?" The procedure can be used to ease the patient into talking. Another nonstandard procedure is for the therapist to take a walk with the patient in place of a formal interview; while they are walking, some patients seem to lose their inhibitions about putting their thoughts into words.

2. *The patient deliberately fabricates or he attempts to manipulate the therapist.*

Generally, the patient is considered to be telling the truth as he perceives it unless the reverse is discovered to be true. At times, the patient's distortions may seem to have all the earmarks of a lie but may actually represent a genuine error. If the patient's *deliberate* distortions are hampering therapy, the therapist has to confront him on this issue. An extremely fruitful area to discuss is why the patient believes he has to misrepresent himself, falsify or withhold crucial information, and deceive the therapist. Such behavior might be the result of a basic mistrust of the therapist, a fear of displeasing him, or it might represent an attempt to manipulate him. Such maneuvers may also be based on the belief that he has to protect himself from being manipulated by the therapist. A discussion in this area could improve patient/therapist relationships and move therapy forward.

3. *The patient develops an incapacitating positive or negative "transference" toward the therapist.*

If there is a "transference" problem, it is good to shift the focus of cognitive therapy to a discussion of the personal issues. The first step is to clarify the problem. One of the ways the therapist can undermine a counterproductive therapist–patient interaction is to investigate the patient's feelings and attitudes.

Often patients will have unverbalized counterproductive ideas about the therapist, and it is good to make them explicit. The patient may think the therapist is too young, too old, or of the wrong sex to help him. Once the problems are pinpointed, they can be discussed and evaluated. If the therapist is too positive and optimistic early in therapy, he sets the stage later for the patient to feel let down and betrayed.

If the patient is furious at the therapist, the therapist can defuse the anger by maintaining a nondefensive attitude, by using humor, or by using distraction: "Has there ever been anyone else in your past life with whom you have gotten as angry as you are with me?" After the anger has diminished, the therapist can engage the patient in exploring its source.

It is better for the therapist to expose and examine the patient's notion that he (the therapist) is rejecting, etc., than to try to prevent such ideas from arising by overwhelming the patient with evidence of dedication, interest, and affection. If the patient's ideas are distorted or exaggerated, they can then be explored and subjected to reality-testing. This not only helps the therapeutic relationship but provides a valuable *in vivo* exercise for the patient in identifying and refuting his faulty interpretations. Even when the patient's observations are accurate, they can provide valuable material for exploring the meaning of these perceptions. For example, a depressed patient may believe that the therapist cannot help him if he regards him as "just another patient"; that if the therapist doesn't regard him highly, he—the patient—is "worthless"; that if the therapist does not feel affection for him then nobody can love him.

The uncovering of such unreasonable beliefs is potentially of great help in demonstrating the patient's "catastrophizing" tendencies and his dichotomous, absolutistic (all-or-nothing) categorizations. It is generally useful to attempt to elicit these dysfunctional beliefs even though the therapist may actually feel warmth and concern for the patient. The therapist can say, "Let's assume, for purposes of illustration, that I feel neutral toward you; what would this mean to you?" Such a probe frequently releases a torrent of dire predictions, such as, "It would be awful. . . . I couldn't stand another rejection." "How can you help me if you don't care for me?" "The only thing that has kept me going was knowing that you wanted to help me. I think I would kill myself if you didn't." These kinds of statements are generally delivered with expressions of considerable pain, and they lead directly to the underlying irrational beliefs.

Some patients develop strongly positive or negative attitudes toward the therapist as a way of diverting attention from painful or embarrassing issues. A few patients, for instance, began to behave negatively toward a therapist because they had developed erotic fantasies about him.

The therapist may avoid sticky positive transference problems with patients of the opposite sex by wearing a wedding ring and by subtly letting the patient know he or she is married. If positive transference takes place, the therapist can tell the patient this kind of feeling is not uncommon in therapy. He can then turn this reaction to therapeutic advantage by investigating why the patient is feeling this way toward him: What else is going on in the patient's life? Perhaps there is a void as far as other relationships go. The therapist should recognize the patient's feelings, encourage their expression, and clarify their sources, but should not make a big issue of them.

4. *The patient talks too much in therapy and goes off on tangents.*

Patients who have been in forms of therapy in which they were expected to talk for the whole session have to be reoriented into cognitive therapy. The therapist can tell the patient that in cognitive therapy, the therapist usually talks part of the time: The therapy is a dialogue, not a monologue (by either patient or therapist).

When the patient tends to wander or become circumlocutory, the therapist should redirect him to the mainstream. The therapist's stance should be that recitation of redundant material takes away from the time needed to cover the crucial material within the limits of short-term therapy. Do not be afraid to interrupt the patient tactfully.

The patient can be told that the amount of potential discussion

314

is practically infinite but that time is finite. The time allowed for the therapy session must be used judiciously, and the session should be paced to distribute time adequately.

More concrete measures may be necessary for some patients. These can include using a timer to limit the amount of time the patient talks. The therapist and patient can agree on some type of cue to indicate that the patient is wandering, such as sounding a buzzer or slapping the desk. In addition to keeping therapy "on target," the last method can help the patient learn to focus his thinking more effectively.

5. The patient abuses telephone privileges.

Telephone calls may be used in three ways in therapy. (1) The therapist as a matter of course gives his home telephone number to the patient and asks him to call if there is a crisis. In the treatment of depressed and suicidal patients this arrangement may save a life. (2) In the early stages of treatment, the therapist may ask the patient to call when an assignment has been completed. This can help motivate the patient to do the task. (3) When the patient cannot come in for treatment or is out of town, therapy can be conducted over the phone. In these cases, the agenda of the sessions has to be structured at the beginning of the call.

When, in rare cases, a patient abuses these telephone privileges, he is probably using the telephone to reduce anxiety. If such is the case, the patient is taught ways to control the anxiety other than by calling. If the pattern continues, the therapist tells the patient that the natural consequence of abusing this privilege is to lose it. Patients usually respond by learning to tolerate anxiety by developing constructive techniques to reduce it.

6. The patient is chronically late and misses appointments.

Our general policy is to let patients finish the remainder of the hour if they come late. The therapist tries to ascertain the reasons for this behavior without sounding accusatory. As a general policy, the therapists maintain tight limits on the mechanics regarding payment and appointments. The general stance of the therapist is that there is too much important work to be done to have available time curtailed by tardiness or other avoidable problems. The patient with these chronic problems is told that if he wants the treatment to be successful he has to follow the rules. If a patient is unavoidably late, the therapist should try to be flexible in providing an opportunity for the patient to make up for the time he missed.

7. *The patient attempts to prolong the interview.*

The therapist should generally be firm in ending the session within the "allotted time." Some patients make the termination seem arbitrary or awkward by not pacing themselves properly or by bringing up important material at the end of the session.

The therapist can help the session to end on a note of completion by prodding the patient with statements such as: "I see we have only about ten minutes left, and I want to move on to the homework assignment." To forestall the patient's leaving important questions to the end of the session, the therapist should make sure that the preparation of the agenda at the start of the interview is sufficiently inclusive. He might say, for instance, "Are you sure that we haven't left out anything important? Because I would hate to have it come up at the end of the session and not have the time to discuss it." Should the patient raise a substantive question at the end of the session, suggest that he write it down with possible solutions and bring in the material to the next session.

If the therapist follows the usual routine of setting time aside— prior to ending the session—to summarize the main points of the session, to obtain feedback from the patient regarding the session, or to make the homework assignment, he will generally find that the patient will fit into the routine.

Chapter 15

PROBLEMS RELATED TO TERMINATION
AND RELAPSE

Preparation for Termination

Because cognitive therapy is time-limited, the problems associated with termination are usually not as complex as those associated with longer forms of treatment. However, much of the benefit of cognitive therapy can be lost through inappropriate or inept closure. For this reason, it is important that the process of completion of therapy be handled as effectively and smoothly as possible. When the conclusion of therapy is handled well, the patient is more likely to consolidate gains and to generalize strategies for handling future problems.

The issue of termination should be touched on periodically throughout therapy. From the beginning the therapist stresses to the patient that he will *not* stay in treatment indefinitely, and that he will be shown how to handle his psychological problems on his own. "Positive transference reactions" are not encouraged; rather, the therapist attempts to present himself realistically in the process of therapy. This "demystification" of therapy has the effect of countering the patient's dependency on the therapist and any belief in the "magic" of therapy. Throughout therapy, the patient is encouraged to become more independent and self-reliant. As therapy progresses, the patient plays an increasingly active role in identifying target problems and choosing strategies. This sets the stage for the patient's becoming his own therapist.

Therapists can further diminish termination problems by emphasizing the educational nature of treatment. The therapist can explain that the patient needs to acquire specialized knowledge, experience, and skill in dealing with certain types of problems; therapy is a training period in which the patient will learn more effectve ways to handle these problems. The patient is not asked or expected to gain

317

complete mastery of these skills in therapy: The emphasis instead is on growth and development. The patient will have ample time after therapy to improve on these cognitive and behavioral coping skills.

Before the final session, patients often express doubts and concerns about leaving therapy. It is best to handle these concerns as soon as they are brought up. One patient, for example, at his twelfth session began to doubt whether he could maintain his improvement once treatment ended (after the fifteenth session). The therapist asked him to list and answer his dysfunctional thoughts about leaving therapy.

The following were his thoughts about ending therapy:

1. "I won't be able to discipline myself after the program ends."
2. "I won't be able to learn therapy well enough and will go back to my old ways."
3. "If I have an anxiety attack, I won't be able to handle it, and I'll forget what I learned."

The following were his answers to these thoughts:

1. "These are thoughts, not facts."
2. "I have some tools to work with now and will have more before I am done with therapy."
3. "I realize that in order to improve on the methods, I must continue to practice them."
4. "Once again I can see I'm still trying to be perfect; if I make a mistake I'll learn something each time I make it."
5. "I am making progress now and I believe I'll be ready to handle anxiety when it comes up."

This is another example of how the therapist can use the patient as a "resource person" to provide answers to troubling thoughts. Whenever possible, it is best to have the patient answer his own dysfunctional thoughts. Responding realistically in this way is an example of the kinds of skills we expect the patient to acquire.

PATIENT'S CONCERNS ABOUT TERMINATION

Despite the groundwork for smooth termination of therapy, various problems associated with termination often arise toward the end of treatment. A common concern expressed by patients is that they are not "completely cured." This is often coupled with the belief that they can't handle their problems without the therapist's help. The therapist has a variety of options in dealing with this issue. One approach is to agree with the patient that "he isn't 100% mentally healthy," but add, "neither is anyone else." The patient's spurious dichotomy of "sick" versus "cured" can then be discussed. The therapist can point out that mental health is not a *dichotomy* but rather a continuum, with many points along the continuum. Using examples from therapy to illustrate how the patient has moved along this continuum during treatment, the therapist can point out incidents in which the patient has handled difficult personal problems on his own.

The therapist can use the patient's dichotomy of "sick versus cured" to illustrate all-or-none thinking and self-defeating, unrealistic standards. The therapist can then review and reinforce the initial goal of therapy: to teach the patient ways to handle his problems more effectively, not to "cure" him or restructure his personality. The patient is told that the best way to improve his skills is to practice them on the inevitable problems he will face. It is best to stress to the patient that he can't expect to have complete mastery over his psychological problems, but that he will learn with each attempt. The therapist can use analogies meaningful to the patient (learning sports, vocational skills, foreign languages, etc.) to show how growth proceeds from an interaction of mistakes, feedback, and success experiences. Thus, each "mistake" can be viewed positively as a bit of information to be utilized in improving one's skill.

The patient may believe he is not ready to end therapy because of an unresolved realistic problem. This could be a problem at work, difficulty in his marriage, or unresolved issues with his parents. If the patient defines these situations realistically, the therapist can reinforce the patient for having learned to separate the real from the pseudoproblems. The therapist should emphasize to the patient that cognitive therapy is not magic and will not prevent or eliminate all problems: To be human is to deal with problems. The cognitive and behavioral procedures that the patient learns in therapy, however, can be used to resolve some of these problems more effectively. The therapist might then ask the patient how he would go about solving the problems he foresees. He should be encouraged to view future problems as challenges that will help him to consolidate his gains.

At times the patient may misinterpret negative fluctuations in his mood and thus make himself even more disturbed. For example, he may have anxiety over having anxiety. This experience can occur near the end of treatment when the patient has doubts about his abilities to handle emotional problems on his own. The patient may misinterpret normal mood shifts as signs that his depression is returning. The strategy, here, is for the patient to realistically appraise his moods and to challenge any depressogenic automatic thoughts.

A frequent concern of a patient is that he will become depressed again after therapy ends. The following is one way this concern can be handled.

> PATIENT: Can you guarantee that I won't become depressed again?
> THERAPIST: You are likely to become depressed again.
> P: How then am I any better off than I was when I started therapy?
> T: What have you learned here?
> P: Well, I've learned to control what causes me to be depressed— my negative thoughts and attitudes.
> T: What you have now are the tools to control how often you get depressed, how severe the depression will be, and how long you will stay depressed.
> P: I never want to become depressed again.
> T: That is certainly understandable, but the nature of depression is such that it's often hard to prevent its occurrence. But the intensity, frequency, and duration are under one's control. In fact, the recurrence of a mild depression could be of benefit . . . What are some of the advantages of becoming depressed after you leave treatment?
> P: I could practice the techniques I've learned . . . I could prove to myself that I can overcome depression and so I won't be afraid that I couldn't handle it.
> T: The way you are describing it, then, is that a mild bout with depression could strengthen you.

The patient's experience of a relapse near the end of treatment may indicate that he is engaged in a form of reality-testing; that is, the patient is testing his ability to cope with depression. This was explicitly spelled out by one patient; he believed that if he could depress himself by thinking negative thoughts and then overcome his depression by applying what he had learned, he would be ready to leave therapy. For a whole day the patient purposely conjured up negative thoughts and consequently became dysphoric. The next day, the patient successfully applied what he learned in therapy to overcome his bleak mood. He then used this experiment as evidence that he was ready to leave therapy.

The therapist can use a similar standard procedure to demonstrate that the patient can control his affect. First, the patient is asked to think as negatively about himself and his future as he possibly can. He is then asked to rate his unpleasant feelings from 0 to 100. Next, the patient answers his negative thoughts with a more balanced point of view, and re-rates his emotions. This procedure often has the effect of counteracting the patient's belief that he won't be able to handle his dysphoria once he leaves therapy.

Another method the therapist can use to provide a smooth closure of therapy is to challenge the patient's progress. In this procedure the therapist plays devil's advocate and presents many of the patient's original negative ideas, while the patient attempts to answer these thoughts. The following is an example of how this technique was used with one patient.

> THERAPIST: You seem to be feeling okay now, but what if you start feeling down and you think, "I'm depressed again. The techniques I learned just don't work." How would you answer this?
>
> PATIENT: I know it works because I was depressed and I got over it before.
>
> T: But this time it's different. No tehnique could get you over this depression.
>
> P: I have no evidence that cognitive procedures won't work this time.
>
> T: Yeah, but you don't have any money, and your health is rotten, and your daughter is unhappy.
>
> P: That doesn't mean that I won't have money in the future, and even if I don't have money, I don't have to be depressed. There's no evidence that my health is really bad. And furthermore, my daughter is responsible for her own happiness.
>
> T: You seem to be able to answer these thoughts.
>
> P: Yes, I seem to be able to carry things I've learned here in my head.

This type of role-reversal procedure can help to inoculate the patient against relapses. The therapist can bring a sense of completion to therapy by summarizing the progress that has been made. An even better method is to have the patient summarize therapy from his perspective by asking him to bring in an essay at the last session which evaluates and summarizes therapy.

At termination a variety of emotions may be felt by the patient. The emotions may range from anger to sadness. Generally, a reflective approach is nonproductive in the early stages of treating depression. However, at the later stages of treatment, when the patient has his depression under control, a reflective approach may be helpful. The therapist can clarify and reflect the feelings the patient may have about ending therapy. The appropriateness of experiencing these feelings can be discussed. The therapist may also choose to discuss his own feeling about ending a very intense relationship.

At times it is helpful to schedule a "booster session" with the patient several weeks after termination and to let the patient know that he can call the therapist if he has any problems. In many cases, just knowing he can call is enough to carry him over difficult times.

PREMATURE TERMINATION

Rapid Relief of Symptoms

At times, patients will respond quickly to treatment and the symptoms of depression will disappear in a few sessions. This may be due to a variety of factors, such as the enthusiasm and expectation of the therapist, or the patient's belief that the therapist can now magically solve all his problems. In some cases, patients have been able to solve realistic problems that have been bothering them, so that they no longer need therapy. It is also possible that the relief of depression simply represents the "natural course of the illness" (spontaneous remission) and is not related to the therapeutic intervention. In most instances, early termination is inadvisable because the psychological factors that predisposed the patient to depression have not been delineated or changed.

There are a variety of ways to handle premature termination. One is to clearly structure from the outset a specific time period for therapy. The therapist can tell the patient that at times people respond quickly to this type of therapy, but it is extremely important to work on the underlying dysfunctional assumptions and belief system. To avoid unscheduled termination, it is helpful to reach an agreement early in treatment that patients will come for a final session *after* they have decided to leave therapy.

Often the patient will not be motivated to continue therapy once he is feeling better. In these cases, the therapist will have to develop other motivators for the patient. This might include other problems the patient wants to work on, such as weight reduction or management of children. If the patient is determined to leave therapy, the therapist can leave it open for the patient to return if he feels the need.

Negative Reactions to the Therapist

The patient may leave therapy prematurely because he is angry at or disappointed in the therapist. Often if the patient leaves for this reason, he may later want to come back but feels too embarrassed to do so. In these cases, a call or letter stating that the patient is welcome to return to therapy at any time in the future provides him with a way to return without shame or embarrassment. If possible, the therapist should also attempt (tactfully) to elicit the specific negative reactions to the therapist and to clarify them.

Lack of Sustained Improvement or Relapse during Treatment

It is unusual for a patient to show a straight-line improvement in therapy. Many patients show frequent fluctuations in the level of their depression, especially during the early weeks of therapy. Other patients may show a marked intensification of symptoms after they have had a period of fairly steady progress. Still other patients may go for eight to ten sessions before they show any tangible benefits from treatment. In each of these cases, the lack of steady improvement or the aggravation of depression may produce a sense of hopelessness and futility and stimulate the patient's desire to drop treatment or to cease performing his homework assignments.

The course of an aggravation of symptomatology runs somewhat as follows: In response to an apparent setback, the patient is likely to apply his typical depressive pattern of thinking (selective abstraction, exaggeration, overgeneralization) and experience such ideas as, "The therapy hasn't helped me at all: It has made me worse"; "I was fooling myself in thinking that I could get better. I am really no better than when I started"; "The therapy hasn't helped at all; I have not made any progress." These negative thoughts then lead to further dysphoria and an increase in sadness and discouragement. The intensification of unpleasant emotions then serves to fuel even more extreme negative thinking and thus the vicious cycle of negative thinking leading to increased dysphoria becomes progressively worse. As mentioned previously, the patient may, at this point, skip appointments, avoid doing homework assignments, or decide to drop out of treatment.

In dealing with this particular problem, the therapist should bear in mind that relapses are to be expected during treatment. Furthermore, the successful handling of such a relapse may be the best way to "immunize" the patient against a serious relapse following termination of treatment. Most treatment programs for a variety of problems (such as obesity, alcoholism, chronic anxiety, etc.) tend to flounder because the treatment gains are not sustained after treatment has been concluded. It is, therefore, crucial to set as a therapeutic object a program that will enable the patient to cope with mild or moderate reversals so that they do not become full-blown relapses. Thus, if the patient does start to slip during treatment, the therapist has a special opportunity to utilize this event to provide him with coping mechanisms which he can then draw on following termination of therapy.

The following procedures should be employed by the therapist in order to deal with the specific problem of relapses or a delayed response to treatment:*

1. In the early interviews, the therapist should prepare the patient to expect fluctuations in the level of depression or even a long period of apparent nonresponsiveness to therapy.

2. The therapist should also explain that learning how to cope with exacerbations of symptoms may be one of the most important learning experiences in therapy and can provide the tools for heading off relapses after therapy is concluded. We strongly advocate that the

---

*For additional discussion of handling the patient's complaint that he is not improving in therapy, see Countertherapeutic Belief No. 11, Chapter 14.

therapist explain this to the patient during the first or second interview.

3. Both therapist and patient should be alert and sensitive to clues that an exacerbation of symptoms is occurring. The patient may be aware of slipping and his scores on one of the symptom rating scales, such as the Depression Inventory, may be increased. Also, patient and therapist may anticipate an exacerbation of symptoms if the patient is about to confront some stress that in the past could have produced aggravation of symptoms. Such stresses might be the anticipation of a possible failure experience, a confrontation with a spouse, close friend, or employer, or an impending serious loss.

4. When such a situation is anticipated, the therapist should give the patient instructions such as those listed below and should then work with him to expand on these further so that he is adequately prepared to practice his coping strategies.

   a. The patient should describe the particular event that may be precipitating his increased depression.
   b. He should remind himself that this relapse was expected and that both he and the therapist are primed to apply remedial techniques.
   c. He should write down negative automatic thoughts elic-ited by the adverse circumstances.
   d. He should also write down some of his "automatic wishes" such as the desire to give up and the desire to drop out of treatment.

In many cases, it is well to prepare the patient prior to an expected increase in symptoms by providing him with a sample of the anticipated negative cognitions and also the rational responses to these cognitions. For instance, the following schematic representation could be written out and given to the patient:

Automatic thought: I am much worse today. The therapy hasn't helped me at all. *Rational response:* Actually I showed a steady improvement until this past week. I have had a lot of troubles this week and it was to be expected that I would feel worse. One or two bad days, however, do not cancel out all of the good days that I have been having during the past month since I started treatment.

Automatic thought: My depression goes up and down. It comes and goes. It's going to be like this for the rest of my life and there is nothing I can do about it. *Rational response:* I now have my depression more under control than I have in the past. Since it is now somewhat worse, I can use this opportunity to apply some of my tools to the negative thoughts that are cropping up again.

Cognitive Rehearsal to Prevent Relapses: If the patient does not experience such exacerbations during therapy, it may still be well for the therapist to rehearse with him the kind of preprogrammed responses listed above so that he can apply them following the treatment. Unless the patient is part of a research study, it may also be well for the patient to call the therapist or come in for a "booster" therapy session should an exacerbation appear to be imminent.

The kind of downward spiral described above is particularly ominous in the suicide-prone patient. As described in the chapter on suicide, it is extremely important for the therapist to train the patient to intervene vigorously at the first sign of discouragement or of the activation of suicidal impulses.

RELAPSE FOLLOWING TREATMENT

Although several outcome studies show that relapse after termination of therapy occurs less frequently after a course of cognitive therapy than other treatments, it is essential for the patient and therapist to be prepared to deal with such an occurrence. Sometimes the recurrence or exacerbation of symptoms may last only a few days and it is well for the patient, after checking with the therapist, to attempt to apply his coping skills in managing the symptoms and relevant problems.

If the depression persists, however, a therapeutic session is indicated. At times, this may be accomplished by telephone, although a personal interview is usually preferable. We have found that even when the severity of the depression at the time of relapse is as severe as it was prior to the initial course of therapy, the patients show a more rapid response than previously. In a way, the relapse may serve a useful purpose: It gives the patient an opportunity to practice his various coping strategies. Furthermore, the relapse may motivate him to concentrate more energy on carrying out his "self-therapy" following termination of the formal treatment program.

We have noted that the frequency and severity of relapses is greatly reduced if the initial course of cognitive therapy is tapered off: For example, two sessions a month, followed by one session a month and gradually extended to a visit every three months. Ultimately, regularly scheduled booster sessions once or twice a year enable the patient to continue to consolidate the gains made in therapy.

Chapter 16

GROUP COGNITIVE THERAPY FOR DEPRESSED PATIENTS

Steven D. Hollon and Brian F. Shaw

INTRODUCTION

The bulk of this volume is devoted to a discussion of the practice of cognitive therapy in the individual treatment of unipolar depression. In this chapter, the utilization of group cognitive therapy sessions will be explored. To the extent that it is effective, the group-treatment format offers a major pragmatic advantage over the individual sessions: More patients can be treated within a given period of time by trained professional therapists than can be treated individually.

This chapter will first focus on the advantages and disadvantages of implementing cognitive therapy in a group format. The second, and major, portion of the chapter will be devoted to a detailed presentation of the actual steps involved in practicing group cognitive therapy. The final portion of the chapter will examine the several studies which have compared group cognitive therapy with (1) alternative types of group therapy, and (2) individual cognitive therapy.

GROUP THERAPY FOR DEPRESSION— GENERAL CONSIDERATIONS

Traditionally, moderately to severely depressed and/or suicidal patients have been considered to be poor candidates for group therapy (Christie, 1970). Concerns regarding such patients have been two-

STEVEN D. HOLLON • Department of Psychology, University of Minnesota
BRIAN F. SHAW • University Hospital, University of Western Ontario

fold. First, it is often feared that the particular, intensive needs of such patients either could not be met in a group context, or, worse, that the condition of such patients might even deteriorate in a group setting. In such a setting, the combination of verbal-performance inhibitions and negative self-adjustments could easily foster unflattering self-comparisons with other group members who are less depressed, more verbal, or less severely disturbed. Second, such patients are also viewed as being potentially destructive to group processes. The self-absorption, unrelieved pessimism, desire for immediate symptom relief, and rejection of others' suggestions, all characteristics of depressed patients, are often regarded as impediments to the generation of therapeutic group processes.

Yalom (1970) has noted that the above considerations may be less of a contraindication for group therapy of depressed patients than a contraindication for the inclusion of depressed patients in groups heterogeneous with respect to the respective targets of treatment. Working with homogeneously depressed patient groups may well prove to be an effective means of circumventing such problems as (1) intensity of focus, (2) negative self-comparisons, and (3) undesirable group-process phenomena. The use of such homogeneous groups has been recommended for both suicidal patients (Farberow, 1972) and depressed patients (Shaw, 1977).

The nature of the therapy utilized, as well as the homogeneity of groups, appears to be a critical consideration. An effort to treat groups of homogeneously depressed patients with traditional psychotherapy was no more effective than a placebo-controlled nontreatment, and less effective than a tricyclic antidepressant (Covi, Lipman, Derogatis, Smith, and Pattison, 1974). Such a finding is hardly surprising, since traditional approaches to psychotherapy have generally proved ineffective in the treatment of acutely depressed patients (Daneman, 1961; Friedman, 1975), or in the prevention of subsequent relapse (Klerman, DiMascio, Weissman, Prusoff, and Paykel, 1974).

As with individual treatments, the structured, time-limited, cognitive–behavioral approaches, such as cognitive therapy, appear to offer the greatest promise in working with homogeneously defined unipolar depressed patients in a group format. Shaw (1977) treated depressed college student outpatients in either cognitive therapy, behavioral therapy, or nondirective therapy groups. All three groups were also compared with a no-treatment waiting-list control cell. Patients treated with group cognitive therapy over a four-week period showed greater symptomatic improvement than all other groups. Further, the symptomatic improvement was maintained through a one-month posttreatment follow-up. Other outcome studies in group cognitive therapy will be described in Chapter 18.

The available evidence favors homogeneous over heterogeneous group composition, and structured, time-limited cognitive–behavioral interventions, such as cognitive therapy, over more traditional approaches to psychotherapy, or strictly behavioral approaches. Given these initial findings, several questions can be raised. Among these questions are the following:

1. What are the special theoretical considerations which must be taken into account when attempting to treat depressed patients in group cognitive therapy?
2. What practical steps are required to adapt individual cognitive therapy, with its combination of cognitive and behavioral techniques unified by a common cognitive theory of depression, to a group-treatment format?
3. How effective is group cognitive therapy in comparison with (or in combination with) antidepressant pharmacotherapy, the current treatment of depressed patients preferred by most practitioners?
4. How effective is group cognitive therapy compared to individual cognitive therapy, which has been found to be even more effective than tricyclic antidepressant pharmacotherapy, both in terms of reduction of acute symptomatology and in the prevention of relapse?
5. What guidelines are available to facilitate the choice between group and individual cognitive therapy for depressed patients?

The remainder of this chapter will be devoted to addressing these issues.

SPECIAL CLINICAL CONSIDERATIONS

Cognitive theory of depression specifies that the operation of a negative cognitive set and systematic misperceptions of the self, the environment, and the future produce the negative affect and behavioral passivity that are major observable components of the depressive syndrome. Working with depressed patients in a group format introduces the possibility of eliciting from the individual patient a variety of negative inferences which would not necessarily come to light during individual therapy sessions. As with any automatic negative thoughts generated by patients, these negative inferences can prove to be either detrimental or beneficial to the course of therapy, depending on how they are handled by the therapist. Left unchallenged by therapist or patient, these automatic thoughts—such as, "I'm not progressing as fast as the other patients in the group"; "Other group members seem so much more intelligent (less depressed) than I"; "There is no point in wasting the group's time with my concerns, my problems are insoluble"— can increase dysphoria and make it increasingly difficult for the patient to participate in therapeutic activities.

When elicited and systematically explored, these negative statements provide excellent opportunities for demonstrating both the relationship between thinking and subsequent feelings or behaviors, and the procedures for identifying, objectifying, and dealing with such idiosyncratic negative cognitions. The difficulties which may develop in the course of group therapy for depressed patients can be traced to three related sources: patients' negative comparisons of themselves with one another, potentially negative effects of interacting among depressed individuals, and potential limitations on the individual's ability to relate the group's examples of negative cognitive processes to his own case.

Negative Self-Comparisons

Depressed patients evidence a marked tendency to view *themselves*, their *worlds*, and their *futures* in a negative, pessimistic way (Chapter 1). Always a major focus in cognitive therapy, automatic negative thoughts are in abundant supply within the framework of group therapy. Patients have other patients and their actions immediately available to compare themselves to; and since they spend a greater portion of time beyond the focus of the therapist's attention, they can more easily slide into silent, negative rumination. If attended to actively and examined by means of the numerous cognitive techniques documented elsewhere in this manual, this propensity may be turned to therapeutic advantage.

Several clinical examples illustrate the technique of capitalizing on negative comparisons. A middle-aged woman was observed to be unusually nonverbal during several group sessions. She would rarely comment directly on either her own concerns or those of other members, appearing to be uncomfortable when invited to do so. She was much more likely to join in the conversation during the periods of more casual conversation preceding or following group sessions. When asked to comment what she thought about expressing herself verbally in the group, she was, after considerable distress and hesitation, able to share her concern that she was "dumb" and would "not be able to say the right things." As evidence, she cited a long history of perceived failures in school when called upon by teachers, despite having received better than average grades. She carried this self-concept into adult social interactions, regarding herself as incompetent to talk about "important things" in group settings. She regarded the therapy sessions as similar in many respects to these earlier experiences. Although she very much wanted to make constructive contributions relating to concerns of various group members, she was firmly convinced that efforts to do so would only expose her as the "dummy" she knew she was.

Once the patient's attitude was articulated, it was possible to test systematically the validity of the thought, both in the group context and by use of structured assignments outside of sessions. The identification of this cluster of thoughts about herself in a group context was particularly interesting in the light of what had been previously revealed (or concealed) in individual sessions. Although, in retrospect, it became apparent that the patient's cognitive self-monitoring during those individual sessions reflected intimations of this particular aspect of her own self-perceptions, her individual sessions had failed to elicit data demonstrating the ubiquitousness of such thoughts in social interactions with peers and their important role in maintaining her negative self-concept.

A patient's invidious comparisons of himself with other group members can provide special opportunities for therapeutic intervention. In another instance, a male group member, a carpenter, expressed a strong concern that he was far less competent than another male group member, a financier, who was temporarily unemployed due to his ongoing depression. The former patient, who had been progressing steadily during his first three weeks in treatment, became profoundly discouraged when the latter patient began to show marked therapeutic improvement. Sample cognitions, once their expression was encouraged, were "I've been working at this for weeks longer than G., yet he's catching on much faster than I am; I'll never get better," or "He's doing this much better than me, I never do anything right." Once identified, these automatic thoughts were then explored and related to similar processes (for example, unwarranted generalizations with respect to time, all-or-none thinking, and selective abstraction) which the patient frequently manifested in his everyday concerns.

In both instances, the group format not only provided situations which brought to light the misinterpretations derived from depressogenic cognitive sets, but also served as an immediate, available context for systematically examining and correcting those negative inferences. As in individual cognitive therapy, while the focus is on events and the cognitions about events that occur outside of therapy, the cognitions that are revealed during the session are often the ones which provide the most compelling demonstrations of both the crucial role of idiosyncratic thinking in depression and the potency of therapeutic techniques in attenuating such dysfunctional thoughts. Group sessions increase the likelihood that negative social comparisons will be triggered. If unattended to, such ideation can undermine the progress of treatment. If identified, such ideation provides opportunities for change which might never arise in the course of individual treatment.

Negative Effects on Other Group Members

Coyne (1976a,b) has presented evidence suggesting that the presence of a depressed individual in a group can in itself increase dysphoria among those who interact with him and can lead to the rejection of the depressed individual. While these studies have involved the effects of depressed individuals' interaction with nondepressed individuals, the dynamics of the phenomenon, if applicable to interactions between depressed pairs, might serve as the basis for a prediction that depressed patients in homogeneous groups raise one another's levels of dysphoria.

Our clinical experience suggests that this is not a major concern. Simply talking about problems or symptoms is, by itself, unlikely to have any tangible effects except perhaps to increase dysphoria—one possible explanation for the fact that traditional expressive psychotherapies have fared so poorly in controlled studies (see Hollon and Beck, 1978). However, in group cognitive therapy, the therapist works actively to focus attention on the examination and reevaluation of these idiosyncratic perceptions as he maintains considerable structure within the sessions. Our experience has been that the behavior of homogeneously depressed groups can be kept task-relevant, and under these circumstances they appear strikingly animated, spontaneous, and active. As in individual cognitive therapy, it is important to realize that many depressions appear "realistic" to the depressed patient. In group cognitive therapy, it appears that focusing on the process by which systematic misconstructions and distortions in information processing combine to make troublesome—but workable—situations appear unresolvable can, with the assistance of other group participants, forestall the type of "contagious" negative affective slide which is apparently attributable to the group's unquestioned acceptance of the depressed patient's pessimistic evaluations.

"Universal" Versus Personal Distortions

While depressed patients appear prone to negative thinking about themselves, their worlds, and their futures, there is evidence suggesting that such distortions are curiously limited to information concerning the depressed individual himself (Chapter 1). It appears that depressives apply to themselves rules quite different from those they apply to others, or, stated another way, that errors in inference and thinking are most evident when the depressed patient is thinking about himself, not when he is thinking about others.

The greater objectivity and flexibility in judging people other than themselves is borne out in our clinical experience with therapy groups. First, a depressed patient generally finds that the recognition of errors in the negative cognitions of other patients and the reevaluation of their thoughts and assumptions is less difficult than the recognition and reevaluation of his own cognitions. Secondly, and of utmost importance, the patient's recognition of the cognitive distortions of others, and his experience with reevaluating them appear to *facilitate the recognition and reevaluation of his own idiosyncratic cognitive sets.* Thus, the members of the group reality-test assumptions, and in so doing, increase their skills in correcting their own maladaptive reactions.

In summary, depressed patients appear capable of functioning within a group format and deriving specific benefits from their group experiences. The focus of discussion and the degree of structure within a cognitive framework, however, appear to be critical determinants of efficacy of group therapy.

FORMAL ASPECTS

The various therapeutic procedures described throughout this monograph can all be utilized in a group format. As in individual cognitive therapy, the fundamental goals of group therapy include an examination and modification of depressed patients' maladaptive belief systems and dysfunctional forms of information processing. Basic techniques include planned behavioral assignments; training in the systematic self-monitoring of cognitions, events, and moods; and training in strategies designed to identify and change distorted cognitive systems. Extensive use is made of a variety of homework assignments, including activity schedules, records of cognitions, and efforts to modify those cognitions. Frequently, patients and therapists collaborate in the design of "experiments" to test views held by the patients.

As in individual cognitive therapy sessions, group sessions are structured, problem-oriented, and focused. Therapists typically are quite active—questioning, challenging, exploring, and instructing. Adapting such procedures to a group format can present a host of specific problems, both in terms of the focus of the sessions and in terms of a number of practical problems which may arise in a group setting. In the following sections, a variety of these issues will be addressed.

Problem-Oriented Versus Process-Oriented Groups

Cognitive therapy is a problem-oriented approach to therapy.

Little emphasis is placed on understanding the interaction between patient and therapist. During the group sessions, attention is focused primarily on the problems of various group members, and, to a lesser extent, on the interaction among the members. Traditional group-therapy topics, such as cohesion, affectivity, dominance, and alliance, are not highlighted in cognitive group therapy. The cognitive sessions often follow a format in which each patient selects a major problem to focus on; patients then take turns commenting on it.

Nonetheless, psychological problems which relate, in part, to group processes will occasionally arise. Most often, these problems are generally consistent with other depressive phenomena and, when detected, lend themselves nicely to a demonstration of the relevance of cognitive principles. They involve such cognitions as, "I am taking up too much of the group's time," "I don't have anything to offer," "I don't fit in," or "I won't get better." Dealing with ongoing cognitions related to group participation serves as a powerful vehicle for learning, much as dealing with negative expectations about individual therapy serves as a useful model for cognitive hypothesis testing in general. The emphasis is on such process-related phenomena for the sake of illustration, however, not for the sake of process itself.

Closed Versus Open Groups

Group therapy similarly requires a decision as to whether to begin a set of patients at the same time and admit no new members thereafter, or whether to add new members on an ongoing basis. Unlike more process-oriented group therapies, cognitive group therapy regards the issue of admitting new members less in a symbolic sense than in a pragmatic sense. Typically, a new patient is quite severely depressed and may require considerable time and attention. Cognitive therapy involves considerable activity on the part of the patient, necessitating an average of twenty to thirty minutes of fairly didactic presentation. Our experience has been that introducing new members can be made less disruptive if several strategies are followed. First, the patient is oriented in a preparatory session, in which he is given an overview of cognitive therapy, reading material (for example, *Coping With Depression*), and training in initial self-monitoring or activity-scheduling. Second, more advanced group members may become involved in the orientation process in a way that provides them with a useful learning experience. Explaining the cognitive A-B-C model or probing for examples of negative automatic thoughts helps ensure that the more experienced patients not only can utilize the procedures themselves, but also understand those procedures well enough to teach them to a new member.

Therapists: Role and Number

As in individual cognitive therapy, working with depressed clients requires considerable activity and structuring on the part of the therapist. Managing several depressed patients at a time requires that he pay particular attention to detail. It is especially important that therapists not allow patients to get "lost" in the group; while much of the time in each session is devoted to intensive focus on one patient at a time, it is important to make sure that each patient is given the chance periodically to air his problems.

The use of multiple therapists, when possible, offers several advantages. While a single therapist can handle a reasonably sized group, (four to six patients), larger groups may necessitate an additional therapist. When there are two therapists, one can be actively working with a given problem and/or patient while the other is attending closely to the reactions of the other group participants. Similarly, patients typically generate a considerable amount of written material between sessions. When two therapists are present the one most directly involved with the topic of the moment can devote his full attention to that discussion, while the other therapist is free to scan the various homework sheets for items of particular interest.

Group: Composition and Number of Patients

At this time, little is known about patient-related factors that either facilitate or retard progress in group cognitive therapy. Certainly, the procedures described throughout this manual are most directly applicable to patients with primary depressive symptomatology. It would appear that any problems for which individual cognitive therapy would be appropriate could also be treated in group cognitive psychotherapy. Severely suicidal and severely withdrawn patients may be exceptions to this guideline, not because the particular advantages of a group treatment do not apply in such cases, but because such patients require more attention than time would permit in a group setting. One arrangement that we sometimes make to accommodate the needs of some patients is to supplement group sessions with individual sessions.

As mentioned above, group size is determined more on the basis of pragmatic than theoretical considerations. The bulk of our experience has involved groups of from four to eight patients led by two therapists. The severity of the problems represented and the experience the various patients have had with therapy are considerations which must be taken into account when a group is formed. A single therapist would be hard pressed to start a group of six or more severely depressed patients at the same time, but one or two such severely depressed patients might appropriately be added to a larger group of patients who had already received varying amounts of specific training. More advanced patients frequently prove helpful in modeling various skills and verbally instructing new patients in basic techniques.

Duration and Frequency of Sessions

A period of two hours of therapy seems to offer a satisfactory compromise between the need to provide adequate in-session time for each patient and yet avoid exhausting either the patients or the therapists. Shorter time periods have been tried (Rush and Watkins, 1978), but there is not sufficient evidence at this time to draw conclusions relating length of session to outcome.

Similarly, there are currently no firm guidelines available to assist in the determination of optimal session frequency. In scheduling sessions for adult outpatients, Shaw and Hollon (1978) conducted them once a week, while Rush and Watkins (1978) held twice-weekly sessions. Treatment efficacy with these two groups appeared roughly comparable, but direct controlled comparisons of the effects of various session frequencies would be desirable.

At this time, clinical experience suggests session lengths from one and one-half to two hours are preferable, while weekly contacts appear to represent a minimum frequency. Systematic consideration of such pragmatic variables is clearly needed.

Time-Limited Contracts

Whether operating in an open- or a closed-group format, the negotiation of explicit, time-limited agreements with each individual patient appears particularly beneficial. Focusing attention on clear, explicit criteria for improvement appears to facilitate both the discussion of expectations and the production of change. Experience suggests that therapy conducted in 12 to 20 sessions, distributed over a period of 12 to 20 weeks is adequate for most outpatient unipolar depressives.

Group Therapy Combined with Individual Therapy

We have found that the moderately to severely depressed patients referred to our outpatient clinic require a varying number of individual therapy sessions even when group therapy appears to be the treatment of choice. In some instances, group therapy serves as a useful adjunct to individual treatment. In other cases, individual treatment is a necessary prelude to assignment to a therapy group. During the preliminary individual session, the therapist is able to gain a comprehensive picture of the patient's problems, personality, background, sensitivities, and coping mechanisms. In addition, he has an opportunity to establish rapport and to familiarize the patient with the concepts and techniques of cognitive therapy.

After the patient has become involved in group therapy, occasional individual sessions may be necessary for a variety of reasons. Since therapy groups are limited in the amount of time devoted to the problems of any specific member of the group, some patients may require the additional focus provided by individual sessions. Other patients may periodically need the kind of specific support and intimate interaction that is characteristic of the dyadic relationship. Further, some patients may be reluctant to risk the possible breach of confidentiality raised by discussing highly sensitive problems in a group.

In research studies comparing cognitive group therapy with other treatment modalities, we have advocated the format of initially alternating individual and group therapy. After the fourth individual therapy session, the patient continues with group therapy exclusively (unless there is a specific indication for special individual sessions). Outcome studies employing exclusively the group format for cognitive therapy have generally concentrated on younger, less severely depressed patients than those observed in our own clinic (Shaw, 1977).

CONDUCTING THERAPY SESSIONS

Preparatory Interviews

Upon entrance into a therapy group, a depressed patient may feel particularly threatened. This apprehension could be reflected in thoughts such as, "I couldn't possibly talk about my problems in front of all of those people," "I get uncomfortable in groups," "I must be an uninteresting patient," or "I must be too sick (or not depressed enough) to benefit from individual therapy." Preparatory interviews scheduled for discussing these or related concerns are helpful.

Sequence of Technical Procedures

Table 2 presents an overview of the recommended structure of group therapy sessions and the progression of topics to be covered and skills to be developed over a period of time. In general, the focus of attention across the sessions shifts from planning and monitoring discrete enactive–behavioral interventions (e.g., activity scheduling, self-monitoring of moods and events, success therapy, graded-task assignment, etc.), to concentrating increasingly on techniques designed to identify, reevaluate, and test various automatic thoughts and underlying assumptions. Similarly, initial cognitive strategies (e.g., the triple-column, reattribution therapy, alternative techniques), are generally aimed at identifying specific automatic thoughts. After several weeks, an increasing amount of time and attention is paid to discerning and altering underlying assumptive systems.

When closed-membership groups are begun, the entire group can be started on the schedule shown in Table 2. In open-membership groups, it is necessary to repeat significant portions of the initial session for each new member, usually in a succinct fashion. Experienced group members can often play a major role in the orientation process: modeling acquired skills and describing relevant theoretical and/or practical aspects of therapy.

1. *Assessing the Syndrome of Depression.* We prefer to begin cognitive group therapy with one or more structured assessments of

TABLE 2
SCHEDULE FOR GROUP COGNITIVE THERAPY

Week		Session Objectives and Methods
0	Diagnostic and/or preparatory session	1. Assess appropriateness for group 2. Assess and discuss expectations 3. Distribute *Coping with Depression*
1	Initial session	1. Measure depression (give BDI) 2. Introduce new members 3. Set agenda 4. Establish ground rules 5. Discuss expectations and review treatment goals 6. Introduce therapeutic rationale and discuss *Coping with Depression* 7. Discuss individual patients' respective concerns 8. Focus on training self-monitoring skills and/or behavioral experiments 9. Homework assignments 10. Assess reactions to session
2–10	Subsequent sessions	1. Measure depression (give BDI) 2. Set agenda 3. Review status since last session 4. Discuss reactions to previous sessions 5. Review homework from last session 6. Introduce new topics and relate material to basic cognitive theory 7. Homework assignments 8. Assess reaction to session
11–12	Termination sessions	1. Measure depression (give BDI) 2. Set agenda 3. Review status since last session 4. Discuss progress to date 5. Discuss expectations regarding termination 6. Assess reactions to session(s)

target problems. The Beck Depression Inventory (see Appendix) provides a brief, well validated self-report measure of syndrome depression. The initial interview, the first group therapy session, and all subsequent group sessions routinely begin with an administration of the Beck Depression Inventory (BDI). Patients who have completed several BDI's may be given a supply to keep at home and may fill out the scale either just before coming or while waiting for the group session to begin.

Such attention to the BDI permits a close monitoring of depression levels, signals any important shifts in discrete symptomatology, such as suicidal ruminations, and clearly keeps the focus on the production of change within the time-limited contract. While depression is generally the major phenomenon of interest, we have at times monitored other relevant processes, such as anxiety, on a regular basis.

2. *Setting Agendas.* At the beginning of each session, it is generally desirable to set a flexible agenda which will allow patients and therapist (s) to target specific areas for discussion. It is frequently useful to poll each participant for suggestions, so that everyone may begin the group session with some kind of active participation. If a new member is being added to an existing group, the therapist will typically use this time to make introductions and to indicate that some time will be set aside for exploring the new member's goals, problems, and current situation. This is also a good time to elicit from experienced group participants any comments they may wish to make on major events or changes in symptomatology over the preceding week. Generally, it is preferable to note a topic, then continue to complete the construction of the agenda, and return to that topic later, rather than risk dwelling too long on any given subject at the beginning of the session. When a new group is starting and before individual patients' concerns are taken up, it is useful to indicate clearly those areas which must be discussed at the first session: e.g., the general structure for sessions, group ground rules, individual goals and expectations, and a general discussion of cognitive therapy.

This approach provides an explicit, formal structure within which the group can function at maximal efficiency. When a therapist is working with depressed patients, it is important that he have such a structure planned in advance and available at all times. Such a strong organizational aid also serves as a precaution against the deadly effects of depressive inertia and pessimism that so readily appear during unfocused moments. The skillful handling of depression-related hesitancy at decision-making points in the session often constitutes a major therapeutic maneuver, and the therapist must have a well-worked-out plan for such contingencies. One patient labeled such an approach in individual therapy "planning my work, then working my plan."

Far from inhibiting spontaneity during the group session, an agreed-upon agenda appears to facilitate spontaneity and involvement on the part of the patients. It seems likely that the apparent poor prognosis for depressed patients in less highly structured groups, or in process-oriented group settings, may be attributed to the failure of such unstructured groups to offset adequately the operation of negative cognitive sets. These negative sets seem to dominate in situations where the lack of structure suggests ambiguities, thereby creating a meaning vacuum for the patients' depressive interpretations to fill.

3. *Establishing Ground Rules.* Early in the initial session, it is useful to discuss basic ground rules and to elicit agreement from all participants. Confidentiality presents special problems in a group setting. We typically approach the issue directly, requesting that each patient agree to respect the other patients' rights to privacy. A general guideline is that all patients are free to discuss their own specific goals, progress, and the procedures they are learning with whomever they choose, but that no other member is ever identified, nor any of their concerns talked about, outside of the group setting. Taking several minutes to discuss these issues and to secure each member's agreement not only draws attention to the importance of the issue, but also appears to facilitate a patient's subsequent disclosure of intimate material about himself.

The second major ground rule that is useful is the notion of "going around," a phrase meaning that the group agrees to structure its time in such a way that each member may have an opportunity to bring up one of his concerns for discussion, that the group may stay with that topic long enough to reach some kind of resolution, and that input will be actively sought from each patient who has not already volunteered comments. This procedure prevents the flow of the discussion from becoming too diffused, while it ensures that no patient gets neglected. Early in any given session and during the first several sessions, it is usually advisable for the therapist to be somewhat more formal in soliciting comments from each member in turn, just as was done in setting the agenda.

Depressed clients typically start therapy identifying with one another's negative perceptions. Initially, comments from other group members often take the form of agreement with the pessimistic view, followed by recounting of idiosyncratic experiences or inferences from the commenting member about his or her own situation. These comments have the effect of diverting attention from the initial problem and the initial speaker. It is unlikely that this process reflects anything more than a spontaneous desire to empathize and/or identify with the first speaker. The therapist can generally redirect the discussion to the initial topic and the initial speaker, then can proceed to examine and work through the initial problem raised.

4. *Assessing Expectations and Reactions to Previous Sessions.* Early in the session(s), the therapist might find it useful to ask each patient what he expects therapy to be like and what he expects will happen in subsequent sessions. The answers to these questions may provide useful indications of unrealistic expectations (generally negative) and may alert the therapist(s) to patients' expectations and assumptions that may not be met during the typical course of cognitive therapy. Patients frequently come into a therapy situation with some notion of how they will fare in treatment and of how treatment is likely to progress. The expectations of homogeneously depressed patients typically tend to be pessimistic, so that eliciting an expression of these expectations from each patient in the first session often demonstrates how negative self-appraisals operate.

For example, near the end of the first session for a new therapy group, we asked each participant separately to rank all group members, including themselves, in terms of whom they thought would benefit the most from the group. Each participant put himself at the bottom of his own list. In the discussion that followed, it became clear that some very striking similarities existed in terms of how participants tended to view themselves *vis-à-vis* the others. Such thoughts as, "Nobody else is as depressed (or as hopeless) as I am," "Everyone else seems so normal; I'm really messed up," "This approach may work for some of the others, but my depression is caused by my husband (or my job, being out of work, my illness, etc.); the way I think has nothing to do with it," were typical.

Pointing out the real similarity in the ways they thought about themselves and their situations facilitated the identification of their negative cognitive distortions.

5. *Initial Statements of Individual Problems.* In the first session for each patient, it is desirable to give that patient an opportunity to discuss the problems that brought him or her into treatment. When starting a new group, we typically go around the group before concentrating on any given patient. The therapist generally uses this period to comment on aspects of these various problems that are consistent with the overall syndrome of depression, and on specific kinds of interventions that will be brought to bear on the problems later in the session.

6. *Presenting Cognitive Theory and Technique.* Cognitive therapy makes several explicit statements about the nature of the relationships between events, ideation, and subsequent affect and behavior. Beginning early in the first session, the therapist attempts to encourage depressed patients to begin examining the way they look at things. Initially, these efforts may take the form of encouraging changes in behavior, despite the patients' misgivings and initial pessimism; more formal cognitive reevaluation techniques are introduced later in treatment.

It is generally useful to make a fairly explicit presentation of cognitive theory, tied closely to examples arising from the patients' presentations of problems. Instead of making a formal abstract presentation, the therapist can use as illustration relevant concrete examples of unwarranted pessimism, self-fulfilling prophecies, and patients' thoughts. Whenever possible, it is desirable to pull one or more relevant examples from each of the patients during that first session. By judicious selection, the therapist can usually demonstrate important aspects of theory and technique, while simultaneously attending to the various needs of each group member.

7. *Homework Assignments.* By the end of each session, every patient should have been assigned at least one explicitly planned activity to execute before the next session. Initially, that assignment will most likely involve some type of specific self-monitoring. For severely depressed patients, the initial assignment might involve carrying out an activity schedule planned during the group meeting. Any of a variety of "experiments" might be designed during the session to help get the patient moving on some therapeutically

relevant task or to test specific beliefs. After a session or two, greater emphasis is placed on regularly monitoring specific thoughts in various situations and systematically reevaluating the beliefs those thoughts reflect.

In general, a basic rule to follow is to assign new homework only as previous assignments are mastered. Similarly, it is most important that the therapist actively attend to assignments at the next session. Nothing so rapidly undermines the motivation to continue utilizing various techniques between sessions as the therapist's neglecting to carefully attend to the work done by the patients.

Specific Management Problems

A variety of specific management problems which are not typically encountered in individual sessions can arise in the group situation. Among these problems are the monopoly of group time by one or more patients, personal attacks on one member by another, lapses into small talk, the development of subgroups, and the development of differing rates of improvement among various group members. In general, each of these problems can be readily handled by an active therapist who does not hesitate to redirect the discussion to more productive topics.

In the case of personal attacks, rephrasing the patient's derogatory comment so that it refers to specific behaviors targeted for group discussion removes the personal "sting" from the comment. Differing rates of improvement may produce therapeutically useful negative reactions. Typically, the distressed patient is responding to someone else's improvement with thoughts like, "He's getting better and I'm not getting better at all; I must really be hopeless." Such inferences provide good material for cognitive reevaluations.

ILLUSTRATIONS OF TYPICAL THERAPEUTIC MANEUVERS

Capitalizing on Interruptions

The following vignette illustrates how the therapist turned to advantage the intrusion of a patient into another patient's description of her problem.

MARY ANN: I've really had a bad week . . . Just nothing seems to have gone well.

THERAPIST: Can you give us an example?

M A: Well, there have been a lot of things. I can't seem to get going, my Mary Beth has been having trouble in school, my idiot brother called my mother and got her all stirred up . . .

T: You mean your mother in the nursing home?

M A: Yes. My brother hasn't lifted a finger to help these last three years . . . but, to hear him tell it, he's always just about ready to come and take her back to Ohio to live with him . . . she gets worked up, then nothing comes from it, then I have to help her handle the disappointment . . .

JOAN: My mother's always interfering, always trying to tell me how to raise my daughter; as if she's the only person who knows how to raise a daughter . . .

T: We've focused on that before, Joan; it's obviously important to you, and, I suspect, shares some important common features with Mary Ann's problems with her brother. Mary Ann, how have you tried to handle the effects of your brother's "promises" on your mother?

M A: I've tried talking to him, but we never get very far. I just get so angry . . . I just don't think it does any good.

J: I used to think that about my mother's nagging, but now I'm not so sure . . . That's what made me think about it just now; it sounds like you've got a problem with your brother that's something like what I've had with my mother.

M A: What do you mean?

J: Well, if it's like my mother, she's trying to be important, even though mostly she's just a pain in the neck . . . but she's trying to be helpful and feel like she knows something. Now, what I always used to do was just get angry with her; I've got enough trouble dealing with my Becky without my mother butting in . . . but when I tried going out of my way to talk things over with her, just to make it easier to get along with her . . .

M A: You mean your mother?

J: Yes, with my mother.

M A: My brother and I could never talk.

T: How do you know?

M A: Well, we never have; we've fought ever since we were old enough to fight.

J: It's worked for me, kind of, and I never thought it would . . .

T: Maybe you could role-play; Mary Ann, would you be willing to take your brother's role?—and Joan, would you be willing to play Mary Ann? Okay?

M A: We're supposed to role-play the kind of argument my brother and I have?

T: Yes, both ways; just a typical interaction, the kind that leads to a fight; then Joan will try to structure her interaction with her brother . . . she initiates and largely guides the topics. That seems to both make your mother happy and keeps her desire to help from becoming a bother, doesn't it?

J: Most of the time; yeah, I think so.

T: Okay. Then, Mary Ann, why don't you start . . .

Role-playing was helpful for both patients in improving their interpersonal skills. By drawing on Joan's interrupting Mary Ann, the therapist was able to utilize Joan's experience to help Mary Ann cope more successfully with her problems. He was then able to lead into an "advanced" and highly therapeutic group technique: role-playing.

Use of Group Members as "Co-Therapists"

Through skillful questioning the therapist can draw a group member into assuming a therapeutic role with another patient.

THERAPIST: Okay. Let's set our agenda for today; Ed, anything to put on?

ED: Well, not specifically. Things have been maybe a little better.

T: We'll want to be sure to go over the self-monitoring you did. Marilyn?

MARILYN: I've got that party coming up Friday . . . I just don't know how I'm going to be able to manage it.

T: That's the party you talked about two weeks ago?

M: Yes, one of us, one of the cousins, has it every year . . . it's my turn this year . . . I just don't think I can do it.

KEN: Why is that, Marilyn?

M: It's too much, I just can't do it . . . I have trouble getting dinners on the table, I have trouble getting out of bed in the morning, I even have trouble getting here to group . . . How can I give a party for a group?

K: What exactly do you have to do?

M: Everything . . . I've got to clean the house, do the shopping, cook the meal, everything . . .

T: Sounds like you're feeling overwhelmed. Ed, if you were Marilyn, how would you try to go about organizing for the party?

Ed: For the party? I don't know . . .

T: I'm thinking about the way you went about getting your apartment cleaned up last week . . .

E: Oh, you mean breaking it up?

T: Yes. You're something of an expert now in chopping big jobs down to size. What kinds of steps might be helpful for Marilyn, do you think?

E: Well, it was helpful to me to make a list of what I needed to do, then check things off as I finished them.

T: You mean actually write things down?

E: Yeah, write out a list. When we did that last time, I just took the list home and went through it.

K: I always try to start with something easy first; that seems to make it easier to get started . . .

T: Marilyn, you look upset; what's going on for you?

M: It just all seems like so much, I'll never be able to do it.

T: That's a good example of an automatic thought, isn't it? Why don't we try listing the things you'll need to do; then we'll see whether or not some of Ed's and Ken's suggestions might not help make it easier.

M: It just seems like too much.

E: It did for me, too. I know just how you feel, like it's all too much. But breaking it up seems to really help.

T: If nothing else, it will give us some good practice both in terms of breaking big tasks up into manageable units, and, help generate some good examples of automatic negative thoughts to practice with; like the one you just had. Ken, will you be the "scribe" here for Marilyn? Ed, what would you want to know from Marilyn about what she needs to do? . . .

In this case, the therapist recognizes that Ken was responding to Marilyn's problems in a therapeutic manner. He then drew Ed into the discussion, and, consequently, both Ken and Ed participated actively as "therapists." Later, he assigned specific therapeutic roles to Ken and Ed. We have found as an interesting byproduct that "patient therapists" show an enhanced capacity to apply these coping skills to managing their own problems and generally become more self-reliant.

EMPIRICAL TRIALS WITH GROUP COGNITIVE THERAPY

How effective is group cognitive therapy? At least five studies speak to this issue, although only one (Rush and Watkins, 1978) has explicitly compared group with individual formats. Treatment efficacy can be evaluated in at least three respects: reduction of initial symptomatology, prevention of relapse, and low incidence of premature termination.

There is now considerable evidence that group cognitive therapy is associated with the reduction of initial symptomatology. Across all five relevant studies, whether involving psychometrically identified depressed volunteers (Gioe, 1975), depressed college student outpatients (Shaw, 1977), or depressed adult outpatients (Morris, 1975; Rush and Watkins, 1978; Shaw and Hollon, 1978), patients treated with group cognitive therapy evidenced significantly lower posttreatment scores on measures of syndrome depression than they had evidenced at pretreatment.

The Shaw study involved comparisons with a strictly behavioral treatment modality modeled after Lewinsohn and colleagues' approach to depression (Lewinsohn, 1974, 1975). Cognitive therapy proved superior both to the strictly behavioral approach, and to a nondirective and a waiting-list control. The relatively weak showing of the strictly behavioral approach in the Shaw study was replicated by Padfield (1976) in a comparison between a Lewinsohn-type behavioral treatment group and a client-centered treatment group with adult outpatients. Given these data, it appears unlikely that positive effects associated with group cognitive therapy can be attributable to either general (nonspecific) factors or to a structured behavioral approach alone.

Shaw and Hollon (1978) treated two consecutive groups of patients in a group format: the first in a closed group format and the second in an open group format. Treatment outcome for the combined groups was compared with those outcomes obtained for patients treated with either individual cognitive therapy or imipramine pharmacotherapy plus brief supportive contacts in a separate clinical trial (Rush et al., 1977). Group cognitive therapy evidenced a treatment response greater than that shown by the pharmacotherapy patients, but less than that shown by the patients treated with individual cognitive therapy, although neither difference was significant. Defining full remission as a posttreatment BDI of 9 or less, 7 of 12 group therapy completers (58%) evidenced a full remission, compared with 15 of 18 individual patients (83%), and only 5 of 17 pharmacotherapy patients (29%). Three of the initial 15 patients assigned to group therapy dropped out of treatment, a 20% dropout, compared with dropout rates of 32% for the pharmacotherapy condition in Rush *et al.*, and 5% for individual cognitive therapy in that latter study.

In the Rush and Watkins study, group cognitive therapy was compared directly with individual cognitive therapy, the latter conducted either with or without antidepressant medication. Despite the fact that treatment was done at a new center located in another region of the country, treatment outcomes were strikingly consistent with those found by Shaw and Hollon. Individual cognitive therapy appeared to produce somewhat greater remission of symptoms than did group cognitive therapy, although all treatment cells were associated with significant pre- to posttreatment reductions in symptomatology. A total of 43% of the group patients showed a full remission, as defined above, by the end of 16 weeks of treatment, while 50% of the individual cognitive therapy patients evidenced a full remission (38% in individual cognitive therapy alone, 72% in individual cognitive therapy plus medication). Interestingly, 18% of the cognitive therapy group patients dropped out of treatment prematurely, compared with 11% in the individual cognitive therapy alone and none (0%) of the individual cognitive therapy plus tricyclic pharmacotherapy cell.

While the results from both the Shaw and Hollon, and the Rush and Watkins comparisons appear to suggest that group cognitive therapy may not be as effective as individual cognitive therapy and may be associated with a higher dropout rate than that latter modality, such a conclusion appears premature at this time. In the Shaw and Hollon study, the various treatment cells were not, strictly speaking, comparable. While patients in the Rush *et al.* study were randomly assigned to either individual cognitive therapy or tricyclic pharmacotherapy, the patients treated in a group format, although drawn from the same research clinic, were not part of that same randomly assigned subject pool. Clinic populations can change in subtle, but important, ways over time. Drawing firm conclusions regarding the comparative efficacy of group cognitive therapy on the basis of what was essentially a quasi-experimental comparison can be hazardous. The findings in that study can be viewed as demonstrating the feasibility of treating adult outpatients in a group cognitive therapy format, but it is not clear that they can be regarded as demonstrating the intermediate effectiveness of group cognitive therapy relative to the less effective tricyclic pharmacotherapy or the more effective individual cognitive therapy.

Similarly, while patients in the Rush and Watkins comparison were randomly assigned to either individual or group cognitive therapy from within the same larger subject pool, treatment in the individual cognitive therapy cell(s) was either combined with tricyclic pharmacotherapy or not. It is not entirely clear what basis was used to determine whether a patient treated in the individual modality received medication or not, but it appears that the decision was left to the discretion of the treating physician. Under these circumstances, it is entirely possible that subtle selective factors related to the physician's judgment may have led to treatment of the potentially more difficult patients in the individual modality with the combination of individual cognitive therapy plus medication. Such circumstances would have produced the pattern of results obtained, with the group cognitive modality doing less well than either individual modality, but with the two individual modalities (no medications versus medications) showing a comparable response to one another, even if group cognitive therapy were, in fact, equally as effective as individual cognitive therapy.

It does appear fair to say that group cognitive therapy appears to be both feasible and practical, and at least as effective as any other modality with which it has been compared, with the exception of individual cognitive therapy, with or without medications. While these data are encouraging, they are not conclusive. Hopefully, these initial studies will spur further, more rigorously controlled comparisons of group cognitive therapy with other viable approaches, especially individual cognitive therapy.

Further, there appear to be few data available at this time to speak to the issue of posttreatment relapse. It is not clear whether group cognitive therapy would have a similar effect, but our expectation is that it would. As with individual cognitive therapy, the long-term efficacy of group cognitive therapy appears to depend upon the execution of a set of skills acquired by the patient during treatment, skills which presumably remain at the patient's disposal long after therapy is over.

CONCLUSIONS

At this time, a number of questions remain to be answered about the nature, parameters, and magnitudes of the effects associated with cognitive therapy as practiced in a group format. It is apparent, after several years of experience, that such groups are both feasible and, perhaps, already better supported by empirical evidence than many of the other approaches already in widespread clinical use. Further, while guidelines can be offered regarding the construction, planning, and implementation of group cognitive therapy, these guidelines are based largely on unsystematic clinical trial and error. Groups based on these principles have been implemented in the ways described above with reasonably satisfying outcomes. However, it seems fair to conclude that group cognitive approaches are still relatively un-developed. While the initial trials have been promising enough to support further clinical experimentation and refinement, it seems likely that such efforts will lead to the development of even more powerful ways of adapting cognitive therapy procedures to the more cost-effective group modality.

Chapter 17

COGNITIVE THERAPY AND ANTIDEPRESSANT MEDICATIONS

INTRODUCTION

Recently, there has been a growing recognition that the terms "depression" and "affective disorder" refer to a heterogeneous group of problems that include a number of distinct psychopathological conditions (Mendels, 1974; Maas, 1975). These conditions appear to be differentially responsive to pharmacotherapy (Baldessarini, 1977). They are also likely to respond differentially to psychotherapy, specifically cognitive therapy. Because the "affective disorders" are heterogeneous with respect to treatment response, the clinician is confronted with the complex problem of selecting the most effective treatment or combination of treatments for a particular patient.

This chapter outlines the indications and contraindications for administering cognitive therapy alone and in conjunction with antidepressant pharmacotherapy. Since clinical research data are scanty in this area, our suggestions are based mainly on clinical experience. A great deal more clinical research is needed to isolate specific predictors for using cognitive therapy alone or in a combined regimen. In addition, this chapter will illustrate how to use cognitive-change techniques specifically in order to increase the degree of compliance with a medication regimen.

Antidepressant medication has been of significant benefit in the treatment of various kinds of depressions, as a large body of literature attests. The tricyclic antidepressants (imipramine, amitriptyline, desipramine, nortriptyline, and protriptyline) and related agents (doxepin) are commonly prescribed for moderate to severely depressed patients. Monoamine oxidase inhibitors (phenelzine, tranylcypromine, nialamide, and others) are also of particular value with specific types of depressions. For both unipolar and bipolar depressions, the tricyclic antidepressants appear to be the most effective chemotherapies for reducing acute depressive symptoms. Furthermore, electroconvulsive therapy (ECT) remains a highly effective, even life-saving procedure for appropriately selected severe depressions. If properly administered, ECT may be used when antidepressant medication is ineffective or when patients cannot tolerate the side effects or risks associated with antidepressants.

Lithium may act as an antidepressant for some patients, particularly those with a personal or family history of mania. Recent studies suggest that lithium is superior to placebo in reducing manic episodes and in preventing either manic or depressive relapses in bipolar affective patients (see Beck, 1973, pp. 90–91). Lithium's usefulness as a prophylactic in nonbipolar depressions is less certain, although a few recent studies do suggest that it has a prophylactic effect (Prien, Caffey and Klett, 1974).

Despite the impressive number of studies showing that the average response rates for antidepressants exceeded those for placebo, and despite the widespread use of antidepressants, the clinician prescribing them must carefully weigh several factors: the degree of the therapeutic response to the drug, its general applicability, and the safety of a particular drug in the treatment of the individual patient. With regard to measurement of the response, most drug–placebo comparisons are conducted over a brief several-week period and reported in terms of relative group averages on various outcome measures. For example, Klerman *et al.* (1974), defined a "significant clinical improvement" as a 50% reduction in initial symptomatology over a 4-week active-medication period. However, a 50% reduction in initial symptomatology may still leave some patients significantly depressed and in need of further treatment. Further, it is not clear whether symptom reduction continues throughout the time that the patient remains on medication. While maximum drug–placebo differences usually emerge between 2 to 10 weeks of treatment, the natural course of the average depressive episode usually lasts from 24 to 56 weeks (Robins and Guze, 1972). Although drugs are clearly associated with relative reductions in symptom levels, they may not produce a complete remission that continues throughout the course of maintenance antidepressant therapy.

Cognitive therapy may well have a place in the treatment of

those patients who fail to obtain complete remission or full prophylaxis from the use of antidepressant medication. In other words, the role of cognitive therapy may be that of enhancing a strong therapeutic response to chemotherapy.

Treatment stability refers to the maintenance of symptom reduction following the termination of active treatment. To an ever increasing extent, clinicians are tending to maintain both unipolar and bipolar depressed patients on permanent medication, much as diabetics are maintained on insulin (Davis, 1976; Klerman et al., 1974; Schou, 1968). Although an estimated 55% of all index cases will have no subsequent episodes (Robins and Guze, 1972), depression has traditionally been considered an episodic phenomenon. In the Boston/New Haven project (Klerman et al., 1974), 36% of the drug responders who were offered no treatment during follow-up relapsed within 8 months after drug termination. Thus, it appears that reliance on the prophylactic use of medication as the sole form of therapy is not indicated in the treatment of many cases of depression. Further, long-term side effects of tricyclic antidepressants and lithium, although infrequent, may be quite severe.

For some types of depressions, cognitive therapy may achieve better treatment stability than chemotherapy (see Chapter 18). We would hypothesize that cognitive therapy helps the patient learn to monitor, reality-test, and modify negative stereotypical thought patterns. Thus, the patient develops new ways of thinking about himself and the .world. If these distorted thought patterns remain unchanged, cognitive theory predicts that they will predispose the patient to experience subsequent relapses.

The potential prophylactic value of cognitive therapy is supported by our recent study of moderate to severely depressed outpatients treated with either tricyclic chemotherapy or cognitive therapy (see Chapter 18). Cognitive therapy patients evidenced a lower risk of relapse and a lower level of self-reported symptoms of depressive symptomatology at one year following termination of treatment. Although additional studies are needed to confirm this finding, cognitive therapy may add to the maintenance of remission once drug treatment is discontinued.

The general applicability of antidepressants is also an important question. Small but important subgroups of depressed patients cannot tolerate various medications due to noxious side effects or to ongoing medical illnesses that preclude the use of antidepressants. Cognitive therapy may be of value to these patients who cannot take antidepressants.

More important numerically is the apparent difficulty of insuring the patient's compliance with medication regimens. While the degree of compliance can probably be increased by more careful handling of the therapist–patient relationship, at least some portion of the drug terminators may be responding to nuisance side effects and/or perceived lack of improvement. Although it is always difficult to determine precisely why a patient terminates treatment prematurely, it is likely that estimates of response rates are inflated by the exclusion of nonresponding dropouts from absolute response calculations.

For some samples of outpatients, cognitive therapy may be more generally applicable than antidepressant treatment. The average dropout rate among patients receiving active medication in controlled outpatient drug studies is generally 25–30%. Cognitive or cognitive-behavior therapies appear to result in a lower dropout rate for depressed outpatients (Rush *et al.*, 1977; McLean and Hakstian, 1978). In addition, cognitive therapy may have an important place in the treatment of depressions that specifically require chemotherapy. We have developed specific cognitive-change techniques to increase adherence to medication regimens and to decrease the incidence of premature termination of biological treatments.

It is important to note that the tricyclic antidepressants have one of the lowest lethal-dosage to therapeutic-dosage ratios of any of the psychotropic medications. Many but not all depressed patients are suicidal, and availability of means is a key factor in suicide attempts. Although their lethal potential does not preclude the use of these medications, it does provide added impetus to develop alternative methods of treatment.

Finally, cognitive therapy can be conducted in the context of the couple or family system (Rush, Shaw, and Khatami, in press). This format can neutralize or even turn to therapeutic advantage the anger or critical attitude of a family member who might otherwise undermine compliance with the medication instructions, and it offers a method for modifying prejudicial or antagonistic social interactions. This modifying effect may both improve prophylaxis and also make possible earlier detection of an impending relapse, thus prompting earlier referral for additional treatment. These speculations are supported by a recent study in which behavioral treatment for obese outpatients resulted in a greater weight loss when spouses were included in the therapy itself (Brownell, Heckerman, and Westlake, 1977).

EVALUATING THE PATIENT

It does appear that with regard to response to treatment, depressions are heterogeneous. The antidepressant chemotherapies are of significant value in the acute treatment and prophylaxis of some depressions. As with any effective treatment, there are specific risks attached to the use of these agents. Then there are, we believe, some depressions which will respond to cognitive therapy alone (Rush, Hollon, Beck, and Kovacs, 1978). For still another group of depressions, there may be clinical justification for use of a combination of both chemotherapy and cognitive therapy. The clinician is confronted with the problem of identifying those patients whose depressions require either cognitive therapy, pharmacotherapy, or a combination of both.

A careful evaluation of each patient is essential before a specific treatment approach is selected. However, with respect to a number of depressed patients, we are currently somewhat limited in our ability to specify the optimal treatment. Although the initial evaluation provides the clinician with information that favors a particular intervention, an empirical trial-and-error approach is often needed. That is, once the treatment is begun, careful evaluations are frequently conducted to determine whether the patient is responding as expected to the prescribed treatment (cognitive therapy, chemotherapy, or a combination). If the patient's response is unsatisfactory, the clinician should either restructure the approach (e.g., change the problem definitions, elevate the dose of medication) or change to a different type of therapy (e.g., add cognitive therapy to pharmacotherapy or *vice versa*). The need for frequent evaluations during treatment becomes clearly evident when the following possibility is considered: Even after a careful evaluation, the clinician may misdiagnose a manic–depressive disorder as depressive neurosis and may therefore initiate cognitive therapy alone. (Recall that there is no evidence that this type of bipolar depression responds to cognitive

·therapy alone. Lithium or tricyclic antidepressant medications continue to be treatments of choice for both symptom relief and prophylaxis.) In this case, the therapist might become aware of this initial error only when the patient fails to respond to cognitive therapy. This failure to respond as expected should alert the clinician to reevaluate both the patient and the treatment selected. On the other hand, recurrent failure to respond to antidepressant medication might indicate that the patient will respond to cognitive therapy alone.

The importance of misdiagnosis should not be underestimated. In a recent study of 100 patients with neurotic depression, extensively evaluated with research and clinical methods, 18% were subsequently found to have a bipolar illness over a 3-to-4-year follow-up period (Akiskal, Bitar, Puzantian, Rosenthal, and Walker, 1978). Furthermore, inadequate treatment of depressed outpatients with antidepressants represents a serious risk to many of these patients. A recent 10-year follow-up study (Robins and Guze, 1972) found that less severe, "neurotic" depressions were least adequately treated with antidepressants and suffered higher mortality as compared to more severely depressed patients.

The combination of antidepressants and cognitive therapy might offer a unique advantage in the treatment of still other types of depression. Unfortunately, we can not yet definitely specify the types of depression for which this combined therapy is most suitable.

What elements are of value in deciding whether to prescribe medication, cognitive therapy, or the combination?

One difficulty in defining depression has been the failure to specify consistent criteria for diagnosing the depressive syndrome. It is often difficult to decide that a clinical problem is not a depression but is another disorder. For example, schizo-affective schizophrenia is considered by some investigators to include patients who, in fact, have a manic–depressive illness. "Masked depression" constitutes another group of potential "depressions" in which the patient does not report feeling sad or "blue" (Lopez-Ibor, 1972).

Although there is yet no common agreement as to what constitutes "depression," the signs and symptoms most commonly seen in patients whom clinicians call depressed can be identified and even subdivided conceptually into affective, behavioral, cognitive, somatic, and motivational clusters (see Beck, 1967, pp. 10–33).

Recent attempts to specify criteria on which to base a diagnosis of depressive syndrome can be of great value to the clinician to assist him in deciding whether a patient has a depressive syndrome. The following criteria are used to diagnose a major depressive disorder (Spitzer, Endicott, and Robins, 1978).

A. One or more distinct periods with dysphoric mood or pervasive loss of interest or pleasure
B. Five or more of the following:
 1. Increase or decrease in appetite or weight
 2. Excessive or insufficient sleep
 3. Low energy, fatigability, tiredness
 4. Psychomotor agitation or retardation
 5. Loss of interest or pleasure in usual activities
 6. Feelings of self-reproach, guilt
 7. Decreased ability to think or concentrate
 8. Recurrent thoughts of death or suicide
C. Duration of dysphoric features for at least two weeks
D. Sought help or sustained functional impairment
E. No other major diagnoses (e.g., schizophrenia)

It is probable that these criteria will be incorporated in the official nomenclature of the American Psychiatric Association. Descriptive diagnoses based on specific criteria are likely to substantially improve reliability.

Minor depressive disorder is diagnosed when there are nonpsychotic episodes of illness in which the most prominent disturbance is a prevailing mood of depression without the full depressive syndrome, although some features are present. This "minor/major" distinction is important because clinical impressions suggest that major disorders are likely to require pharmacotherapy. However, some major depressive disorders may respond to cognitive therapy alone or to the combined approach, while the minor disorders may be more responsive to cognitive therapy without added antidepressant medication. These clinical impressions should be tested with additional research studies.

It is important to bear in mind the limitations of a descriptive diagnostic approach. Although such a system provides a basis for determining whether a patient *is* or *is not* suffering from a depressive syndrome, certain types of depression may be arbitrarily excluded by this scheme. In other words, the validity of this scheme for all types of depression has yet to be established. In addition, a number of factors can influence the frequency and configuration of the signs and symptoms presented by the patient. Age, sex, ethnicity, socioeconomic background, premorbid personality, level of intelligence, and severity of illness may all influence how a specific patient appears and feels when he or she is depressed. For instance, older patients are likely to have a greater preponderance of somatic symptoms (sleep, appetite, weight, and libidinal losses). The timing and actual conduct of the diagnostic interview itself can also significantly influence this descriptive diagnosis. For example, a patient whose depressive episode is spontaneously ending or just beginning may have only a few of the expected signs and symptoms that occur at peak severity of the depressive illness.

Even though a patient fits the criteria for depressive syndrome, he is not necessarily a candidate for cognitive therapy. Recall that depressions are a heterogeneous group of problems—heterogeneous with respect to etiology and response to therapy. First of all, a number of medications are known to cause the depressive syndrome (for an excellent review, see Lipowski, 1975). Drugs such as reserpine, alphamethyldopa (an antihypertensive), propranolol (cardiac drug), birth-control pills, and steroids can cause the depressive syndrome. The obvious treatment, if medically safe, is to discontinue these medications; it is not to administer cognitive therapy.

Secondly, a number of studies indicate that psychiatric patients frequently have medical illnesses that are undetected at the time of referral. Even in a medical setting (such as a clinic or hospital) patients who have psychiatric complaints should be thoroughly evaluated for the presence of occult or contributing medical disorders. Koranyi (1972) found 50 of 100 consecutive psychiatric outpatients had evidence of physical illness, half of which were *not* diagnosed at the time of the referral.

On the other hand, a number of specific medical disorders are associated with various kinds of psychopathology, particularly symptoms of the depressive syndrome (Schwab, Bialow, Brown, and Holzer, 1967). These disorders include thyroid, adrenal and parathyroid dysfunctions, pernicious anemia, viral infections, cancer, epilepsy, vitamin deficiencies, hysterectomy, and rheumatoid arthritis, among others. In addition, physical illness often precipitates a psychiatric disorder, particularly depression. Studies of precipitating events related to the onset of severe depressions rate physical illness as the fifth most common cause (Leff, Roatch, and Bunney, 1970; Paykel, Klerman, and Prusoff, 1970). Because treatment of the physical illness usually relieves the depressive syndrome, the clinician should obtain a careful medical history, and a history of current medications, as well as the report on physical examination, in order to identify potential medical causes of the depressive syndrome. Without such an evaluation, cognitive therapy or antidepressant medication may be inappropriately administered.

Finally, other psychiatric disorders may be misdiagnosed as depressive syndrome. These include schizo-affective schizophrenia (Kasanin, 1944) and borderline syndrome (Grinker, Werble, and Drye, 1968; Gunderson and Singer, 1975). There are no controlled outcome data or case reports to suggest that these syndromes *do* or *do not* respond to cognitive therapy. However, it is our clinical impression that patients with more severe impairments in reality-testing are less likely to respond to cognitive therapy alone. There is a real need for further studies to determine whether cognitive treatment is efficacious with the borderline syndrome schizo-affective schizophrenia.

Assuming that medical causes of the depressive syndrome have been ruled out, the clinician still must decide whether to prescribe cognitive therapy and/or antidepressant medication. This decision rests on our capacity to identify which depressions are likely to respond to one or the other treatments. Various attempts to subdivide the affective disorders may have a bearing on this decision (Becker, 1974; Klerman, 1971; Robins and Guze, 1972).

The 1968 *Diagnostic and Statistical Manual* of the American Psychiatric Association (DSM-II) recognizes a single nonpsychotic depression (depressive neurosis) and five types of psychotic depression (psychotic depressive reaction; involutional melancholia; and manic–depressive illness, manic, depressed, and circular types). Several studies show that both neurotic and psychotic depressions respond to medication.

In Great Britain, psychosis refers to a severe impairment in reality-testing, as manifested by hallucinations and delusions. According to this definition, only 15% of all depressions are psychotic depressions (Klerman and Paykel, 1970). However, in the United

States, the use of the term "psychotic depression" depends upon the severity of symptoms and degree of functional impairment.

Current practice dictates that these psychotic depressions, according to DSM-II, are most effectively treated with biological methods. The treatment of choice for involutional melancholia remains electroconvulsive therapy (ECT). Psychotic depressive reactions and manic–depressive illness, manic or circular types, are best treated with lithium, antidepressants, or, sometimes, antipsychotic medications (Freedman, Kaplan, and Sadock, 1975). We do not know whether manic–depressive illness, depressed type, responds to cognitive therapy, although it does respond significantly to appropriate antidepressant drugs. Perhaps cognitive therapy can heighten the efficacy of biological treatments for psychotic depressions, either by increasing the degree of adherence to medication regimen or by correcting associated dysfunctional attitudes and thought patterns. Given our current state of knowledge, we would *not* recommend cognitive therapy as the *sole treatment* for these psychotic depressions.

Let us consider the nonpsychotic depression, depressive neurosis, a diagnosis given to a majority of outpatients with depression. Although patients suffering from depressive neurosis do, in general, appear to respond to cognitive therapy, this group of patients may also include some depressions that are not particularly responsive to the cognitive approach. In fact, a growing body of data indicates that depressive neurosis refers to a spectrum of problems. Further, a number of these patients may benefit from antidepressant medication.

Although other attempts have been made to subclassify depressions (e.g., endogenous–reactive; endogenomorphic–nonendogenomorphic; primary–secondary), the relevance of these dichotomous groupings for predicting response to cognitive therapy is untested. The initial dualistic distinction between "reactive" depressions and "endogenous" or "autonomous" depressions was meant to differentiate depressions triggered by response to environmental events from those without a perceptible precipitant. Advocates of this dichotomy contend that endogenous depressions respond to antidepressant drugs or to electroconvulsive therapy, whereas reactive depressions fare better with psychotherapy. However, recent evidence suggests that patients who initially report no precipitating stress will subsequently identify one or more stresses in the course of careful interviewing (Leff *et al.*, 1970). Other investigators have also found evidence to suggest that the simple presence or absence of reported stress is of little value in predicting response to chemotherapy (Klein, 1974; Akiskal *et al.*, 1978). We, in turn, would suggest that the presence or absence of stress is also of little value in predicting response to cognitive therapy.

The unipolar–bipolar distinction is important because bipolar depressions (those associated with a history of mania or hypomania) are best treated with lithium and/or tricyclic medication (Freedman *et al.*, 1975). Many nonpsychotic unipolar depressions appear to respond well to cognitive therapy, and it is likely that others will respond to antidepressant medication in combination with cognitive therapy or to antidepressant medication alone (Rush *et al.*, 1977).

Klein (1974) has coined the term "endogenomorphic depression" to designate a disorder characterized by inhibition of the pleasure/ reward system to such an extent that the patient no longer has the capacity for enjoyment. There may or may not be an apparent environmental precipitant or stress. Inhibition of the pleasure mechanism leads to a "profound lack of interest in the environment, with inability to enjoy food, sex, or hobbies." He hypothesizes that these patients cannot experience pleasure either from current sensory input or via anticipated or recollective imagery. Often these patients have dramatic abnormalities in psychomotor activity and somatic rhythms (sleep, appetite, weight maintenance, libido). They may be delusional. All bipolar and some unipolar depressives are included in this "endogenomorphic" group. Klein believes that endogenomorphic depressions respond well to antidepressant drugs or to electroconvulsive treatment and that they are difficult to treat with psychotherapy alone.

There is some evidence (Mendels and Cochrane, 1968) that the presence of profound somatic symptoms are good predictors of response to biological interventions (e.g., ECT). Severe somatic symptoms do appear to increase the probability of a therapeutic response to antidepressants. Thus, we would recommend that the clinician give greater consideration to using antidepressants in treating patients with more severe somatic symptoms. For example, a weight loss of 15 pounds or more over 3 months should be considered a very suggestive clinical indicator of the need for including antidepressants in the treatment plan.

There is a lack of sufficient research data to test Klein's

hypothesis. However, in our study of 44 patients assigned to either cognitive therapy alone or to imipramine with brief supportive therapy (see Chapter 18), we found that cases with a preponderance of endogenomorphic symptoms were associated with a better end-of-treatment status for either treatment, as compared to those cases with fewer such symptoms (Hollon, Beck, Kovacs, and Rush, 1977). Thus while somatic symptoms may be of some value in determining type of treatment, their relevance is not sufficiently specific to predict degree of response to either antidepressant medication or cognitive therapy.

In addition, cognitive therapy may be a useful treatment for endogenomorphic depression when combined with antidepressant medication. Antidepressants may increase the capacity of some of these patients to participate in psychotherapy; then, cognitive therapy may be rendered even more effective by combining it with medication. Further research is needed to determine whether the combined therapy is of specific value for these endogenomorphic depressions.

In summary, "depression" refers to a heterogeneous group of problems. Biological interventions are very effective treatments for some depressions and should be judiciously administered when indicated. Further, cognitive therapy appears to be of value for some types of depression. Our ability to specify those depressions that are responsive to cognitive therapy is limited by the lack of a commonly agreed-upon system for classifying depressions and by a lack of needed research data. However, improvements in descriptive diagnosis and biological and psychological assessment may be of help in identifying depressions that require medication and in selecting depressions for cognitive therapy.

We can offer a number of suggestions based on available research data and our clinical impressions. These suggestions should be regarded as general impressions rather than specific rules. They go beyond currently available data and, as such, remain subject to revision as greater clinical experience and research findings accrue.

Certain kinds of depressions appear to respond relatively well to biological treatments. They include bipolar depressions (those with mania or hypomania) and psychotic depressions (those with hallucinations or delusions). There is no evidence that patients with psychosis (delusions or hallucinations) or those with a history of mania or hypomania will respond to cognitive therapy alone. Given our current state of knowledge, exclusive treatment with cognitive therapy is contraindicated for these persons. However, the addition of cognitive therapy to medication treatment may strengthen the overall response of a number of these patients.

The "neurotic depressions" (diagnosed according to the criteria of DSM-II or those of Klein, 1974) as a group appear likely to respond to cognitive treatment alone. However, some DSM-II neurotic depressions also appear to respond to medication alone. Whether cognitive therapy in combination with, or following, chemotherapy offers any advantage in either symptom relief or prophylaxis for these neurotic depressions remains a matter for further study. Patients with minor affective disorders are more likely to be candidates for cognitive therapy alone, whereas more of the major affective disorders will require either medication or the combined approach.

Whether patients with obvious somatic symptoms (decreased sleep, appetite, weight, and libido) and anhedonia (Klein's "endogenomorphic" depressions) are likely to respond to cognitive therapy remains unclear. One study suggests that some of these depressions respond to cognitive therapy (Rush *et al.*, 1977). Until further studies are available, we suggest that severe somatic symptoms in nonhallucinating, nondelusional, nonbipolar depressions provide a good justification for including antidepressants in the treatment plan, since the evidence that antidepressants are effective for these depressions is substantial. We would recommend that "severe" be operationalized as 15 pounds or more weight loss over 3 months, and/or 2 hours or more early-morning insomnia.

Other potential indicators of response to cognitive therapy have been suggested but are untested in controlled research studies. High reactivity to environment events and a history of gradual onset of the depressive syndrome may indicate a better respone to cognitive therapy. A history of short, less severe episodes of depression may predict a good response to either psychological or biological treatments.

The following criteria would justify the administration of cognitive therapy alone:

1. Failure to respond to adequate trials of two antidepressants
2. Partial response to adequate dosages of antidepressants
3. Failure to respond or only a partial response to other psychotherapies

366

4. Diagnosis of minor affective disorder
5. Variable mood reactive to environmental events
6. Variable mood that correlates with negative cognitions
7. Mild somatic disturbance (sleep, appetite, weight, libidinal) symptoms
8. Adequate reality-testing (i.e., no hallucinations or delusions), span of concentration, and memory function.
9. Inability to tolerate medication side effects, or evidence that excessive risk is associated with pharmacotherapy

The following features suggest that cognitive therapy alone is not indicated:

1. Evidence of coexisting schizophrenia, organic brain syndromes, alcoholism, narcotic abuse, mental retardation
2. Patient has medical illness or is taking medication that is likely to cause depression
3. Obvious memory impairment or poor reality-testing (hallucinations, delusions)
4. History of manic episode (bipolar depression)
5. History of family member who responded to antidepressant
6. History of family member with bipolar illness
7. Absence of precipitating or exacerbating environmental stresses
8. Little evidence of cognitive distortions
9. Presence of severe somatic complaints (e.g., pain)

The features listed below are indications for combined therapies (medication plus cognitive therapy):

1. Partial or no response to trial of cognitive therapy alone
2. Partial but incomplete response to adequate pharmacotherapy alone
3. Poor compliance with medication regimen
4. Historical evidence of chronic maladaptive functioning with depressive syndrome on intermittent basis
5. Presence of severe somatic symptoms and marked cognitive distortions (e.g., hopelessness)
6. Impaired memory and concentration and marked psychomotor difficulty
7. Severe depression with suicidal danger

8. History of first-degree relative who responded to antidepressants
9. History of mania in relative or patient

We do not assert that each patient who receives medication should also receive cognitive therapy nor do we believe that only a lack of response to cognitive therapy stands as a clear indication that biological intervention is necessary. Rather, we are trying to suggest a rough set of guidelines for determining whether antidepressant medication alone, cognitive therapy alone, or cognitive therapy in combination with antidepressants will provide a course of treatment with the greatest potential for success. Currently there are insufficient clinical research data upon which to base these decisions for each depressed patient. Thus, we are in a phase of development of this body of knowledge in which clinical experience and available research data must be continually reappraised to provide for the most rational selection of treatment(s).

Over the next several years, we anticipate further advances in the area of pharmacotherapy. We hope that these advances will improve the efficacy, safety, and general applicability of medication for patients in need of biological treatment. Similarly, we might expect further improvements in cognitive therapy as well. The development of additional cognitive therapy techniques for specific formats (e.g., couples or groups) and/or for other subgroups of patients may also improve its efficacy and applicability. Thus, the guidelines we offer will need revision as these advances are made and as additional research data accrue.

As we pointed out previously, regardless of how carefully one assesses a depressed patient before selecting a treatment, initial evaluations can be misleading or incorrect (Akiskal et al., 1978). Thus, every initial "diagnosis" is only a hypothesis upon which to base treatment selection. However, as with other hypotheses, it is subjected to empirical testing in treating the patient. If the response pattern does not show significant effects after an adequate trial of the intervention(s), the initial diagnosis and/or treatment program must be reconsidered, and, in many cases, altered.

The treatment(s) chosen should be based upon: (1) the formulation of a descriptive diagnosis from current and past signs and symptoms; (2) the identification of cognitive distortions that seem to be amenable to cognitive change methods and/or responsive to environmental events; (3) a calculation of the relative risks and benefits that appeared to accompany each treatment.

The clinician's selection of treatment must be based on a careful assessment and on the anticipated response of the patient to treatment. Furthermore, the treatment itself should be tailored to the individual patient. There are patients who cannot or will not accept medication for medical or philosophical reasons, patients for whom depth psychotherapy is an anathema, and patients for whom certain components of cognitive therapy are unacceptable. Thus, the clinician must adapt the treatment to the patient without sacrificing potential efficacy.

In some cases, the judicious use of more than one psychotherapeutic approach is indicated; that is, cognitive therapy may be combined with other nonbiological adjuncts to treatment. For example, consider the patient suffering from chronic pain and depression. It is our clinical impression (as yet unsupported from controlled research) that specific adjuncts to treatment (e.g., relaxation and/or biofeedback training) are sometimes of help to these patients. Furthermore, the addition of specific instructions to the family or changes in the structure and function of the patient's social system may also add to the efficacy of cognitive therapy for some of these patients (Khatami and Rush, 1978). Thus, the clinician must carefully consider the various therapeutic modalities available and must weigh the advantages and disadvantages of combining cognitive therapy with other psychotherapeutic interventions or with medication with respect to each patient.

However, we firmly believe that a helter-skelter approach to treatment, in which multiple therapies are applied simultaneously with insufficient rationale and/or incomplete evaluation, will result in confusion, poor outcome, and possibly increased depression. We believe that patients should be treated with as few techniques or medications at a time as are clinically indicated. In this way, an adequate trial of one modality or one set of techniques can be obtained before turning to an alternative, second approach.

The following case highlights some of the problems that indicate the combined treatment approach.

A 23-year-old widowed white female was seen in the intensive-care unit following a suicide attempt by overdose. The apparent precipitant was the death of her 27-year-old husband from acute leukemia 2 months previously. She had no previous psychiatric history or treatment.

On mental status examination, the patient presented evidence of impaired reality-testing and poor impulse control. She reported auditory and visual hallucinations in the weeks prior to her suicide attempt. In addition, for several weeks following her husband's death, she had been hitchhiking across the country, attempting to "cheer myself up."

Although she did not feel that she was personally defective, she expressed feelings of emptiness, loneliness, and being abandoned. Hostile and belligerent, she denied wanting to see a psychiatrist. Furthermore, she had marked somatic symptoms of the depressive syndrome (sleep, appetite, weight loss, and libidinal disturbances). She had no history of mania or hypomania and no family history of depression or mania. This patient was diagnosed as having a psychotic depressive reaction.

Treatment: Psychotropic medication (low doses of antipsychotics and antidepressants) was administered. The patient's marked difficulty with sleep (she slept less than an hour per night), her defective reality-testing, and poor impulse control were the targets for this biological treatment.

Her Beck Depression Inventory score was initially 48. She was discharged from the hospital after one week. After a total of 3 weeks of medication her BDI score was 24. At this time, the patient had become less hostile and was beginning to accept the prospect of psychotherapy. Furthermore, she had no further hallucinations and her impulse control had improved significantly. She seemed more amenable to the scheduling of twice-weekly sessions of cognitive therapy, which she began as an outpatient.

At first her negative cognitions about accepting psychiatric treatment and medication were elicited and neutralized sufficiently to increase her adherence to the recommended treatment. The cognitions that were directed against her accepting treatment included the following: "There is nothing anyone can do to help me, and I should be dead." "Life is not worth living without my husband." Although this patient continued to require extensive cognitive therapy (15 months) and psychotropic medication (12 months) following this crisis, she gradually began to confront her negative cognitions and to reorganize her conceptualization of her relationship to her deceased husband.

This case illustrates the importance of differential diagnosis. Specifically, the evidence of poor reality testing (hallucinations) and poor impulse control, as well as marked somatic symptoms and the high potential for suicide, all indicated that medication would be of significant value. The initial target of cognitive therapy was to help this patient accept both medication and psychotherapy. It seemed that as she responded to medication, more extensive cognitive therapy was feasible. Her extended treatment demonstrates how severe depressions may require a sustained therapeutic effort over a prolonged period of time.

INCREASING ADHERENCE TO MEDICATION THROUGH COGNITIVE-CHANGE TECHNIQUES

The importance of gaining patients' adherence to both psychotherapeutic and medical regimens is a topic that has been receiving greater attention. Some studies indicate that less than half the patients follow medication regimens that require daily adherence over several months (Sackett and Haynes, 1976). These figures suggest that adherence may be the most critical factor in contributing to a weak (or strong) response.

It is clinically well-known that the depressed patient may be difficult to involve in treatment. The cognitive model would predict that cognitive distortions contribute significantly to this "paralysis of will" or "poor motivation." The depressed patient may believe that he is hopelessly ill, that therapy will be ineffective, and that the roads to a depression-free life are either nonexistent or totally blocked. Given these fixed ideas, it is not surprising that such a patient would lack the motivation necessary for adherence to a prescribed course of treatment.

A lack of careful attention to the patient's attitudes and perceptions about pharmacotherapy may lead the clinician to misdiagnose him as "unmotivated" when it is the patient's negative distortions that are the real problem. The depressed patient's "negative view of the world" may further distort his already negative views about pharmacotherapy, particularly psychotropic medication.

371

In the initial phase of treatment the patient's depression, and consequently his cognitive distortions, are usually most severe. Furthermore, the majority of patients drop out of treatment (whether cognitive therapy or chemotherapy) in this initial phase. By targeting the patient's negative conceptualizations of treatment, the clinician can often strengthen adherence to the treatment plan (e.g., medication).

In dealing with poor adherence, we have elicited from the patient a variety of cognitions about the medication *before* it is taken, cognitions about actual effects of the medication (both therapeutic and side effects) *while* it is taken, and cognitions about the depression. A sample of these cognitions are presented in Table 3.

TABLE 3
EXEMPLAR COGNITIONS CONTRIBUTING TO POOR ADHERENCE TO MEDICATION
PRESCRIPTION

Cognitions about the medication (before taking it)
1. It's addicting.
2. I am stronger if I don't need medicine.
3. I am weak to need it (a crutch).
4. It won't work for me.
5. If I don't take medication, I'm not crazy.
6. I can't stand side effects.
7. I'll never get off medication once I start.
8. There's nothing I need to do except take medicine.
9. I only need to take medication on "bad days."

Cognitions about medication (while taking it)
1. Since I'm not perfectly well (any better) after days or weeks, the medicine isn't working.
2. I should feel good right away.
3. The medicine will solve all my problems.
4. The medicine won't solve problems, so how can it help?
5. I can't stand the dizziness (or "fuzziness") or other side effects.
6. It makes me into a zombie.

Cognitions about depression
1. I am not ill (I don't need help).
2. Only weak people get depressed.
3. I deserve to be depressed since I am a burden to everybody.
4. Isn't depression a normal reaction to the bad state of things?
5. Depression is incurable.
6. I am one of the small percentage that does not respond to any treatment.
7. Life isn't worth living so why should I try to get over my depression?

A patient's distorted cognitions about the medication and its effects may be extremely negative during an acute episode of depression. Patients who are acutely depressed may selectively attend to news media and personal reports from family and friends that reinforce his notion that medication is ineffective or dangerous. They also appear to selectively attend to and/or magnify unpleasant side effects of the medication once they have begun to take it. Their selective attention (as well as magnification, arbitrary inference, etc.) may also lead to the erroneous conclusion that the medication is either not working or is causing severe problems.

The therapist should bear in mind that the negative cognitive set of depressed patients warps their beliefs about medication and their reported experiences while taking medication. With this understanding, the therapist is more likely to elicit these counterproductive cognitions and to provide corrective information.

A 47-year-old white female, mother of two, was self-referred for complaints of severe chronic depression over the previous 10 years. At evaluation, she complained of significantly decreased sleep, appetite, weight, and sexual drive. She also reported suicidal preoccupation, difficulty in concentration, intermittent panic and anxiety attacks, and several specific phobias. She was not hallucinating or delusional. She had no history of mania or hypomania, although she did have a family history of depression.

The patient complained of intermittent severe headaches, abdominal distress, mild intermittent chest pains (without evidence of coronary artery disease), and intermittent ankle and knee pain that was diagnosed as early arthritis. These somatic complaints appeared to covary in severity with other symptoms of the depressive syndrome. They had first appeared *after* the onset of her depression 10 years ago.

The patient was vague about the initial stress that led to her first hospitalization; however, she did report multiple daily environmental stresses that seemed to contribute currently to her depressed mood. The most recent stresses included her husband's loss of employment, which resulted in significant financial hardship on the family, and her 14-year-old son's recent trouble with school and legal authorities.

Her previous treatment included three psychiatric hospitalizations, during the first two of which electroconvulsive therapy (ECT) was given. Although her first course of ECT had been quite successful, the second ECT treatment provided only partial relief for one or two months.

Previous medications included antipsychotics (chlorpromazine and thioridazine) and antidepressants (amitriptyline, doxepin, imipramine, and protriptyline). These various medications had led to only partial, poorly sustained relief, although several antidepressants had not been adequately tried (i.e., she did not take large enough doses over a long enough time to accurately test whether the medication would have been effective). Although she partially responded to some of these antidepressants, she had never felt completely like her "normal self" for the past 10 years.

Furthermore, she participated in roughly 100 weekly sessions until her insurance had been depleted. About half of these sessions were primarily supportive in nature, as the therapist had tried to direct her toward managing current problems and issues. She also had about 40 once-weekly psychodynamically oriented sessions, but again without significant relief in symptoms.

At evaluation, she was taking the following medications: an antidepressant (doxepin), antipsychotics (chlorpromazine and thioridazine), an anxiolytic (diazepam), a sleeping pill, an addicting analgesic, thyroid medication, and arthritis medication. She also intermittently took massive doses of megavitamins that had been prescribed in the past by another therapist. She believed that she had multiple allergies and had been on various types of food restrictions in the previous several months in hopes of reducing her depressive symptoms of several years' duration.

Treatment: Treatment was both complex and extended. It consisted of several stages.

Step 1: Developing a Therapeutic Alliance and Combating Negative Expectations about Treatment

At first, establishment of a therapeutic relationship was the top priority. At evaluation, she was so anxious that she was almost unable to give a description of her previous treatments. Part of her anxiety centered on the idea that she would be committed to a hospital and subjected to ECT again because of her suicidal ideation. The therapist uncovered this idea during evaluation while trying to establish a cognitive basis for her anxiety. The therapist simply asked the patient what sort of feelings and ideas she had while sitting in the waiting room before the evaluation.

As the patient's history unfolded, she supplied data with which to counter these cognitions (e.g., most of her time while depressed was not spent in the hospital but as an outpatient; evidence was that ECT had been only partially and transiently effective and had not even been used in her most recent hospitalization).

Furthermore, the therapist raised the *possibility* (but not the promise) of successful treatment for her depression by informing her about various treatment alternatives. She had assumed that no medication would be of any value because she had had only partial responses to some antidepressants. Her poor responses to two types of psychotherapies in the past also contributed to her pessimism. The therapist discussed other psychotherapeutic approaches that might prove of value.

Her history of chronic, "treatment-resistant" depression led the therapist to formulate and discuss a treatment plan that included alternative treatments to be considered if the initial approach was ineffective. Initial discussions were designed to help the patient develop an attitude of "let's see what might be of use" and give less credence to the idea that "nothing will work."

Step 2: Simplifying Medications

The next objective consisted of simplifying her medication regimen without sacrificing therapeutic benefit. To accomplish this, the therapist elicited the patient's beliefs about her medications. She thought that all her medications were necessary and, in fact, that added medication would be of further value. In order to test the validity of these beliefs, a behavioral task was used to help clarify for the patient the actual effect of each medication, as well as to identify which changes in medication would be of value.

First, as homework, she made a written record on a daily basis of her medication ingestion (type, dose, and time of each medication ingestion). In addition, she recorded her somatic and mood com-plaints at the time of each ingestion.

Next, changes in the medication regimen were made on a gradual basis. First, her megavitamin treatment was discontinued completely since it appeared to have produced no relief in the previous several months. Next, the frequency of the medication ingestions was reduced by combining medications where appropriate (e.g., her thyroid medication was combined with an antipsychotic agent in the morning). This reduced the actual frequency of ingestion from eight to four times per day.

Her symptom records of intermittent anxiety with panic attacks, tremulousness, and rapid heart rate revealed that these symptoms were most severe between 11 a.m. and 7 p.m. Careful questioning revealed she was drinking some 22 cups of coffee per day, and a preliminary diagnosis of caffeinism was made. Decaffeinated coffee substitution was made on a graduated schedule over the next several weeks. She continued to record her symptoms without changing other medications. This record provided the patient with evidence that coffee was probably the cause of many of her anxiety symptoms, since a 70% decrease in symptoms resulted from the substitution.

Next, diazepam was decreased as the dosage of a single antipsychotic (thioridazine) was increased. The chlorpromazine was discontinued over the same time period. To accomplish this, thioridazine was prescribed four times a day independent of her symptoms at the time, and diazepam was taken at specific times rather than on an "as needed" basis. Thus, the patient was put on a time-based dosage schedule for all medications. It was hoped that this schedule could weaken the association she had made between feeling upset and taking medication. The patient was seen twice a week while these medication changes were made (over the next four to five weeks of treatment).

Eventually, she was on a schedule of thioridazine 50 mg three times per day and 100 mg at bedtime, thyroid medication, arthritis medication, and one analgesic pill every other day. Her sleeping medication was no longer necessary. The diazepam had been discontinued, as well as her megavitamins. Finally, the antidepressant (doxepin) was fixed at a twice-per-day dosage of 75 mg. She was drinking three or less cups of caffeinated coffee per day. Her BDI score (initially 40) had dropped to 24 by the end of this medication management phase. In addition, her complaints of intermittent anxiety and sleep-onset insomnia had decreased but not disappeared.

Step 3: Maximizing Benefit from Medication

To maximize the potential therapeutic benefit from the simplified psychotropic medication regimen, the antidepressant was increased to 250 mg/day over the next several weeks. At this dose, she complained of relatively severe side effects (e.g., dry, pasty taste in her mouth, mild blurred vision, and slight dizziness on standing without measurable orthostatic hypotension). While increasing the antidepressant dose, her BDI score did not improve (range 22–24). Thus, the antidepressant was discontinued, after which the BDI showed no worsening of her symptoms.

Step 4: Identifying Negative Cognitions

While medication changes were being made, cognitive therapy techniques were used to address target symptoms of the depressive syndrome. The patient collected her cognitions that revealed themes consistent with both anxiety and depression. She tended to see danger and rejection in most situations, and she felt personally powerless to influence either her husband or her son significantly. She believed she was a failure, and she construed multiple, even minor, environmental stimuli in ways that reinforced her belief in her own ineffectiveness. She saw that her intermittent hostile outbursts were associated with her tendency to attribute cause for her difficulties with her family and her occupation to those around her.

Step 5: Correcting Negative Cognitions

Subsequently, additional cognitive-change techniques (e.g., triple-column method) were used to elicit and reality-test the evidence that supported specific cognitive distortions. For example, this patient was a particularly intelligent, highly motivated person who felt that she was not making a contribution to anyone and that her life was without meaning. The therapist and patient reviewed her previous occupational successes. The reasons for her current occupational problems were isolated by asking for a record of cognitions. Her fear of failing at a new job was thereby identified.

Subsequently, behavioral experiments to test the validity of these thoughts were conducted by persuading the patient to have several interviews for new jobs. In addition, her husband was interviewed. He stated that he could see that she showed a partial response to treatment so far and that he supported her in pursuing new occupational opportunities. Previously he had been so worried about her condition and the potential for suicide that he had stayed at home and not looked for a new job himself. This behavior had led the patient to conclude that he did not want to work any more. She felt she was to be the sole bread winner.

Step 6: Final Readjustment of Medication

As cognitive therapy proceeded, she learned to identify, then reality-test and modify her cognitions. She began to see how this skill resulted in immediate improvement in her mood. It was hypothesized that the dose of thioridazine could be further reduced; in fact, the patient had begun to express concern about taking so much medication for such a long period of time. Subsequently, thioridazine was decreased to a final dose of 25 mg three times a day. She continued her thyroid medication in the morning and continued to abstain from caffeinated coffee. She had discontinued her analgesic, although she continued her arthritis medicine.

Steps 7–10

Cognitive therapy continued over a course of nearly eight months. The patient was initially seen twice a week for the first four months and subsequently once weekly for the remainder. Several additional phases of treatment ensued. They included: identification and correction of silent assumptions; behavioral experiments; acting on new assumptions (role rehearsal); and several couples sessions to clarify her marital relationship, with identification and correction of silent assumptions held by both partners. Family-counseling sessions were also used to identify problems in her 14-year-old son, to restructure family interaction, and to resolve some of these issues.

By the end of treatment, the patient's Beck Depression Inventory score was 15 and had been in the 10–15 range for approximately four months prior to termination of treatment. The patient's husband and the patient had obtained employment.

At one year follow-up, this patient's BDI score was 5. During that time period her daughter had been divorced. Although the patient did not enter a depressive episode, she did participate in three "booster" sessions of cognitive therapy to deal with this upsetting and distressing life event.

At two-year follow-up her BDI score remained in the normal range. Although she continued to take thioridazine (50 mg/day), she was taking no other psychotropic agents. Her somatic complaints (which had markedly decreased by the end of active treatment) continued to be very infrequent at follow-up. In fact, she discontinued her arthritis medication after consulting with her family physician. The BDI scores at specified intervals are listed below.

Week	1	2	3	4	5	6	7	8	9	10	11	12
BDI	40	32	43	38	37	36	36	14	26	26	19	22

Week	13	14	15	16	17	18	19	20	21	22	40	52
BDI	24	24	24	24	24	24	24	24	24	13	15	14

1-year follow-up: 5
2-year follow-up: 8

This example illustrates how complex the treatment of some depressions can be. The first problem, that of adherence to prescribed treatment, was combatted by eliciting and correcting cognitions expressed very early in the course of therapy. Although she believed that no medication would be of help, she felt she needed more medication after having experienced incomplete relief with previous pharmacologic agents.

Secondly, as medication changes were made, cognitive and behavioral techniques were used to demonstrate to the patient the actual effects of these changes on her symptoms. In this way, the patient was shown that a great deal of apparently "needed" medicine was not of value.

Cognitive-change techniques were easily applied once the patient's medication was stabilized. This step was facilitated by training the patient in record-keeping before cognitive therapy was used (i.e., when the medication changes were ongoing).

Furthermore, this example illustrates the potential value of involving the social system (husband and son) in the treatment. Her husband provided external validation of progress, and the couple's meetings allowed for correction of various cognitive distortions within the relationship.

The "booster" sessions were of value to help the patient continue to apply these techniques when a significant opportunity (a stressful life event in this case) occurred. These sessions in essence provided further practice in applying the techniques that the patient had already learned.

This patient required an extensive amount of cognitive therapy compared to the usual patient. It seemed that her more chronic history of depression made it difficult for her to recollect times when she was not depressed. Also, cognitive therapy was judiciously structured to include sessions with her family (husband and son) because her social system seemed to be contributing to the maintenance of her depressive symptomatology.

Her initial reluctance to engage in psychotherapy seemed to subside after she derived benefit from a partial response to psychopharmacologic treatment. While her medications were being simplified, she had learned to pay careful attention to and actually record her behavior, thoughts, and mood. This skill was then used as part of subsequent cognitive-change strategies (e.g., triple-column technique).

Thus, cognitive therapy was used to obtain compliance with a course of medication, to change specific depressogenic cognitions and silent assumptions, and to modify the social system. Finally, this case illustrates that continued improvement may follow termination of active treatment without the addition of further psychotropic medication. Thus, this patient's social and occupational functioning continued to improve at one- and two-year follow-ups.

There are several techniques that can be employed to strengthen adherence to medication regimens and to correct cognitive distortions that weaken adherence. We can begin to combat these ideas with information. First, the patient is asked to read (and later discuss with the therapist) the introductory pamphlet, Coping with Depression (Beck and Greenberg, 1974). This explains how cognitive distortions are part of a depression (just as chest pain is part of a heart attack). As these unrealistically negative views are changed, the patients can expect to be more realistically optimistic about themselves, their future, and the treatment.

In addition to printed information, the therapist can use

cognitive-change techniques to directly combat negatively distorted cognitions that contribute to poor adherence. The therapist should discuss the basis for negative cognitions about medication and the specific positive and negative effects that the patient anticipates. We find it much more useful to *first* elicit the cognitions, *then* elicit the basis for these thoughts, and *finally* to provide corrective information. This method is to be distinguished from the common clinical approach of simply telling the patient about the medication and its expected effects, without eliciting the patient's ideas about it first.

This method can be implemented by asking the patient such questions as: "Have you ever taken antidepressant medication before? What was your experience with that? What do you believe is likely to happen to you as a consequence of taking this medication? How did you come to believe that?" Sometimes patients have the mistaken notion that antidepressant drugs (mood normalizers) are similar to stimulating drugs such as amphetamines—that they are addicting and that they produce immediate euphora. Other patients believe that medication is a crutch and that taking medication is evidence that they are particularly weak or lazy. Thirdly, because of previous experience with either inadequate or inappropriate medication treatment, many patients, assuming that all antidepressants are the same, believe that since one medication failed to produce complete relief, all other medications and dosage schedules will also be ineffective. Furthermore, some patients have the notion that if they do not take medication, it is proof of their mental health, whereas the ingestion of medication is evidence of severe mental illness. This notion often is related to experience with relatives or acquaintances who have taken antipsychotic medication but who continued to have repeated hospitalizations. These experiences may lead the patient to believe erroneously that taking medication increases the likelihood of hospitalization (it is the step in treatment that precedes hospitalization).

Other patients believe that antidepressants are prescribed for a lifetime. The idea of lifetime treatment is often supported by the mistaken notion that antidepressants are addicting.

Poor adherence to a course of antidepressants may also result from previous experience with anxiolytic medications. Many patients have taken "anti-anxiety" agents (e.g., diazepam, chlordiazepoxide, etc.) on an as-needed basis. Thus they have decided that any dysphoric emotion (feeling upset) is an indication for taking medication. Because they have taken medication when they felt anxious, they try to take antidepressants when they feel sad. Although anxiolytics do relieve acute anxiety, antidepressants are not indicated for sadness. The patient should be instructed to take antidepressants according to a fixed time schedule and not on an "as needed" basis. Thus, a "good day" is not an indication that the medication should be discontinued. These ideas can often be corrected with simple direct information. Sometimes the importance of obtaining a specific blood level of the drug is of value in dispelling the idea that an episode of dysphoria is a cue for medication ingestion.

Finally, depressed patients often erroneously believe that medication will produce "horrible" side effects. This idea may come from an interaction of their negative cognitive bias with reports of bad side effects from the media and friends. Many educated depressed patients have obtained a *Physician's Desk Reference* or other book which enumerates not simply the most common side effects but virtually *all* of the side effects ever reported in the research literature. The actual frequency and severity of these side effects are usually not specified. The patient (due to cognitive distortion) will focus on the most severe or esoteric-sounding side effects and assume that they are very likely to occur as a result of the currently prescribed medication. Sometimes specific correction of these cognitions will involve a review of the literature that the patient has already read to help the patient develop a realistic perspective—a sense of the actual probability of various side effects.

Certain unrealistic expectations may also contribute to poor adherence. Some patients have the expectation that they should feel total improvement right away after one or two days on antidepressants. They often do not recall that they were told that antidepressants require three to four weeks to produce a therapeutic effect *after* the correct dose is obtained. Therefore, they are likely to conclude incorrectly that medication will not work after a trial of a few days. Their negative cognitive set (e.g., selective attention to the lack of effect) will increase the probability of poor adherence.

Furthermore, a negative cognitive set will lead patients to focus on persisting problems while they fail to report actual partial improvements in some symptoms that do remit early in the course of medication treatment (e.g., improved sleep). A symptom inventory

(Beck Depression Inventory) is very useful in helping to assess improvement and to avoid relying simply on verbal reports.

Some patients have the expectation that *all* of their life problems will be solved by taking the medicine. When the problems persist, these patients construe this as evidence that the medication is valueless. Thus, persistent marital or occupational problems, which generally require some time to resolve and which may necessitate psychotherapy, are viewed by the patient as evidence that the medication is not effective. Consequently, the patient's willingness to take the medication may decrease.

On the other hand, the patients may believe that antidepressant medication will not solve *any* of their problems or change their ability to resolve any of these problems. This view is also incorrect, as antidepressants are known to improve concentration, decrease hopelessness, guilt, suicidal preoccupation, and easy fatigability. Thus, for selected patients medication is likely to help the patient to function at a more effective level and, thereby, to efficiently confront more complex interpersonal issues.

More frequent visits seem to be of value in improving adherence. By seeing the patient once a week (or in severe cases, twice a week), the therapist and patient can collaborate to monitor side effects and therapeutic effects. This routine also allows for ongoing correction of cognitive distortions. Negative attitudes and distorted ideas that occur while actually taking the prescribed medication can be elicited and corrected. Once medication is stabilized, less frequent visits are needed.

A number of patients are already on a complex medication regimen. Often, a complex medication schedule may be the result of having consulted many physicians, each of whom prescribed various agents without attempting to simplify the schedule of administration for the patient. The interactions among multiple medication agents are, in general, poorly studied.

For most depressed patients, multiple psychopharmacologic agents are generally not needed and should be avoided unless specifically indicated for specific treatment-resistant depressions. As illustrated above, cognitive methods can be used to simplify medication regimens. The patient records the specific symptoms, frequency, and dose of medications being used for a week or two. This record allows both physician and patient to monitor changes in symptoms as they occur while medication schedules are adjusted. Further, it helps the patient realize that the adjustments are effective rather than harmful. Finally, it confirms the fact that the patient is actually making the changes recommended.

Keeping schedules can also be of value in assessing side effects. A number of patients tend to label as "side effects" symptoms of depression that were present before taking medication. A written daily record sometimes offers convincing proof to the patient that these symptoms are *not* side effects. This realization often seems to result in stronger adherence.

In addition, if the patient begins to experience side effects (not an unusual development at the initiation of antidepressant treatment), his cognitions about the side effects (the somatic stimuli) can be identified and corrected with such a written record. For example, he may experience a dry mouth that can be quite severe at the initiation of treatment. As this occurs, the therapist can reassure the patient that continued ingestion at the same dose is likely to lead to decreased severity in the side effect over time as the patient accommodates to the medication.

Telephone calls can be of great value in improving adherence, particularly early in treatment. The patient should be told to call the therapist first, rather than independently make medication changes. Side effects, negative cognitions, and unrealistic expectations often contribute to poor self-management of medication regimens. Telephone calls provide a method for both eliciting and correcting these cognitions before they lead to poor adherence or premature treatment termination.

The above suggestions for using cognitive methods to strengthen adherence are based mainly on clinical experience. The cognitive approach allows for the development of additional methods to improve adherence. Clearly, further research is needed to determine how effective these methods are and for which patients these methods are indicated.

In summary, this chapter has focused on issues of differential diagnosis, combined therapy (cognitive therapy plus medication), and adherence. On the basis of the available research data and our clinical experience, we have offered a set of guidelines which undoubtedly will change as greater knowledge accrues. The area of cognitive-change techniques to increase adherence is one deserving of further research. It is important to bear in mind that the negative cognitive set in depression can contribute to poor adherence and that it is important to correct these ideas at both the outset and during the course of whatever treatment has been prescribed.

Chapter 18

OUTCOME STUDIES OF COGNITIVE THERAPY

Chapter 1 briefly presented the cognitive model of depression. This theory forms the basis for developing the specific techniques of the cognitive therapy of depression. Cognitive therapy is derived from this formulation: The source of the depression is a hypervalent set of negative concepts; therefore, the correction and damping down of these schemas may be expected to alleviate the depressive symptomatology. As we have detailed in previous chapters, the cognitive therapist and patient work together to identify distorted cognitions, derived from dysfunctional beliefs. Logical analysis and empirical testing are used to correct these distorted negative cognitions. Through the assignment of specific tasks, the patient learns to realign his thinking with reality and to master problems and life situations which he previously considered insuperable.

The cognitive model appears to make "sense," and it allows for the development of specific therapy techniques. However, whether cognitive therapy is in fact of value in treating depressed patients is a matter of empirical study. In addition, studies of the efficacy of cognitive therapy offer an indirect test of the cognitive model. If techniques to correct cognitions offer no specific advantage over no treatment or nonspecific treatment controls, we might conclude that negative cognitions, although present in association with a depressed mood, may simply be a secondary effect of the mood itself, or an epiphenomenon, rather than having a causal relationship to the disorder. Secondly, if (as the theory predicts) dysfunctional attitudes contribute to a predisposition to depression, and if these attitudes are corrected with cognitive therapy, then patients treated with cognitive therapy should be afforded some prophylaxis against relapse compared to no treatment or perhaps to other treatments. Once again, empirical studies can test this notion directly.

A number of the reports in the literature which support the use of cognitive or behavioral techniques involve case reports and analog studies. For example, Rush, Khatami, and Beck (1975) reported the treatment of three patients with chronic relapsing depression using a combination of cognitive and behavioral techniques. The main behavioral modality consisted of the use of activity schedules. The cognitive approach was directed at exposing and correcting the patients' negative distortions of the activities undertaken. These patients, who had not been substantially helped by drug therapy, showed prompt and sustained improvement with therapy as reflected by their scores on clinical and self-report measures.

SYSTEMATIC STUDIES: DEPRESSED VOLUNTEERS

Recently, a number of studies using controlled research designs have evaluated the relative efficacy of cognitive and behavioral procedures, alone and in combination. While the studies must be viewed as preliminary, due to research issues such as the sample size and the severity of symptomatology in the population studied, it is notable that treatments which focus on cognitive and behavioral targets have been effective in alleviating depression. Furthermore, they appear to be more efficacious than nondirective and supportive approaches.

Shipley and Fazio (1973) demonstrated that an individual-treatment approach which provided functional problem-solving alternatives resulted in significantly greater improvement in *depressed student volunteers* than an interest-support control group. Twenty-four treatment subjects and 25 controls were seen for 3 one-hour sessions in a period of 3 weeks by one therapist. In addition to the significant treatment effects, the authors also found that the effects were not contingent on the initial expectancies of the subjects.

Taylor (1974; Taylor and Marshall, 1977) conducted a controlled treatment comparison among groups which received cognitive modification, behavior modification, cognitive *and* behavior modification, and a waiting-list group. One therapist treated seven *depressed college student volunteers* in each group. Taylor (1974) concluded that the *depressed student volunteers* in the treatment groups showed significant improvement in depression, as compared to the waiting-list control subjects. Furthermore, the combination treatment was superior to either the cognitive or the behavioral treatment alone.

Gioe (1975) compared a modified cognitive modification treatment in combination with a "positive group experience," a cognitive modification treatment, a treatment consisting of a "positive group experience" alone, and a waiting-list control. Using a group therapy modality with 10 *depressed student volunteers* in each group, Gioe (1975) found that the combination treatment package was clearly superior in alleviating depressive symptomatology.

Hodgson and Urban (1975) demonstrated that both a behavioral–interpersonal skills procedure and a treatment program which altered the interpersonal perceptions of *depressed college student volunteers* were significantly more effective than no treatment. In addition, they found the behavioral procedures to be more effective than the interpersonal–perception techniques.

Results from two outcome studies conducted by Rehm and his colleagues (Fuchs and Rehm, 1977; Rehm, Fuchs, Roth, Kornblith, and Romano, 1978) indicated the efficacy of a behavioral self-control therapy program with *depressed female volunteers.* In the first study, the self-control group and a nondirective placebo group produced changes in depression which were significantly different from a waiting-list control. These changes were maintained at a six-week follow-up. In the second study the self-control group was compared with a social-skills-training group. Two pairs of therapists treated one therapy group in each condition during six weekly sessions. While subjects in both conditions improved with therapy, the self-control group showed greater improvement with respect to the symptoms of depression.

SYSTEMATIC STUDIES: DEPRESSED CLINIC PATIENTS

Note: Although the use of volunteers scoring above a certain cutoff point on a variety of depression scales is important in presenting a tightly controlled research design and provides preliminary evidence of the efficacy of a particular type of therapy, the generalizability of these findings to a *clinically depressed* population seeking help has to be demonstrated. This principle is underscored by community surveys that show that individuals diagnosed as neurotic but who do not seek help fare much better than similar individuals who seek and receive psychiatric help.

Increased confidence in the applicability of cognitive procedures to a clincal sample resulted from a study by Shaw (1975; 1977). He treated depressed students who had sought help at a University Health Service and were assessed by psychometric ratings and independent clinical evaluations by two psychologists. Again, a group-therapy format was employed with one therapist treating eight subjects in each group. Cognitive therapy was found to be significantly more efficacious than behavior (interpersonal skills training) therapy, nondirective therapy and a waiting-list control. The behavioral and nondirective procedures were significantly better than no treatment.

In a study of depressed female outpatients (*not* college students), Morris (1975) compared a "didactic cognitive behavioral program," an "insight-oriented therapy" (an experiential and unstructured program which focused on self-understanding), and a waiting-list control group. Four therapists were used to treat two discreet subgroups within the treatment conditions. Twenty-two subjects were in the cognitive–behavioral group, 17 were in the insight group, and 12 served as controls. Morris (1975) found that the cognitive–behavioral treatment was as effective in a 3-week period as a 6-week period when the number of sessions (6) remained constant. This finding is important, since one of the notable features of the cognitive approach is that significant change can occur during a time-limited intervention period.

Using a single subject, multiple-baseline design, (A–B–A), Schmickley (1976) reported significant improvement in a sample of 11 depressed outpatients at a Community Mental Health Center as a direct result of a cognitive–behavioral treatment intervention. Each subject was seen individually by a therapist for 4 one-hour sessions. Four therapists (but not the author) participated. Changes in the direction of improvement were found on 11 of 12 psychometric and behavioral measures following treatment. The patients had baselines of varying durations prior to starting treatment; a subsequent follow-up period of two weeks was controlled for spontaneous remission. In brief, no change occurred during baseline period; patients improved significantly as a result of the 2-week treatment intervention; they relapsed when treatment was withdrawn. The reinstitution of treatment at this point would have followed the accepted A–B–A–B paradigm and the results would have been more convincing.

An intensive pilot study at the University of Pennsylvania (Rush, Beck, Kovacs, and Hollon, 1977) was undertaken to assess the relative efficacy of cognitive therapy and an antidepressant drug (imipramine hydrochloride) in the treatment of 41 depressed outpatients. Cognitive therapy was found to be more effective than imipramine.

This study has been extended to 44 depressed outpatients, and follow-up data are now available. All patients were self-referred psychiatric outpatients who satisfied research diagnostic criteria for the depressed syndrome (Feighner, Robins, Guze, Woodruff, Winokur, and Munoz, 1972). All had a diagnosis of depressive neurosis according to the *Diagnostic and Statistical Manual–II*. As a group they were mostly white, partially college-educated, and in their mid-thirties.

Their past histories and Minnesota Multiphasic Personality Inventories indicated a substantial degree of psychopathology. In general, the patients had been intermittently or chronically depressed almost 9 years, and one-fourth of these patients had been hospitalized for depression in the past. On the average, the patients had seen more than two previous therapists prior to the study. The average current episode of depression had been present for just less than 12 months at the time of entering the study. All patients were moderately to severely depressed at initiation of treatment by self-report (Beck Depression Inventory), observer evaluation (Hamilton Rating Scale), and therapist rating (Raskin Scale). Seventy-five percent reported significant suicidal ideation at the start of treatment. Thus, the population of unipolar depressed patients generally had a substantial degree of psychopathology *and* a history of *poor* response to other *psychotherapies*. (Patients who had shown a previous poor response to chemotherapy were excluded, and in this way the sample was biased against psychotherapy.)

Patients were randomly assigned either to individual cognitive therapy or to pharmacotherapy (imipramine hydrochloride) for 12 weeks of treatment. Prescribed psychotherapy consisted of twice-weekly hour-long cognitive therapy sessions for a maximum of 20 visits. Pharmacotherapy consisted of not less than 100 or more than

250 mg/day of imipramine prescribed in 20-minute, once-weekly visits for a maximum of 12 weeks.

The methodology of cognitive therapy was specified in a 100-page treatment manual. The therapists were systematically supervised on a weekly basis by three experienced clinicians. All sessions were audio-recorded and spot-checked for adherence to protocol. Therapists consisted mainly of psychiatric residents who had treated only two "practice" cases with supervision prior to treating research cases.

Both treatment groups were equivalent with respect to demographic characteristics, histories of illness, treatment and mean severity of depression at the start of treatment. Of 19 patients assigned to cognitive therapy, 18 completed treatment over a mean period of 11 weeks. Of 25 patients assigned to pharmacotherapy, 17 completed treatment over the same mean period of time.

By the end of active treatment, both treatment groups showed statistically significant decreases ($p<.001$) in depressive symptomatology according to self-reports, observer evaluations and therapist ratings. The response rate to both pharmacotherapy and cognitive therapy exceeded the reported ranges for placebo response in depressed outpatients (Morris and Beck, 1974). By the end of treatment, cognitive therapy resulted in significantly greater improvements than did pharmacotherapy on self-reports and observer-based clinical ratings of depression ($p<.01$).

Of the cognitive therapy patients, 78.9% showed marked improvement or complete remission by the end of therapy, whereas only 20.0% of those who completed pharmacotherapy showed a similar degree of response. Both treatments resulted in substantial decreases in subjective reports and interviewer-based ratings of anxiety.

The dropout rate during active treatment was significantly greater with pharmacotherapy than with cognitive therapy ($p<.05$). However, even when these dropouts were eliminated from the data analysis, cognitive therapy patients showed a significantly greater improvement in depressive symptomatology than did the pharmacotherapy patients ($p<.05$).

Follow-up data at 6 months past termination indicate that treatment gains were maintained for both groups. A significantly greater number of the drug-treatment group returned to treatment during the follow-up period. Patients assigned to cognitive therapy showed significantly lower levels of depression at 3 and 6 months of follow up. Considering only those who completed treatment, the cognitive therapy patients had significantly lower levels of depression at 3 months ($p<.05$ and a trend ($p<.10$) toward lower levels of depression at 6 months following treatment.

Follow-up of the completers revealed that although many patients had an intermittently symptomatic clinical course, both groups still showed maintenance of their treament gains 12 months after protocol termination. However, self-rated depressive symptomatology was significantly lower for cognitive-therapy-treated patients than for the chemotherapy completers. In addition, imipramine-treated patients had twice the cumulative relapse rate of those treated with cognitive therapy (Kovacs, Rush, Beck, and Hollon, 1978).

This is the first controlled outcome study to show the superiority of any psychological or behavioral intervention over pharmacotherapy in moderate–severely depressed outpatients. Obviously, additional studies will be needed to determine which form of therapy is most effective for a given subgroup of depressives.

Finally, a study that suggests that cognitive therapy alone may be effective in the treatment of hospitalized depressed patients was conducted by Dr. Brian Shaw at the University Hospital of the University of Western Ontario. The patients were drawn from two sources: (a) depressed patients, hospitalized on a metabolic ward for endocrine studies, who were assigned to treatment with cognitive therapy since the research procedure precluded the use of drug therapy, and (b) depressed patients who had proven to be refractory to antidepressant medication. The mean age of the 11 patients was 40 years, with a range of 29 to 66. There were 6 females and 5 males in the study. All of the patients had the diagnosis of primary depression.

The mean Depression Inventory score was 29.8 (with a range of 19 to 41) at the time of admission to the hospital. The mean BDI score at discharge was 15.6. The mean number of weeks in the hospital was 8.1. Ten of the 11 patients showed appreciable improvement. At the time of discharge, depression scores (of those who improved) were in the normal range for 3, in the mild range for 5, and in the moderate range for 2. At follow-up at 4 to 6 weeks, the mean BDI was 13.5; thus, it is apparent that the improvement was sustained.

Cognitive Therapy Compared to Combined Cognitive Therapy and Amitriptyline. A recent study by our group compared the effect of (1) cognitive therapy alone with the effect of (2) the combination of cognitive therapy and amitriptyline prescribed according to a flexible dosage schedule providing maximum efficacy of the drug. The admission criteria for the study were similar to those in the Rush *et al.* (1977) study with the exception that schizoaffective patients were accepted into the more recent study to determine whether the addition of antidepressant medication would be beneficial to these patients. Thirty-three patients were assigned randomly to each of the treatment conditions and were treated in individual sessions according to the procedure described in the study by Rush *et al.* Of the 18 patients assigned to cognitive therapy alone, 4 patients were discontinued from the study because of a breach of research protocol (as a result of missed appointments or a decision on the part of the head of the clinic either to increase the frequency of appointments or to add medication). One of these patients showed a schizophrenic decompensation and was given a phenothiazine. The 3 discontinued patients in the combined treatment group did not show satisfactory adherence to the drug regimen.

With the discontinued cases eliminated, there were 14 patients in the cognitive therapy alone and 12 in the combined therapy condition. The cognitive therapy group showed a reduction in their scores on the Beck Depression Inventory from 31.0 to 8.64 at the termination of treatment. The combined cognitive therapy and amitriptyline group showed a reduction in scores from 29.9 to 9.83. The ratings on the Hamilton Depression Scale (HRS-D) for the cognitive therapy group decreased from 22.0 to 6.00; the combined group showed a drop of from 20.08 to 5.55. Thus both groups showed a highly significant and clinically substantial improvement. At 6-month follow up, these treatment gains were partially sustained (BDI 12.8 and HRS 9.0 for cognitive therapy alone; BDI 14.4 and HRS 8.75 for the combined treatment). No significant differences between the two groups were found at termination of therapy or during the follow-up period. Thus, the following conclusions can be reached from this study:

TABLE 4. STUDIES OF COGNITIVE/BEHAVIORAL

Study	Population	Sex	Age	Main measures	Treatment comparisons
Shipley and Fazio (1973)	College student volunteers	M&F	18 to 33	Zung MMP	1. Functional problem solving (cognitive) 2. Supportive 3. Wait list control
Taylor and Marshall (1977)	College student volunteers	M&F	18 to 26	BDI D-30	1. Cognitive modification 2. Behavior modification 3. Combined CM & BM 4. Wait list control
Gioe (1975)	College student volunteers	M&F	?	BDI	1. Cognitive modification 2. Positive group experience (PGE) 3. Combined CM & PGE 4. Wait list control
Fuchs and Rehm (1977)	Community volunteers	F	18 to 48	BDI MMPI-D	1. Self-control therapy 2. Nonspecific therapy 3. Wait list control
Hodgson and Urban (1976)	College student volunteers	M&F	?	Lubin, Zung	1. Interpersonal perception (cog.) 2. Interpersonal skills (beh.) 3. Nontreatment wait list control
Shaw (1977)	Student health patients	M&F	18 to 26	BDI HRSD	1. Cognitive modification 2. Behavioral modifification 3. Nondirective (ND) 4. Wait list control
Morris (1975)	Clinic patients	F	18	BDI Zung	1. Cognitive program Insight-oriented 3. Wait list control
Schmickley (1976)	Clinic patients	F	22 to 53	BDI HRSD	1. Cognitive therapy 2. Pharmacotherapy (imipramine)

THERAPY OF DEPRESSION

Modality		Number of sessions (italics), length, weeks, total time	Therapists (* author)	N (Com- pleters)	Dropouts	Success %	Conclusions
Group	3,	1-hr sessions	1 Grad. student*	13	—	100%	FPS>S>WLC
		3 weeks		14	—	15%	
		= 3 hrs		11		0%	
Individual	6,	40-min sessions	1 Grad. student*	7	—	Not	CM&BM>CM
		3 weeks		7	—	reported	CM&BM>BM
		= 3½ hr		7	—		CM = BM
				7	—		Each>WLC
Group	5,	½-hr sessions	1 Grad student*	10	—	Not reported	CM&PGE>CM
		1 week		10	—		CM&PGE>PGE
		= 2½ hr		10	—		CM = PGE
				10	—		Each>WLC
Group	6,	2-hr sessions	2 Grad. students*	8	33%	100%	SC>NS>WLC
		6 weeks		10	17%	30%	
		= 12 hr		10	17%	0%	
Group	8,	2-hr sessions	1 Grad. student*	8	—	63%	CM>BM
		4 weeks		8	—	25%	CM>ND
		= 16 hrs		8	—	25%	BM = ND
				8	—	0%	Each>WLC
Group	6,	1½-hr sessions	3 M.S.W.'s and	22	19%	Not reported	CM>10
		3 weeks	1 grad student*	17	57%		Each>WLC
		= 9 hr		12	14%		
Individual	4,	1-hr sessions	4 Grad. students	11	—	Not reported	Significant treatment effects
		4 weeks					
		= 4 weeks					
Individual		C.T. = max. 20 50- min. sessions Drug = 12 20-min. sessions	18 Psychiatrists, psychologists, residents, or interns	18 14	4% 36%	83% 36%	CM>drug

1. The cognitive therapy group (with the exception of the schizoaffective patients) responded approximately as well in this study as in the Rush *et al.* study.

2. The addition of amitriptyline to cognitive therapy did not enhance the efficacy of cognitive therapy in that treatment condition.

However, this finding does not preclude the possibility that for a given individual, the addition of an antidepressant drug might have an additive effect to cognitive therapy. In fact, in our clinical experience we have noted that in the case of a few patients (not included in the research study) who did not seem to be responding to cognitive therapy, the addition of antidepressant medication seemed to have an almost immediate effect in breaking the impasse in therapy.

SUMMARY

A review of published reports of controlled studies of psychotherapy of depression showed significant superiority of cognitive or behavioral (or combined cognitive–behavioral) treatments over control or comparison groups. Of these, six (6) studies used volunteers, either students or individuals solicited from the community; four (4) studies applying cognitive therapy, or some variation of this approach, used actual clinical populations (see Table 4).

An unpublished study suggests that cognitive therapy *without* antidepressant medication may be a powerful treatment for a large proportion of hospitalized depressed patients. Another study suggests that the addition of antidepressant medication does not enhance the effectiveness of cognitive therapy alone.

In summary, the available evidence indicates the efficacy of cognitive therapy on a continuum of depressed individuals ranging from subclinically depressed college students to depressed hospitalized inpatients.

APPENDIX: MATERIALS

BECK INVENTORY

Name _____ Date _____

    On this questionnaire are groups of statements. Please read each group of statements carefully. Then pick out the one statement in each group which best describes the way you have been feeling the <u>PAST</u> <u>WEEK</u>, <u>INCLUDING</u> <u>TODAY</u>! Circle the number beside the statement you picked. If several statements in the group seem to apply equally well, circle each one. <u>Be sure to read all the statements in each group before making your choice.</u>

1   0 I do not feel sad.
    1 I feel sad.
    2 I am sad all the time and I can't snap out of it.
    3 I am so sad or unhappy that I can't stand it.

2   0 I am not particularly discouraged about the future.
    1 I feel discouraged about the future.
    2 I feel I have nothing to look forward to.
    3 I feel that the future is hopeless and that things cannot improve.

3   0 I do not feel like a failure.
    1 I feel I have failed more than the average person.
    2 As I look back on my life, all I can see is a lot of failures.
    3 I feel I am a complete failure as a person.

4   0 I get as much satisfaction out of things as I used to.
    1 I don't enjoy things the way I used to.
    2 I don't get real satisfaction out of anything anymore.
    3 I am dissatisfied or bored with everything.

5   0 I don't feel particularly guilty.
    1 I feel guilty a good part of the time.
    2 I feel quite guilty most of the time.
    3 I feel guilty all of the time.

6   0 I don't feel I am being punished.
    1 I feel I may be punished.
    2 I expect to be punished.
    3 I feel I am being punished.

7   0 I don't feel disappointed in myself.
    1 I am disappointed in myself.
    2 I am disgusted with myself.
    3 I hate myself.

8   0 I don't feel I am any worse than anybody else.
    1 I am critical of myself for my weaknesses or mistakes.
    2 I blame myself all the time for my faults.
    3 I blame myself for everything bad that happens.

9   0 I don't have any thoughts of killing myself.
    1 I have thoughts of killing myself, but I would not carry them out.
    2 I would like to kill myself.
    3 I would kill myself if I had the chance.

10 0 I don't cry anymore than usual.
    1 I cry more now than I used to.
    2 I cry all the time now.
    3 I used to be able to cry, but now I can't cry even though I want to.

11 0 I am no more irritated now than I ever am.
   1 I get annoyed or irritated more easily than I used to.
   2 I feel irritated all the time now.
   3 I don't get irritated at all by the things that used to irritate me.

12 0 I have not lost interest in other people.
   1 I am less interested in other people than I used to be.
   2 I have lost most of my interest in other people.
   3 I have lost all of my interest in other people.

13 0 I make decisions about as well as I ever could.
   1 I put off making decisions more than I used to.
   2 I have greater difficulty in making decisions than before.
   3 I can't make decisions at all anymore.

14 0 I don't feel I look any worse than I used to.
   1 I am worried that I am looking old or unattractive.
   2 I feel that there are permanent changes in my appearance that make me look unattractive.
   3 I believe that I look ugly.

15 0 I can work about as well as before.
   1 It takes an extra effort to get started at doing something.
   2 I have to push myself very hard to do anything.
   3 I can't do any work at all.

16 0 I can sleep as well as usual.
   1 I don't sleep as well as I used to.
   2 I wake up 1-2 hours earlier than usual and find it hard to get back to sleep.
   3 I wake up several hours earlier than I used to and cannot get back to sleep.

17 0 I don't get more tired than usual.
   1 I get tired more easily than I used to.
   2 I get tired from doing almost anything.
   3 I am too tired to do anything.

18 0 My appetite is no worse than usual.
   1 My appetite is not as good as it used to be.
   2 My appetite is much worse now.
   3 I have no appetite at all anymore.

19 0 I haven't lost much weight, if any lately.
   1 I have lost more than 5 pounds.   I am purposely trying to lose weight
   2 I have lost more than 10 pounds.   by eating less. Yes ____ No ____
   3 I have lost more than 15 pounds.

20 0 I am no more worried about my health than usual.
   1 I am worried about physical problems such as aches and pains; or upset stomach; or constipation.
   2 I am very worried about physical problems and it's hard to thing of much else.
   3 I am so worried about my physical problems, that I cannot think about anything else.

21 0 I have not noticed any recent change in my interest in sex.
   1 I am less interested in sex than I used to be.
   2 I am much less interested in sex now.
   3 I have lost interest in sex completely.

SCALE FOR SUICIDE IDEATION
(For Ideators)

Name_____ Date_____

Day of   Time of Crisis/Most
Interview   Severe Point of Illness

I. Characteristics of Attitude Toward Living/Dying

( )   1. Wish to Live   ( )
           0. Moderate to Strong
           1. Weak
           2. None

( )   2. Wish to Die   ( )
           0. None
           1. Weak
           2. Moderate to Strong

( )   3. Reasons for Living/Dying   ( )
           0. For living outweigh for dying
           1. About equal
           2. For dying outweigh for living

( )   4. Desire to Make Active Suicide Attempt   ( )
           0. None
           1. Weak
           2. Moderate to Strong

( )   5. Passive Suicidal Attempt   ( )
           0. Would take precautions to save life
           1. Would leave life/death to chance (e.g., carelessly crossing a busy street)
           2. Would avoid steps necessary to save or maintain life (e.g., diabetic
               ceasing to take insulin)

If all four code entries for Items 4 and 5 are "0," skip sections II, III, and IV, and
enter "8" - "Not Applicable" in each of the blank code spaces.

II. Characteristics of Suicide Ideation/Wish

( )   6. Time Dimension Duration   ( )
           0. Brief, fleeting periods
           1. Longer periods
           2. Continuous (chronic), or almost continuous

( )   7. Time Dimension: Frequency   ( )
           0. Rare, occasional
           1. Intermittent
           2. Persistent or continuous

( )   8. Attitude toward Ideation/Wish   ( )
           0. Rejecting
           1. Ambivalent; indifferent
           2. Accepting

Copyright © 1978 by Aaron T. Beck, M.D.

SSI   -2-

| Day of Interview | | | Time of Crisis/Most Severe Point of Illness |

( ) 9. Control over Suicidal Action/Acting-out Wish   ( )
         0. Has sense of control
         1. Unsure of control
         2. Has no sense of control

( ) 10. Deterrents to Active Attempt (e.g., family, religion; serious   ( )
          injury if unsuccessful; irreversible)
          0. Would not suicide because of a deterrent
          1. Some concern about deterrents
          2. Minimal or no concern about deterrents

          (Indicate deterrents, if any:_____

          _____

( ) 11. Reason for Contemplated Attempt   ( )
          0. To manipulate the environment, get attention, revenge
          1. Combination of "0" and "2"
          2. Escape, surcease, solve problems

                  III. Characteristics of Contemplated Attempt

( ) 12. Method: Specificity/Planning   ( )
          0. Not considered
          1. Considered, but details not worked out
          2. Details worked out/well formulated

( ) 13. Method: Availability/Opportunity   ( )
          0. Method not available; no opportunity
          1. Method would take time/effort; opportunity not really available
          2a. Method and opportunity available
          2b. Future opportunity or availability of method anticipated

( ) 14. Sense of "Capability" to Carry out Attempt   ( )
          0. No courage, too weak, afraid, incompetent
          1. Unsure of courage, competence
          2. Sure of competence, courage

( ) 15. LEAVE BLANK   ( )

( ) 16. Expectancy/Anticipation of Actual Attempt   ( )
          0. No
          1. Uncertain, not sure
          2. Yes

( ) 17. LEAVE BLANK   ( )

401

SSI   -3-

Day of   Time of Crisis/Most
Interview   Severe Point of Illness

IV. Actualization of Contemplated Attempt

( ) 18. Actual Preparation   ( )
          0. None
          1. Partial (e.g., starting to collect pills)
          2. Complete (e.g., had pills, razor, loaded gun)

( ) 19. Suicide Note   ( )
          0. None
          1. Started but not completed or deposited; only thought about
          2. Completed; deposited

( ) 20. Final Acts in Anticipation of Death (insurance, will, gifts, ( )
          etc.)
          0. None
          1. Thought about or made some arrangements
          2. Made definite plans or completed arrangements

( ) 21. Deception/Concealment of Contemplated Attempt   ( )
          0. Revealed ideas openly
          1. Held back on revealing
          2. Attempted to deceive, conceal, lie

V. Background Factors

( ) 22. Previous Suicide Attempts   ( )
          0. None
          1. One
          2. More than one

( ) 23. Intent to Die Associated with Last Attempt   ( )
          (if N/A enter "8")
          0. Low
          1. Moderate; ambivalent, unsure
          2. High

DAILY RECORD OF DYSFUNCTIONAL THOUGHTS

DATE	SITUATION Describe: 1. Actual event leading to unpleasant emotion, or 2. Stream of thoughts, daydream, or recollection, leading to unpleasant emotion.	EMOTION(S) 1. Specify sad anxious angry, etc. 2. Rate degree of emotion, 1-100.	AUTOMATIC THOUGHT(S) 1. Write automatic thought(s) that preceded emotion(s). 2. Rate belief in automatic thought(s). 0-100%.	RATIONAL RESPONSE 1. Write rational response to automatic thought(s). 2. Rate belief in rational response, 0-100%.	OUTCOME 1. Re-rate belief in automatic thought(s), 0-100%. 2. Specify and rate subsequent emotions, 0-100.

EXPLANATION: When you experience an unpleasant emotion, note the situation that seemed to stimulate the emotion. (If the emotion occurred while you were thinking, daydreaming, etc., please note this.) Then note the automatic thought associated with the emotion. Record the degree to which you believe this thought: 0%=not at all, 100%=completely. In rating degree of emotion: 1=a trace; 100=the most intense possible.

4/79 ATB,JY

Competency Checklist for Cognitive Therapists

Therapist_____ Patient_____ Date of Session_____
Session Number_____ Rater_____ Date of Rating_____
Clinic_____ Circle one: One-way mirror   Videotape   Audiotape

Coding Key: √ = appropriately included   0 = optionally omitted
                   — = inappropriately omitted   NA = not applicable

Part I. GENERAL INTERVIEW PROCEDURES

1. Collaboration and Mutual Understanding
_____a. Therapist worked with patient even when using primarily educative role.
_____b. Therapist asked for feedback.
_____c. Patient gave feedback.
_____d. Therapist asked for suggestions and/or offered choices.
_____e. Patient offered suggestions and/or made choices.
_____f. Therapist responded to patient's feedback and/or suggestions; did not ignore or
           negate them.
_____g. Therapist checked periodically for his understanding of key points made by patient
           (e.g., gave brief summaries of patient's verbalizations--"What I hear you say is
           . . . ." to ascertain whether he is tuned into patient).
_____h. Therapist periodically summarized his key points to determine whether patient was
           tuned into him.

2. Established Agenda (not applicable for first session)
_____a. Therapist and patient established agenda for session.
_____b. Agenda items were specific and problem-oriented, rather than vague or general
           topic areas.
_____c. Priorities for agenda items were established.
_____d. Agenda was appropriate for time allotment (neither too ambitious nor too limited).
_____e. At some point, patient discussed events during the week since the last session.

3. Elicited Reactions to Interview and Therapist
_____a. Elicited patient's feelings and reactions to present interview.
_____b. Elicited feedback regarding previous interview.

4. Structured Therapy Time Efficiently
_____a. Therapist covered most items on agenda and rescheduled unfinished business.
_____b. Therapist was flexible enough to include important issues that arose during
           session but were not on the agenda.
_____c. Therapist limited time spent on peripheral or tangential topics.
_____d. Therapist limited unproductive discussion on relevant topics.

5. Focused on Appropriate Problem
_____a. Therapist identified specific problem(s) to focus on.
_____b. Identified problems were central, rather than peripheral, to patient's distress.
_____c. Identified problems were appropriate for treatment at this time.
_____d. Identified problems were the key ones to focus on; the major problem was not overlooked.
_____e. Therapist concentrated on one or two problems instead of skipping around.

6. Questioning
_____a. Therapist skillfully blended questions to elicit data regarding symptoms, life situation, current experiences, thoughts, feelings, and past experiences (when applicable).
_____b. Used open-ended questions appropriately.
_____c. Minimal use of questions requiring yes or no responses.
_____d. Avoided rapid-fire questioning.
_____e. Interspersed questions with reflective statements, illustrative examples, or capsule summaries.
_____f. Used questions to show incongruities or inconsistencies in patient's conclusions without demeaning patient.
_____g. Used questions to help patient explore the various facets of a problem.
_____h. Used questions to examine patient's arbitrary conclusions or assumptions.
_____i. Used questions to elicit alternative ways of solving a problem.
_____j. Used questions to consider alternative explanations.
_____k. Used questions to predict positive and negative consequences of a proposed action (e.g., doing homework assignments, resigning from a job, or having a personal confrontation).

7. Provided Periodic Summaries during Interview
_____a. Therapist periodically recapitulated or reformulated problems being worked on in session.
_____b. Therapist explained rationale for specific techniques to be utilized in dealing with problems.
_____c. Therapist summarized progress made on identified problems during the session (problem closure).

8. Assigned Homework
_____a. Therapist carefully reviewed previous week's homework.
_____b. Therapist summarized conclusions derived, or progress made, from previous homework.
_____c. Therapist assigned new homework.
_____d. Homework assignment was appropriate for identified problems.
_____e. Therapist explained rationale for homework assignment.
_____f. Homework was specific and details were clearly explained.
_____g. Therapist asked patient if he/she anticipated problems in carying out homework.

Part II. SPECIFIC COGNITIVE AND BEHAVIORAL TECHNIQUES

9. Appropriateness and Application of Techniques
_____a. Techniques used were generally appropriate for identified problems.
_____b. Techniques used were the most appropriate for identified problems (e.g., preferable techniques were not overlooked).
_____c. Therapist executed techniques successfully.
Comments explaining inappropriate or incorrect application of techniques:

10. Elicited Automatic Thoughts
_____a. Specific automatic thoughts were identified.
_____b. Therapist helped patient identify thoughts rather than repeatedly pointing out automatic thoughts to patient in a didactic fashion.
_____c. Therapist used appropriate techniques to elicit automatic thoughts (check techniques used):
            inductive questioning   mood shifts during session
            imagery   dysfunctional thought record
            role-playing
_____d. Therapist helped patient recognize connection between affect and specific cognitions.

11. Tested Automatic Thoughts
_____a. Tested or questioned automatic thoughts in systematic manner.
_____b. Did not use exhortation or argument to "talk patient out of automatic thoughts."
_____c. Helped patient set up specific, testable hypotheses.
_____d. Helped patient collect valid evidence systematically concerning hypotheses.
_____e. Helped patient evaluate evidence and draw conclusions from evidence.

12. Identified and Tested Underlying Assumptions
_____a. Specific underlying ("silent") assumptions were identified.
_____b. Therapist helped patient discover relevant assumptions from a joint analysis of automatic thoughts.
_____c. Therapist did not rely solely on didactic counterarguments to evaluate assumptions.
_____d. Therapist helped patient analyze validity of assumptions (e.g., by inductive questioning or by listing advantages and disadvantages).

13. Other Basic Cognitive and Behavioral Techniques
    a. Techniques used:
        _____reattribution   _____role-playing
        _____alternative technique   _____diversion procedures
        _____ascertaining meaning of an event   _____assertive training
        _____cognitive rehearsal   _____other, specify:_____
        _____focussing and concentration practice _____
        _____activity scheduling   _____
        _____mastery and pleasure ratings
        _____graded task assignments

    b. Specific instruments, materials and devices:

_____Daily Record of Dysfunctional Thoughts	_____autobiographies
_____activity schedule: summary	_____diary
_____activity schedule: planning	_____wrist counter
_____mastery and pleasure ratings	_____videotape of session for patient
_____written list of main points of	to observe
interview for patient	_____audiotape of session for patient
_____reading assignment	to listen to
_____Dysfunctional Attitude Scale	_____Depression Inventory
_____other:	

Part III. PERSONAL AND PROFESSIONAL CHARACTERISTICS OF THERAPIST

14. Genuineness
_____a. Therapist seemed to be saying what he sincerely felt or meant. Seemed honest and "real."
_____b. Therapist seemed open rather than defensive.
_____c. Therapist did not seem to be holding back impressions or information, or evading patient's questions.
_____d. Therapist did not seem patronizing or condescending.
_____e. Therapist did not seem to be playing the role of a therapist. Did not sound contrived or rehearsed.

15. Warmth
_____a. Therapist's tone of voice and non-verbal behavior conveyed warmth and interest.
_____b. The content of what the therapist said communicated concern and caring.
_____c. The therapist did not criticize, disapprove, or ridicule the patient's behavior.
_____d. The therapist did not seem cold, distant, or indifferent.
_____e. The therapist did not seem effusive, possessive, or overinvolved.
_____f. The therapist responded to or displayed humor when appropriate.

16. Accurate Empathy
_____a. The therapist accurately summarized what the patient explicitly said.
_____b. The therapist accurately summarized the patient's most obvious emotions (e.g., sadness, anger).
_____c. The therapist accurately summarized more subtle nuances of feeling or implicit belief.
_____d. The therapist communicated through his verbal and non-verbal behavior that he/she understood the patient's feelings and was responding to them.

17. Professional Manner
_____a. Therapist's tone of voice and non-verbal behavior conveyed confidence.
_____b. Therapist made clear statements without frequent hesitations or rephrasings.
_____c. Therapist was in control of the session; he was able to shift appropriately between listening and leading.
_____d. Therapist seemed relaxed and did not seem to be anxious or "trying too hard."

18. Rapport
_____a. Patient and therapist seemed comfortable with each other.
_____b. Eye contact maintained.
_____c. Good affective interaction (e.g., when one smiles, the other smiles).
_____d. Flow of verbal interchanges was smooth.
_____e. Neither patient nor therapist appeared overly defensive, cautious, or restrained.

This form was developed by Jeffrey Young, Karen El Shammaa and Aaron T. Beck. A syllabus and guide for the Competency Checklist for Cognitive Therapists may be obtained from Aaron T. Beck, M.D., Center for Cognitive Therapy, Room 602, 133 South 36th Street, Philadelphia, PA 19104.

POSSIBLE REASONS FOR NOT DOING SELF-HELP ASSIGNMENTS
(To be completed by patient)

The following is a list of reasons that various patients have given for not doing their self-help assignments during the course of therapy. Because the speed of improvement depends primarily on the amount of self-help assignments that you are willing to do, it is of crucial importance to pinpoint any reasons that you may have for not doing this work. It is important to look for these reasons at the time that you feel a reluctance to do your assignment or a desire to put off doing it. Hence, it is best to fill out this questionnaire at that time. If you have any difficulty filling out this form and returning it to the therapist, it might be best to do it together during a therapy session. (Rate each statement with a "T" (True) or "F" (False). "T" indicates that you agree with it; "F" means the statement does not apply at this time.)

1. It seems that nothing can help me so there is no point in trying.___
2. I really can't see the point of what the therapist has asked me to do.___
3. I feel that the particular method the therapist has suggested will not be helpful. It doesn't really make good sound sense to me.___
4. "I am a procrastinator, therefore, I can't do this." Then I end up not doing it.___
5. I am willing to do some self-help assignments, but I keep forgetting.___
6. I do not have enough time. I am too busy.___
7. If I do something the therapist suggests it's not as good as if I come up with my own ideas.___
8. I feel helpless, and I don't really believe that I *can* do anything that I choose to do.___
9. I have the feeling that the therapist is trying to boss me around or control me.___
10. I don't feel like cooperating with the therapist.___
11. I fear the therapist's disapproval or criticism of my work. I believe that what I do just won't be good enough for him.___
12. I have no desire or motivation to do self-help assignments or anything else. Since I don't feel like doing these assignments, it follows that I can't do them and I should not have to do them.___
13. I feel too bad, sad, nervous, upset (underline appropriate word(s)) to do it now.___
14. I am feeling good now and I don't want to spoil it by working on assignment.___
(15) Other Reasons (Please write them in)

_____
_____
_____
_____

This form was developed by David Burns, M.D. and Aaron T. Beck, M.D.

RESEARCH PROTOCOL FOR OUTCOME STUDY
AT CENTER FOR COGNITIVE THERAPY

A. Preliminary Evaluation
   1. Complete Clinical Evaluation: Mental Status, History of Present Illness, Past History.
   2. Schedule of Affective Disorders and Schizophrenia (SADS: Spitzer and Endicott).
   3. Diagnosis according to Research Diagnostic Criteria and Feighner criteria.
   4. Clinical Scales: Hamilton Scale for Depression; Hamilton Scale for Anxiety; Scale for Suicide Intentionality (SSI).
   5. Psychometric Tests: Minnesota Multiphasic Personality Inventory, Spielberger State–Trait Anxiety Scale, Symptom Checklist–90 (Hopkins); Beck Depression Inventory.
   6. Special Scales: Self-Concept Test; Dysfunctional Attitude Scale; Hopelessness Scale; Picture Order Test; Story Completion Test.
B. Assignment of patient to therapist
C. First therapeutic interview (to be scheduled within 3 days of intake evaluation)
D. Frequency and duration of interviews and duration of treatment: Maximum of 20 visits over a 12-week period; duration of each interview, 50 minutes; interviews scheduled twice a week until patient is ready for once-a-week treatment.
   Treatment schedule for average case (15 visits): Weeks 1, 2, and 3: 2 visits per week; Weeks 4–12: visits once a week.

First Interview
   1. Establish rapport
   2. Inquiry regarding expectations of therapy
   3. Elicitation of negative attitudes regarding self, therapy, or therapist
   4. Pinpointing most urgent and accessible problem (e.g., hopelessness, suicidal wishes, loss of functioning, severe dysphoria)
   5. Explanation of cognitive–behavioral strategies with emphasis on the rationale for behavioral assignments and homework
   6. Review form for recording activities until next interview
   7. Give patient *Coping with Depression* to read
   8. Inquiry regarding reactions to interview. *Note:* Most patients feel better by the end of the first interview; if not, therapist should probe for reasons for adverse reaction

Second Interview
   1. Inquiry regarding effect of first interview
   2. Review of form for recording schedule of activities
   3. Review of reactions to *Coping with Depression*
   4. Discussion of problems and accomplishments since previous interview
   5. Scheduling of activities until next interview
   6. Discussion of recording "Mastery" and "Pleasure" ratings on schedule for recording activities (optional)

7. Preparation of agenda and focus on the problem(s) to be discussed
8. Inquiry to reactions toward present interview

Third Interview
1. Preparation of agenda
2. Inquiry regarding effects of first interview
3. Review of homework assignments
4. Discussion of reactions to previous interview
5. Discussion of automatic negative thoughts (optional)
6. Demonstration of the use of the wrist counter for clicking negative automatic thoughts (optional)
7. Preparation of homework assignments
8. Feedback regarding today's session
9. Request that patient write a biographical sketch or autobiography for next interview

Fourth Interview
1. Follow same general format as in third interview
2. Further instruction in identifying negative automatic thoughts (use "induced fantasy" or role-playing if indicated)
3. Explanation of how these automatic thoughts represent distortions of reality and are related to other symptoms of depression
4. Elicitation of automatic thoughts, specifically relationship to homework assignments

Fifth Interview
1. Follow same general format as in previous interview
2. Review schedule of activities with a special reference to mastery and pleasure
3. Review and discuss automatic negative thoughts
4. Demonstrate to the patient ways of evaluating and correcting cognitive distortions (automatic thoughts)
5. Instruction in using the Daily Recording of Dysfunctional Thoughts, explain columns 4, 5, and 6 ("Rational Response," etc.)
6. Use of wrist counter for monitoring automatic thoughts

Interviews 6, 7, and 8
1. Same format as above
2. Continue to remove psychological blocks to return to premorbid level of functioning
3. Continue to identify negative automatic thoughts
4. Further demonstration of rational responses to automatic thoughts
5. Further homework assignments
6. Discussion of the concept of Basic Assumptions (Chapter 12)

Interviews 8–12
1. Increasing delegation of responsibility for setting the agenda to the patient
2. Increase responsibility for homework to the patient
3. Identification and discussion of Basic Assumptions. Testing validity of the assumptions

Closing Interviews 13–15 (up to 20)
1. Preparation of patient for termination of therapy
2. Emphasis on continuation of homework assignments and practicing other strategies after the termination; emphasis on psychotherapy as a learning process that continues throughout the individual's life
3. Delineating of anticipated problems and rehearsal of coping strategies.

Further Materials and Technical Aids

The preceding tests and forms, and other materials related to the cognitive therapy of depression, are available from the Center for Cognitive Therapy.

Available materials include the following:
Videotapes and cassettes demonstrating techniques of cognitive therapy
Audio cassettes demonstrating techniques of cognitive therapy
Transcripts of videotaped demonstration interviews
Treatment manual for cognitive therapy of anxiety and phobic disorders
Treatment manual for cognitive therapy of drug abuse
Coping with Depression (booklet for patients)
Daily Record of Dysfunctional Thoughts
Beck Depression Inventory
Hopelessness Scale
Suicidal Intent Scale
Scale for Suicide Ideation
The Center will consider requests for any of these training aids. However, as supplies are limited in some cases, priority is given to investigators engaged in outcome studies of cognitive therapy.

If interested, please write to the Center for Cognitive Therapy, 133 South 36th Street, Philadelphia, Pennsylvania, 19104, and state the purpose for which you would like to receive materials.

The wrist counters mentioned in Chapter 8 may be obtained from the Behavior Research Company, Box 3351, Kansas City, Kansas, 66103.

REFERENCES

Adler, A. *What life should mean to you* (A Porter, Ed.). New York: Capricorn, 1958. (Originally published, 1931.)

Akiskal, H. S., Bitar, A. H., Puzantian, V. R., Rosenthal, T. L., and Walker, P. W. The nosological status of neurotic depression. *Archives of General Psychiatry,* 1978, *35,* 756–766.

Alexander, F. *Psychosomatic medicine: Its principles and applications.* New York: Norton, 1950.

American Psychiatric Association. *Diagnostic & Statistical Manual, II.* Washington: American Psychiatric Association, 1968.

Baldessarini, R. J. *Chemotherapy in psychiatry.* Cambridge, Mass.: Harvard University Press, 1977.

Bandura, A. *Social learning theory.* Englewood Cliffs, N.J.: Prentice Hall, 1977.

Beck, A. T. Thinking and depression: 1, Idiosyncratic content and cognitive distortions. *Archives of General Psychiatry,* 1963, *9,* 324–333.

Beck, A. T. Thinking and depression: 2, Theory and therapy. *Archives of General Psychiatry,* 1964, *10,* 561–571.

Beck, A.T. *Depression: Clinical, experimental, and theoretical aspects.* New York: Hoeber, 1967. (Republished as *Depression: Causes and treatment.* Philadelphia: University of Pennsylvania Press, 1972).

Beck, A. T. *The diagnosis and management of depression.* Philadelphia: University of Pennsylvania Press, 1973.

Beck, A.T. *Cognitive therapy and the emotional disorders.* New York: International Universities Press, 1976.

Beck, A. T. *Depression inventory.* Philadelphia: Center for Cognitive Therapy, 1978.

Beck, A. T., and Greenberg, R. L. *Coping with depression* (a booklet). New York: Institute for Rational Living, 1974.

Beck, A. T., Kovacs, M., and Weissman, A. Hopelessness and suicidal behavior: An overview. *Journal of the American Medical Association,* 1975, *234,* 1146–1149.

Beck, A. T., Kovacs, M., and Weissman, A. Assessment of suicidal intention: The Scale for Suicidal Ideation. *Journal of Consulting and Clinical Psychology,* 1979, *47,* 2, 343–352.

Beck, A. T., Resnik, H. L. P., and Lettieri, D. (Eds.). *The prediction of suicide.* Bowie, Md.: Charles Press, 1974.

413

Beck, A. T., and Rush, A. J. Cognitive approaches to depression and suicide. *In* G. Serban (Ed.), *Cognitive defects in the development of mental illness.* New York: Brunner-Mazel, 1978.

Beck, A. T., Weissman, A., Lester, D., and Trexler, L. The measurement of pessimism: The Hopelessness Scale. *Journal of Consulting and Clinical Psychology,* 1974, *42,* 861-865.

Becker, J. *Depression: theory and research.* Washington, D.C.: V. H. Winston and Sons, Inc., 1974.

Berne, E. *Transactional analysis in psychotherapy: A systematic individual and social psychiatry.* New York: Grove Press, 1961.

Berne, E. *Games people play.* New York: Grove Press, 1964.

Binswanger, L. [The case of Ellen West: An anthropological-clinical study.] (W.M. Mendel and J. Lyons, trans.). In R. May, E. Angel, and H.F. Ellenberger (Eds.), *Existence: A new dimension in psychology and psychiatry.* New York: Basic Books, 1958. (Originally published, 1944–45.)

Bowers, H.S. Situationism in psychology: An analysis and critique. *Psychological Review,* 1973, *80,* 307–336.

Breger, L., and McGaugh, J.L. Critique and reformulation of "learning theory" approaches to psychotherapy and neurosis. *Psychological Bulletin,* 1965, *63,* 338–358.

Brownell, K., Heckerman. C.L., and Westlake, R.J. *The effect of couples training and spouse cooperativeness in the behavioral treatment of obesity.* Paper presented at the annual meeting of the Association for Advancement of Behavior Therapy, Atlanta, December 1977.

Cautela, J., and Kastenbaum, R. A reinforcement survey schedule for use in therapy, training, and research. *Psychological Reports,* 1967, *20,* 1115–1130.

Chassell, J.O. *The "basic model" of psychotherapy.* Paper presented at the meeting of the American Psychoanalytic Association, New York, December 1953 (revised, March 1977).

Christie, G.L. Group psychotherapy in private practice. *Australian and New Zealand Journal of Psychiatry,* 1970, *43,* 43–48.

Covi, L., Lipman, R., Derogatis, L., Smith, J., and Pattison, I. Drugs and group psychotherapy in neurotic depression. *American Journal of Psychiatry,* 1974, *131,* 191–198.

Coyne, J. C. Depression and the response of others. *Journal of Abnormal Psychology,* 1976, *85,* 186–193. (a)

Coyne, J. C. Toward an interactional description of depression. *Psychiatry,* 1976, *39,* 28–40. (b)

Daneman, E. A. Imipramine in office management of depressive reactions (a double-blind study). *Diseases of the Nervous System,* 1961, *22,* 213–217.

Davis, J. M. Overview: Maintenance therapy in psychiatry: II. Affective disorders. *American Journal of Psychiatry,* 1976, *133,* 1–13.

Dember, W. N. Motivation and the cognitive revolution. *American Psychologist,* 1974, *29,* 161–168.

Ellis, A. Outcome of employing three techniques of psychotherapy. *Journal of Clinical Psychology,* 1957, *13,* 344–350.

References

Ellis, A. *Reason and emotion in psychotherapy.* New York: Lyle Stuart, 1962.

Ellis, A. *Growth through reason: Verbatim cases in rational–emotive psychotherapy.* Palo Alto: Science & Behavior Books, 1971.

Ellis, A. *Humanistic psychotherapy: The rational–emotive approach.* New York: McGraw-Hill, 1973.

Ellis, A., and Harper, R. A. *A new guide to rational living.* Englewood Cliffs, N.J.: Prentice-Hall, 1975.

Emery, G. Cognitive vs. behavioral methods in weight reduction with college students. (Doctoral dissertation, University of Pennsylvania, 1977). *Dissertation Abstracts International,* 1978, *38,* 5563B-5564B. (University Microfilms No. 7806578)

Emery, G. Self-reliance training for depressed patients. In D. P. Rathjen and J. P. Foreyt (Eds.), *Social competence: Interventions for children and adults.* New York: Plenum, in press.

Farberow, N. L. Vital process in suicide prevention: Group psychotherapy as a community concern. *Life threatening behavior,* 1972, *2,* 239–251.

Feighner, J. P., Robins, E., Guze, S. B., Woodruff, R. A., Winokur, J., and Munoz, R. Diagnostic criteria for use in psychiatric research. *Archives of General Psychiatry,* 1972, *26,* 57–63.

Frank, J. *Persuasion and healing.* Baltimore: Johns Hopkins Press, 1961.

Frankl, V. *Man's search for meaning.* New York: Washington Square Press, 1963.

Freedman, A. M., Kaplan, H. I., and Sadock, B. J. (Eds.). *Comprehensive textbook of psychiatry—II.* Baltimore: Williams and Wilkins, 1975.

Freeman, A. The use of dreams and imagery in cognitive therapy. *In* G. Emery, S. Hollon, and R. Bedrosian (Eds.), *New directions in cognitive therapy: A casebook.* New York: Guilford Press, in press.

Freud, S.[*The interpretation of dreams*] (J. Strachey, Ed. and trans.). In the *Standard edition of the complete psychological works of Sigmund Freud, V.* London: The Hogarth Press and the Institute of Psychoanalysis, 1953. (Originally published, 1900.)

Friedman, A. S. Interaction of drug therapy with marital therapy in depressive patients. *Archives of General Psychiatry,* 1975, *32,* 619–637.

Fuchs, C., and Rehm, L. P. A self-control behavior therapy program for depression. *Journal of Consulting and Clinical Psychology,* 1977, *45,* 206–215.

Gioe, V. J. Cognitive modification and positive group experience as a treatment for depression. (Doctoral dissertation, Temple University, 1975). *Dissertation Abstracts International,* 1975, *36,* 3039B-3040B. (University Microfilms No. 75-28, 219)

Goldfried, M. R., and Davison, G. C. *Clinical behavior therapy.* New York: Holt, Rinehart, and Winston, 1976.

Green, R. A., and Murray, E. J. Expression of feeling and cognitive reinterpretation in the reduction of hostile aggression. *Journal of Consulting and Clinical Psychology,* 1975, *43,* 375–383.

Greenwald, H. *Direct decision therapy.* Los Angeles: Knapp, 1973.

Grinker, R. R., Sr., Werble, B., and Drye, R. C. *The borderline syndrome.* New York: Basic Books, 1968.

Gunderson, J. G., and Singer, M. T. Defining borderline patients: An overview. *American Journal of Psychiatry*, 1975, *132*, 1–10.

Hodgson, J. W., and Urban, H. B. *A comparison of interpersonal training programs in the treatment of depressive states.* Unpublished manuscript, Pennsylvania State University, 1975.

Hollon, S.D., and Beck, A.T. Cognitive therapy and suicide. In E.C. Kendall and S.D. Hollon (Eds.), *Cognitive–behavioral interventions. Theory, research, and procedures.* New York: Academic Press, in press.

Hollon, S. D., Beck, A. T., Kovacs, M., and Rush, A. J. *Cognitive therapy vs. pharmacotherapy of depression: Outcome and followup.* Paper presented at the annual convention, American Psychological Association, Madison, August 1977.

Hollon, S. D., and Beck, A. T. Psychotherapy and drug therapy: Comparison and combinations. In S. L. Garfield and A. E. Bergin (Eds.), *Handbook of psychotherapy and behavior change: An empirical analysis* (2nd ed.). New York: Wiley, 1978.

Horney, Karen. *Neurosis and human growth: The struggle toward self-realization.* New York: Norton & Co., 1950.

Janov, A. *The primal scream: Primal therapy, the cure for neurosis.* New York: G. P. Putnam's Sons, 1970.

Jaspers, K. [*General psychopathology*] (J. Joenig and M. W. Hamilton, trans.). Chicago: University of Chicago Press, 1968. (Originally published, 1913.)

Kasanin, J. The acute schizoaffective psychoses. *American Journal of Psychiatry*, 1944, *13*, 97.

Kazdin, A. E., and Wilson, G. T. *Evaluation of behavior therapy: Issues, evidence, and research strategies.* Cambridge, Mass.: Ballinger, 1978.

Keith-Speigel, P., and Spiegel, D. E. Affective states of patients immediately preceding suicide. *Journal of Psychiatric Research*, 1967, *5*, 89–93.

Kelly, G. *The psychology of personal constructs* (Vols. 1 and 2). New York: Norton & Co., 1955.

Khatami, M., and Rush, A. J. A pilot study of the treatment of outpatients with chronic pain: Symptom control, stimulus control and social system intervention. *Pain*, 1978, *5*, 163–172.

Klein, D. F. Endogenomorphic depression. *Archives of General Psychiatry*, 1974, *31*, 447–454.

Klerman, G. L. Clinical research in depression. *Archives of General Psychiatry*, 1971, *24*, 305–319.

Klerman, G. L., DiMascio, A., Weissman, M., Prusoff, B., and Paykel, E. Treatment of depression by drugs and psychotherapy. *American Journal of Psychiatry*, 1974, *131*, 186–191.

Klerman, G. L., and Paykel, E. S. Depressive pattern, social background and hospitalization. *Journal of Nervous and Mental Disease*, 1970, *150*, 466–478.

Koranyi, E. K. Physical health and illness in psychiatric outpatient department populations. *Canadian Psychiatric Association Journal*, 1972, *17*, 109–113.

Kovacs, M., Beck, A. T., and Weissman, A. The Use of Suicidal Motives in the Psychotherapy of Attempted Suicides. *American Journal of Psychotherapy*, 1975, *29*, 363–368.

Kovacs, M., Rush, A. J., Beck, A. T., and Hollon, S. D. *Comparative efficacy of cognitive therapy and pharmacotherapy in treatment of depressed outpatients: A 12-month follow-up.* Unpublished manuscript, University of Pittsburgh, 1978.

Kuhn, T. S. *The structure of scientific revolutions.* Chicago: University of Chicago Press, 1962.

Lazarus, A. *Behavior therapy and beyond.* New York: McGraw-Hill, 1972.

Lazarus, A., and Fay, A. *I can if I want to.* New York: William Morrow and Co., Inc., 1975.

Lazarus, R. *Psychological stress and the coping process.* New York: McGraw-Hill, 1966.

Leff, M. J., Roatch, J. F., and Bunney, W. E. Environmental factors preceding the onset of severe depressions. *Psychiatry,* 1970, *33,* 293–311.

Lerner, M. J. Deserving versus justice: A contemporary dilemma. Paper presented at the Symposium on Freedom, Justice, and Social Responsibility of the American Psychological Association, Washington, September 1969.

Lewinsohn, P. M. A behavioral approach to depression. *In* R. M. Friedman and M. M. Katz (Eds.), *The psychology of depression: Contemporary theory and research.* Washington, D.C.: Winston-Wiley, 1974.

Lewinsohn, P. M. The behavioral study and treatment of depression. *In* M. Hersen, R. M. Eisler, and P. M. Miller (Eds.), *Progress in Behavior Modification,* Vol. 1. New York: Academic Press, 1975.

Lipowsky, Z. J. Psychiatry of somatic diseases: Epidemiology, pathogenesis, classification. *Comprehensive Psychiatry,* 1975, *16,* 105–124.

Lopez-Ibor, J. J. Masked depressions. *British Journal of Psychiatry,* 1972, *120,* 245–258.

Low, Abraham. *Mental health through will-training.* Boston: Christopher, 1950.

Maas, J. W. Biogenic amines and depression: Biochemical and pharmacological separation of two types of depression. *Archives of General Psychiatry,* 1975, *32,* 1357–1361.

MacPhillamy, D. J., and Lewinsohn, P. M. *Pleasant events schedule.* Unpublished manuscript, University of Oregon, 1971.

Mahoney, M. J. *Cognition and behavior modification.* Cambridge: Ballinger, 1974.

Mahoney, M. J. Reflections on the cognitive-learning trend in psychotherapy. *American Psychologist,* 1977, *32,* 5–13.

Mahoney, M. J., and Mahoney, K. *Permanent weight control—A total solution to the dieter's dilemma.* New York: Norton & Co., 1976.

Maultsby, M. C. *Handbook of rational self-counseling.* Madison, Wisconsin: Association for Rational Thinking, 1971a.

Maultsby, M. C. Systematic written homework in psychotherapy. *Psychotherapy: Theory, Research, and Practice,* 1971b, *8,* 195–198.

Maultsby, M. C. *Help yourself to happiness through rational self-counseling.* Boston: Esplanade Books, 1975.

McFall, R. M., and Twentyman, C. T. Four experiments on the relative contributions of rehearsal, modeling, and coaching to assertion training. *Journal of Abnormal Psychology,* 1973, *81,* 199–218.

McLean, P. D., and Hakstian, A. R. *Clinical depression: Comparative efficacy of outpatient treatments.* Paper presented at the annual meeting of the Society for Psychotherapy Research, Toronto, June 1978.

McMullin, C., and Casey, B. *Talk sense to yourself.* Lakewood, Colorado: Jefferson County Mental Health Center, Inc., 1975.

Meichenbaum, D. B. *Cognitive-behavior modification: An integrative approach.* New York: Plenum, 1977.

Mendels, J. Biological aspects of affective illness. In S. Arieti and E. B. Brady (Eds.), *American handbook of psychiatry.* New York: Basic Books, 1974.

Mendels, J., and Cochrane, C. The nosology of depression: The endogenous-reactive concept. *American Journal of Psychiatry,* (Supplement), 1968, *124,* 1–11.

Morris, N. E. A group self-instruction method for the treatment of depressed outpatients. (Doctoral dissertation, University of Toronto, 1975). National Library of Canada, Canadian Theses Division, No. 35272.

Morris, J. B., and Beck, A. T. The efficacy of antidepressant drugs: A review of research (1958 to 1972). *Archives of General Psychiatry,* 1974, *30,* 667–674.

Novaco, R. *Anger control: The development and evaluation of an experimental treatment.* Lexington, Mass.: Heath & Co., 1975.

Padfield, M. The comparative effects of two counseling approaches on the intensity of depression among rural women of low socioeconomic status. *Journal of Counseling Psychology,* 1976, *23,* 209–214.

Paykel, E. S., Klerman, G. L., and Prusoff, B. A. Treatment setting and clinical depression. *Archives of General Psychiatry,* 1970, *22,* 11–21.

Piaget, J. [*Psychology of Intelligence*] (M. Piercy and D. E. Berlyne, trans.). New York: Harcourt, Brace & Co., 1950. (Originally published, 1947.)

Piaget, J. [*The moral judgment of the child*] (M. Gabain, trans.). Glencoe, Ill.: Free Press, 1960. (Originally published, 1932.)

Prien, R. F., Caffey, E. M., Jr., and Klett, C. J. Factors associated with treatment success in lithium carbonate prophylaxis. *Archives of General Psychiatry,* 1974, *31,* 189.

Raimy, V. *Misunderstandings of the self.* San Francisco: Jossey Bass, 1975.

Rehm, L. P., Fuchs, C. Z., Roth, D. M. Kornblith, S. J., and Romano, J. M. A *Comparison of self-control and social skills treatments of depression.* Unpublished manuscript, Cornell University, 1978.

Robins, E., and Guze, S. Classification of affective disorders: The primary–secondary, the endogenous, and the neurotic–psychotic concepts. In *Recent advances in the psychobiology of depressive illness.* Washington, D.C.: U.S. Department of Health, Education and Welfare Publication No. 70-9053, 1972.

Robinson, F. P. *Principles and procedures in student counseling.* New York: Harper & Brothers, 1950.

Rogers, C. *Client-centered therapy.* Boston: Houghton Mifflin Co., 1951.

Rush, A. J., Beck, A. T., Kovacs, M., and Hollon, S. Comparative efficacy of cognitive therapy and imipramine in the treatment of depressed outpatients. *Cognitive Therapy and Research,* 1977, *1,* 17–37.

Rush, A. J., Beck, A. T., Kovacs, M., Khatami, M., Fitzgibbons, R., and Wolman, T. *Comparison of cognitive and pharmacotherapy in depressed outpatients: A preliminary report.* Presented at meetings of the Society for Psychotherapy Research, Boston, Mass., 1975.

Rush, A. J., Hollon, S. D., Beck, A. T., and Kovacs, M. Depression: Must pharmacotherapy fail for cognitive therapy to succeed? *Cognitive Therapy & Research*, 1978, 2, 199–206.

Rush, A. J., Khatami, M., and Beck, A. T. Cognitive and behavioral therapy in chronic depression. *Behavior Therapy*, 1975, 6, 398–404.

Rush, A. J., Shaw, B., and Khatami, M. Cognitive therapy of depression: Utilizing the couples system. *Cognitive Therapy and Research*, in press.

Rush, A. J., and Watkins, J. T. *Specialized cognitive therapy strategies for psychologically naive depressed outpatients.* Paper presented at meeting of the American Psychological Association, San Francisco, August 1977.

Rush, A. J., and Watkins, J. T. *Group versus individual cognitive therapy: A pilot study.* Unpublished manuscript, Southwestern Medical School (Dallas), 1978.

Sackett, D. L., and Haynes, R. B. *Workshop symposium on compliance with therapeutic regimens*, McMasters University, 1974. Baltimore: Johns Hopkins University Press, 1976.

Saul, L. J. *Emotional maturity.* Philadelphia: Lippincott, 1947.

Schmickley, V. G. *The effects of cognitive-behavior modification upon depressed outpatients.* (Doctoral dissertation, Michigan State University, 1976).

Schou, M. Special review: Lithium in psychiatric therapy and prophylaxis. *Journal of Psychiatric Research*, 1968, 6, 67–95.

Schreiber, M. T. Depressive cognitions (letter to the editor). *American Journal of Psychiatry*, 1978, 135, 1570.

Schuyler, D., and Katz, M. M. *The depressive illnesses: A major public health problem.* Washington, D.C.: U.S. Government Printing Office, 1973.

Schwab, J. J., Bialow, M., Brown, J. M., and Holzer, C. E. Diagnosing depression in medical inpatients. *Annals of Internal Medicine*, 1967, 67, 695–707.

Secunda, S. K., Katz, M. M., Friedman, R. J., and Schuyler, D. *Special report: 1973—The depressive disorders.* Washington, D.C.: U.S. Government Printing Office, 1973.

Shapiro, A. K., and Morris, L. A. Placebo effects in medical and psychological therapies. In S. L. Garfield and A. E. Bergin (Eds.), *Handbook of psychotherapy and behavior change: An empirical analysis* (2nd ed.). New York: Wiley, 1978.

Shaw, B. F. *A systematic investigation of three treatments of depression.* (Doctoral dissertation, University of Western Ontario, Canada, 1975.)

Shaw, B. F. Comparison of cognitive therapy and behavior therapy in the treatment of depression. *Journal of Consulting and Clinical Psychology*, 1977, 45, 543–551.

Shaw, B. F., and Hollon, S. D. *Cognitive therapy in a group format with depressed outpatients.* Unpublished manuscript, University of Western Ontario (London), 1978.

Shelton, J. L., and Ackerman, M. J. *Homework in counseling and psychotherapy.* Springfield, Ill.: Charles C. Thomas, 1974.

Shipley, C. R., and Fazio, A. F. Pilot study of a treatment for psychological depression. *Journal of Abnormal Psychology*, 1973, 82, 372–376.

Spitzer, R. L., Endicott, J., and Robins, E. Research diagnostic criteria: Rationale and reliability. *Archives of General Psychiatry*, 1978, 36, 773–782.

Straus, E. W. *Phenomenological Psychology: Selected Papers.* New York: Basic Books, 1966.

Sullivan, H. S. *Interpersonal theory of psychiatry.* New York: Norton & Co., 1953.

Taylor, F. G. *Cognitive and behavioral approaches to the modification of depression.* (Doctoral dissertation, Queen's University, Kingston, Ont., 1974.)

Taylor, F. G., and Marshall, W. L. Experimental analysis of a cognitive–behavioral therapy for depression. *Cognitive Therapy and Research,* 1977, *1,* 59–72.

Weimer, W. B., and Palermo, D. S. (Eds.). *Cognition and the symbolic processes.* Hillsdale, N.J.: Lawrence Erlbaum, 1974.

Wolfe, J., and Fodor, I. A cognitive–behavioral approach to modifying assertive behavior in women. *The Counseling Psychologist,* 1975, *5,* 45–52.

Yalom, I. D. *The theory and practice of group psychotherapy.* New York: Basic Books, 1970.

Yessler, P. G., Gibbs, J. J., and Becker, H. A. Communication of suicidal ideas. *Archives of General Psychiatry,* 1961, *5,* 12–29.

INDEX

Absolutistic (all-or-nothing) thinking, 14, 99, 129, 153, 194–196, 228, 234
Ackerman, M. J., 276
Activity schedule(-ing), 5, 99, 106–108, 120–131, 188, 197, 200, 202, 266, 275, 277, 283–286, 293
Adherence to medication, 371–385
Adler, Alfred, 8–9
Affect, 3, 8, 11, 147–148, 156–157
Affective symptom(s), 8, 96, 169–182
Agenda of sessions, 105, 106, 315, 342–343
Amitriptyline, 354, 393, 396
Anger, 36, 43, 151, 171, 179–80, 313
Antidepressant(s), 2, 24, 27, 144, 354–385, 393, 396
Anxiety, 23, 24, 36, 111, 113, 156–57, 180–82, 304, 315, 320, 374, 376, 381–382
Appetite disturbance, 205–206
Assertive(-ness) training, 83, 110, 112, 137–139, 185
Assumption(s), 3, 4, 9, 24, 30, 55–6, 80, 104, 113, 185, 227, 244–271, 287, 304, 307, 334, 378
Attitude(s), 3, 12, 48, 51–54, 57, 63, 76, 155, 279, 298, 308, 314, 332, 371, 375, 383, 386
Authoritarianism, 103, 280, 305, 308, 310
Automatic thought(s), 30, 79, 83, 87, 111, 134, 147, 150–57, 165–166, 192, 199, 230, 247, 253, 287–289, 303–304, 308, 325–326, 331–333
Auxiliary (co-)therapists, 33, 85, 163, 308, 348–349
Avoidance, 120, 182–83, 197–203, 207, 279

Bandura, A., 17, 22
Beck Depression Inventory (BDI), 37, 89, 93, 104–16, 168ff, 287, 307, 342, 370, 376–379, 383, 392–393
Behavior(-al) change, 3, 17, 58, 64, 76, 110, 117–120
Behavioral symptom(s), 97, 141, 197–204
Behavioral technique(s), 5, 97, 99, 117–141, 169, 204, 259
Belief(s), 4–7, 9–12, 14, 16, 31–32, 37, 55, 59, 61–63, 72, 114, 118, 119, 130, 133, 134, 153, 154, 193, 216–217, 220, 231, 248, 249, 253, 269, 274, 297–311, 381, 383
Berne, E., 10
Bipolar depression, 23, 27, 356, 358–359, 364, 365
Blame, 64, 151, 157, 171, 190, 249–250
Booster therapy, 6, 322, 327, 380
Bowers, H. S., 9

Capsule summaries, 83–84, 101
Casey, B., 290
Chemotherapy, 3, 358, 392
Clinic patients, 388–394
Cognition(s), 3–4, 8, 9, 12, 36, 48, 55, 64, 79, 104, 108–110, 119, 147–150, 157, 166, 253, 276, 297, 333, 371–373
Cognitive-change technique(s), 117–120, 357, 371–385
Cognitive model, 4, 8–20, 22, 29, 371
Cognitive revolutions, 20–22
Cognitive symptom(s), 97, 185–197

421

Index

Index